P9-DMU-114

THE skinnytaste COOKBOOK

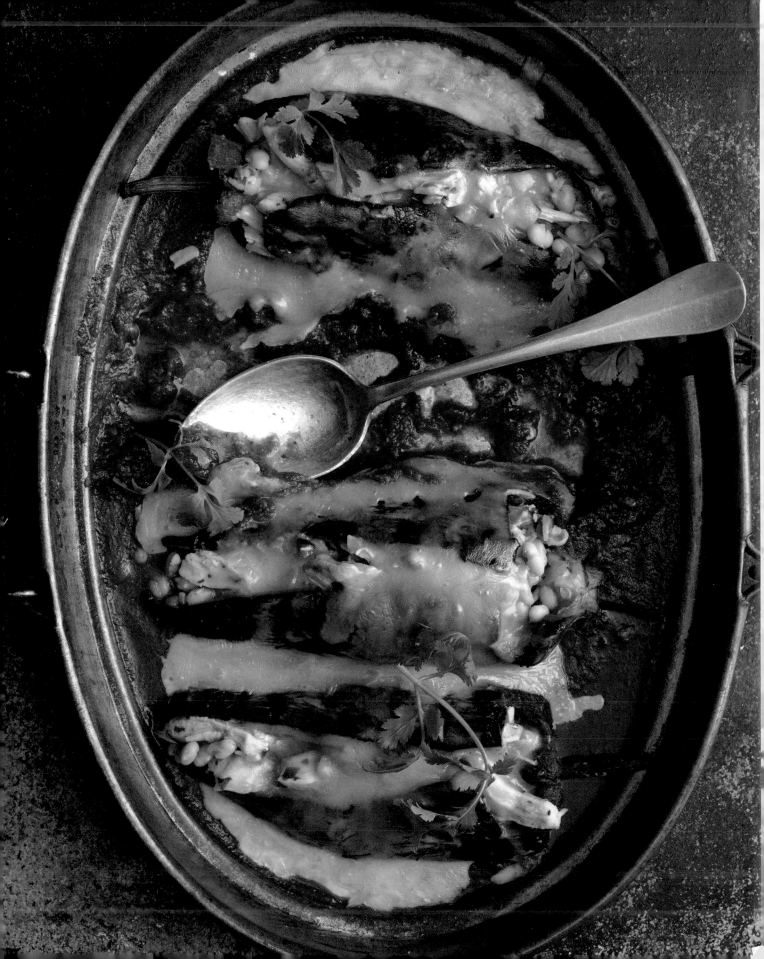

THE skinnytaste COOKBOOK

light on calories, big on flavor

GINA HOMOLKA

with Heather K. Jones, R.D.

CLARKSON POTTER/PUBLISHERS

NEW YORK

Copyright © 2014 by Gina Homolka
Photographs copyright © 2014 by Penny De Los Santos
Selected recipes first appeared on skinnytaste.com

Library of Congress Cataloging-in-Publication Data
Homolka, Gina.
    The skinnytaste cookbook / Gina Homolka. — First
edition.
        pages cm
    Includes index.
1. Reducing diets. 2. Low-fat diet—Recipes.
3. Low-calorie diet—Recipes. I. Title.
    RM222.2.H5865 2014
    641.5'635—dc23
2013050608

ISBN 978-0-385-34562-0
eBook ISBN 978-0-385-34563-7

Printed in the U.S.A.

Book design by Stephanie Huntwork
Jacket design by Stephanie Huntwork
Jacket photographs by Penny De Los Santos

10 9

First Edition

To all of my Skinnytaste fans, this book is dedicated to you. Without your loyalty and support, this book would never have been possible.

To my favorite taste-testers—my husband, Tommy, and my two girls, Karina and Madison—thanks for trying all my cooking experiments (the good and the bad!) and for your love throughout this amazing journey.

And to my mom and dad: you shared your love of cooking and taught us the joys of being in the kitchen. I am eternally grateful.

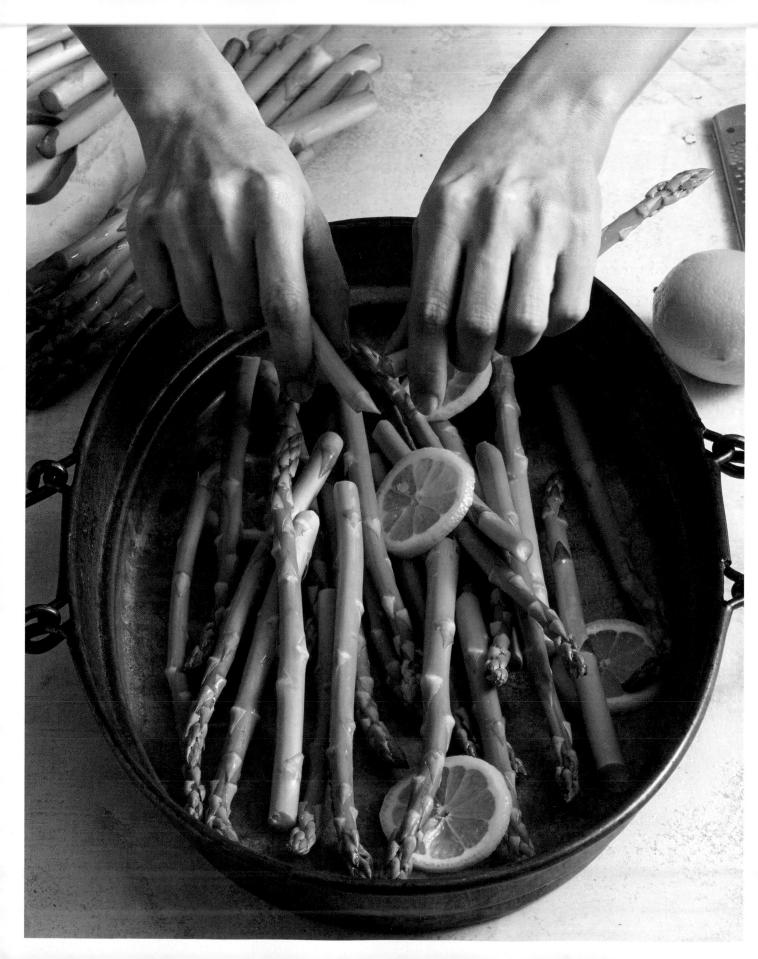

CONTENTS

INTRODUCTION

Struggling to shed some pounds while still eating healthfully and feeding your family meals that they will love? Considering that nearly 130 million American adults are overweight or obese, and families are looking for meals they can all enjoy together, the answer for most is yes. The problem is that too many people get sucked into the "diet" trap, buying processed, so-called "weight loss" food that is nothing more than junk (some of it isn't even *food*) loaded with artificial ingredients that can actually make you sick. Well, I'd like to offer a better suggestion: Head to the kitchen and get cooking!

Okay, I know what you're thinking. You're running through a list of reasons you just can't do it. Maybe you don't have time, or it's too expensive, or it takes too much effort. Perhaps you have no idea what you're doing in the kitchen or you believe healthy food tastes bland. I'm sure you have a ton of reasons—and I've heard most of them.

I'm going to bust all the excuses that keep you out of your kitchen, and show you that cooking—even cooking healthy, nutritious food—is quick, easy, and, dare I say it, painless. It's not nearly as pricey as buying processed, packaged junk food, or, down the line, treating the diseases caused by obesity, including cancer, heart disease, and diabetes. Cooking at home is both delicious and satisfying—and it can encourage healthy habits in your family, too.

Still skeptical? Doubt I can change your mind about healthy cooking? If you don't believe me, just take it from the millions of readers of my recipe and healthy-eating blog, Skinnytaste.com. Since 2008, I've been converting the most reluctant eaters, and I'm hoping you'll be next on my list! I'm thrilled (and so humbled) by the incredible number of Skinnytaste success stories—people who have turned to my site for inspiration, advice, and help in creating delicious meals that enable them to lose weight and keep it off. Speaking of success stories, I consider myself one, too.

THE ORIGINAL SKINNYTASTE SUCCESS STORY

I was one of those skinny teens who could eat whatever I wanted and never gain a pound (I actually used to try to *put on* weight). But like all good things, it didn't last. Once I was in my twenties, those days of eating whatever I wanted without worrying about weight gain soon came to an end, as pregnancy, children, a slower metabolism, and a love for eating out led to weight gain. Like many, I turned to lots of fad diets, which inevitably didn't stick. My turning point was trying Weight Watchers, which is really more of a lifestyle than a diet. The program gave me the tools to learn how to eat right, which helped me form a healthy relationship with food.

But still I found myself faced with a huge hurdle: I couldn't find any healthy and tasty recipes that supported my lifestyle. Sure, there were plenty of so-called "diet" recipes out there, but many of them used processed foods or they tasted, well, diet-y. I realized that Weight Watchers—or any other diet plan, for that matter—wouldn't work for me unless I found a way to love the food I was eating.

I've always loved to cook, and I love a challenge, so I set my mind to figuring out how to make some of my favorite meals lighter. I

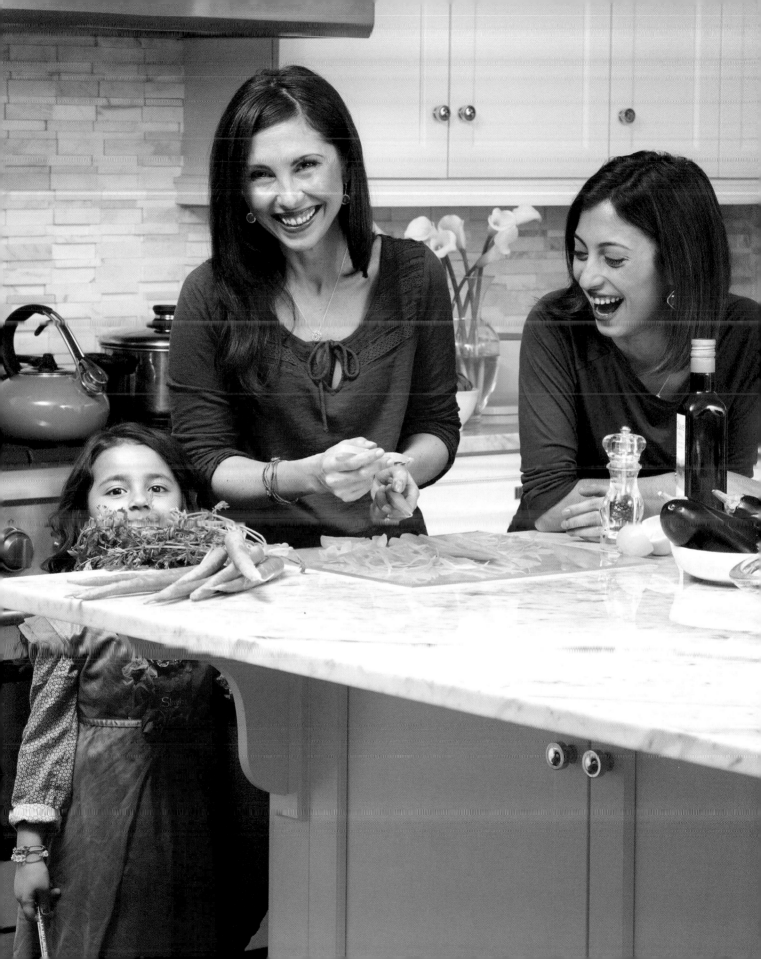

was thrilled when I discovered that many of my favorite dishes could easily be tweaked to lower the fat and calorie content. But here's the thing: It wasn't enough that the dishes tasted good and were good for me—they also had to appeal to my family. After all, having to make a meal for myself and then a separate meal for the rest of the family was not an option. Really, who has the time for that?

Happily, my kitchen experiments worked. I uncovered the secret formula to kitchen and waistline success: If you skinny-fy (that is, put a healthy spin on) dishes you already love, you'll feel satisfied as you slim down—no sacrificing or deprivation necessary. And a big bonus, my family loved the meals I prepared.

Needing a place to house all of my skinny creations, I started Skinnytaste.com purely for fun. As a graphic designer, my blog allowed me to marry several of my passions: creating fabulous skinny meals, design, and photography. As my blog grew more popular, the feedback started pouring in. It was incredibly gratifying to read weight-loss stories from Skinnytaste fans and receive heartfelt letters from people who were slimming down cooking my recipes (and loving them!). I was touched by their praise, and this motivated me to keep my pots in action! Skinnytaste.com is now my full-time job—one that I love. (Can someone please pinch me?)

SO, WHAT'S YOUR EXCUSE?

Now that you know a little about me, let's talk about you. What is keeping you from whipping up healthy, homemade meals? If you're not sure, take a quick look at some of the following reasons people struggle to embrace cooking. Do any sound familiar? This book is going to help you get beyond those excuses.

you don't have the time

I hear you—really, I do. For those who just can't seem to find the time, I've created loads of recipes that you can pull together in 30 minutes or less—those recipes are all labeled with a Q symbol for quick. I've also cooked up a bunch of slow-cooker meals, so you can throw everything together in the morning and then forget about it until it's time to eat that night. Those recipes are all marked with the SC symbol. In addition, you'll find recipes you can double up on and freeze for future use; look for the FF for freezer-friendly.

it's too much work

The little effort I put into prepping and cooking my meals is nothing compared with the rewards. Nothing makes me happier than having my family and friends sitting around my dinner table, laughing, eating, and enjoying my food. I want you to get to a point where you're comfortable enough in the kitchen that cooking becomes not only easy but also enjoyable. You can get there, and I'm here to help.

Recipe Key

Look for these helpful icons throughout the book:

V – Vegetarian

GF – Gluten-Free

Q – Quick (ready in 30 minutes or less)

FF – Freezer-Friendly

SC – Slow Cooker

it costs too much

At first glance, the meal deal at your local fast-food joint seems to be the better buy. But fresh ingredients go beyond one meal—you can stretch them out over the course of several days or more in a variety of meals. Another problem: Many people buy fresh ingredients, only to throw them out because they go bad too fast. If that happens to you, I can see why you think it's more expensive to eat healthfully. I'll show you how to buy the right things and plan ahead so you use it all without wasting.

you don't know the difference between broiling and braising

Not a kitchen pro? Don't sweat it. You'll find a number of simple dishes with easy-to-follow, step-by-step directions for cooks of all levels. And don't be afraid to make mistakes—they provide some of the best lessons.

healthy food sounds about as appetizing as eating paper

I don't know about you, but crispy Buttermilk Oven "Fried" Chicken (page 151), creamy Too-Good-to-Be-True Baked Potato Soup topped with bacon (page 58), and cheesy Kiss My (Shrimp and) Grits (page 219) don't sound like diet food at all. Lucky for you, I'm completely obsessed with figuring out ways to make the dishes I just can't live without skinnier and healthier, and yet unbelievably tasty. I also stay away from artificial ingredients and fake sweeteners and, instead, use what the earth has provided: Quality ingredients, fresh herbs, spices, and seasonal produce that will tantalize your taste buds.

my family won't eat healthy stuff

Can't get anything green past your two-year-old? Have a meat-and-potatoes husband who won't even entertain the idea of chicken, or, gasp, fish? Or maybe your family eats pretty healthfully but doesn't need to lose any weight? There is something for everyone in this book, from picky kids to those with upscale palates. And I haven't forgotten those with food allergies or eating limitations. Gluten-free recipes are marked **GF**; I've also given suggestions on how to adapt various recipes. Vegetarian options are marked with a **V**.

But it's not all about the recipes. This book is filled with easy-to-understand advice that simplifies healthy eating and cooking. And as a special bonus, I've partnered with registered dietitian Heather K. Jones to provide healthy food facts and useful nutritional information, so you can feel good about enjoying the recipes you love.

So step into my kitchen and cook yourself skinny with me!

Salt Solution

All salt is not created equal. Different brands (such as Morton's or Diamond Crystal) and different types (such as table or kosher) vary not only in sodium content but also in taste. To avoid under or (even worse) oversalting a recipe from this book, stick with my preferred salt, Diamond Crystal Kosher. Or just go easy with the shaker and adjust as need be.

THE SKINNY BASICS

create a good-for-you kitchen and lifestyle

Be honest with yourself: Aren't you over all the excuses? What have they done for you, besides keep you from achieving your goals and creating a better life for yourself? By picking up this book, you've already taken the first step to end the excuses. Congratulations! You are now officially on the path toward your goals and a healthier life.

I can assure you that every single recipe in this book will help you on your road to a leaner lifestyle. How do I know this? I've tested and retested every recipe for accuracy in the Skinnytaste test kitchen, which has a staff of just two, my aunt and me. My aunt is a baker, so she's accustomed to following a recipe precisely as written. She catches any blunders and she doesn't overlook small details, so we make the perfect team. (Plus, she lives only minutes away from me.) As you can imagine, testing recipes for a book while also creating new recipes for my blog every day left me with A LOT of extra food at the end of the day. Each afternoon, my aunt and I had a Skinnytaste lunch together, and I would send her home with more food to eat for dinner each night. All this food, and yet there was not a single pound gained. In fact, as the months passed, my aunt dropped 37 pounds and went from a size 12 to a size 4. At first, she thought there might be something wrong, so she went to her doctor to get a full checkup.

The good news: Her doctor said she was in the best shape of her life, her cholesterol was great, and she had more energy than ever. Her doctor asked her secret, and she happily told him to visit Skinnytaste.com. I can't even tell you how great it makes me feel that she is another Skinnytaste success story!

The pages that follow will hopefully make you one, too. I will show you that cooking—even cooking healthy, nutritious food—is quick, easy, and even FUN. It's time to get back into the kitchen, where you can start improving and refining your healthy cooking skills while you simultaneously make your way back into your skinny jeans. And guess what? It's not as hard as you think. Here's how to whittle your waist without skimping on taste, Skinnytaste style.

PLAN AHEAD AND EAT HEALTHY ALL WEEK

Whipping up a week's worth of light, filling, and family-friendly meals is as easy as one, two, three:

1 **Plan your menu for the week.**

2 **Make a shopping list.**

3 **Head to the grocery store to shop for all the ingredients you need.** You can choose one or two freezer-friendly recipes to make on your day off; these will serve as more than one meal so you can have leftovers for lunch or dinner later in the month.

TAKE CHARGE OF YOUR KITCHEN

The bottom line: When *you're* in charge of the cooking, you can control what you eat and what you put into your food. The benefits of home cooking are too many to list, but one that's worth repeating is the fact that making your own meals and snacks is the easiest way to control the types of ingredients and the amount of calories you consume.

Don't be intimidated! You don't have to put together elaborate four-course meals, you don't have to spend hours in front of the stove, and you don't have to use recipes that feature ingredients you can't even pronounce. Just get in the kitchen and start cooking. No matter what your comfort level, these recipes will work for you. And if you make a mistake, it's okay! That's the best way to learn. Cut yourself some slack and enjoy the process (and the results)!

DUMP THE JUNK

The road to Skinny isn't paved with processed food. And yet, supermarket shelves are jam-packed with them. What's the draw? They may help save a little time and effort, but try to read the label—there will be a long list of ingredients you've never even heard of or can't pronounce. Even the so-called "healthy" foods can be loaded with sodium, calories, sugar, and fat. If that's what's in your fridge, freezer, or pantry, the road to Skinny will be a bumpy one.

Having a properly stocked kitchen, on the other hand, can help set you up for weight loss success. (See "A Skinny Kitchen Makeover," page 17.) Whenever a snack attack strikes, you'll be fully prepared with healthy snacks.

FALL IN LOVE WITH REAL FOOD

My eating philosophy is built on utilizing in-season, whole foods—those that are in their unprocessed and natural state. Whole foods are healthier and there's no doubt they taste better. Not only that, when you cook with whole foods, you know exactly what you're putting into your body. Head to your local farmers' market, check

out the organic and produce sections of your neighborhood supermarket, or visit a health food store to stock up on the freshest, tastiest, most nutritious ingredients. Another option, if it's available in your area: a CSA (community supported agriculture). When you join one, you'll get a weekly box of fresh produce and other foods delivered from a local farm. It's a win-win: You'll be supporting local farmers and you'll get the opportunity to experiment with new foods. It's time to reconnect with real food.

KEEP IT SIMPLE

If you're intimidated by healthy eating, you're not alone. But there's no need to stress, because I like to keep things simple. I base my meals largely on nutrient-packed, energy-boosting vegetables, fruits, beans, whole grains, and healthy fats. You'll eat fish and only modest amounts (if you choose to) of lean meat and dairy products. You'll also cut back on salt, refined sugars, white flour, and partially hydrogenated oils. That's it!

FORGET THE FADS

Here's a Skinny secret: Typical fast-fix diets don't work. I've tried several diets that either required me to eat the same bland, tasteless food every day or that required me to cut out carbs completely. Sure, those diets may help you lose weight in the short-term, but they very rarely keep the pounds away for good. In fact, more often than not, they lead to dangerous yo-yo dieting, which could permanently damage your relationship with food. To really shrink your waistline—and keep it that way—you must alter your eating habits and lifestyle in a way that's easy to stick with in the long run.

SERVE UP PERFECT PORTIONS

If you stick to the recipes in this book, your portions will automatically be controlled. Of course, that's not the case if you're making a different recipe or you're dining out.

A good guideline that always helps me at home: Picture a plate divided in half. Fill one half with salad and veggies, one fourth with whole grains, and the last fourth with lean protein. You can mix up your food options at each meal to maximize your nutrient intake and shake things up for your taste buds. Another trick to use at home is to eat on smaller plates; studies show you'll eat less but you will still feel full.

When you eat out, try to use a few tricks to keep portion sizes under control. For instance, pass on the bread basket (it's too easy to lose track of slices), order an appetizer as your full meal, split an entrée with a dining companion, or take half the meal home for lunch the next day.

Make Your Calories Count

While all food contains calories, some are better than others at helping your body look and feel its best. In other words, the quality of your calories counts as much as the quantity. These "high-quality calories" come from healthy fats, lean protein, and high-fiber carbohydrates.

While exact calorie needs depend upon a variety of factors (height, weight, activity levels, etc.), an intake of around 1,500 to 1,600 calories per day will lead to a healthy weight loss of about two pounds per week for most women. (For extra help keeping track, use a free calorie counter app, such as myfitnesspal.com.)

An ideal meal combines at least two of these three groups to help you feel full, maintain normal blood sugar levels, stop you from overeating, and promote a healthy glow from the inside out. Create your own meals and snacks by picking foods from at least two of these three categories:

healthy fats
Monounsaturated and polyunsaturated fats help improve blood cholesterol levels, which reduces your risk of heart disease. Plus, they're filling, so they contribute to weight control.

TRY: olives, avocados, hummus, peanut butter, hazelnuts, almonds, cashews, pumpkin seeds, sesame seeds, and olive oil

lean protein
Lean protein is super-satisfying and low in saturated fat, which is a huge help for weight loss and heart health. Protein also provides building material for muscles, and muscles are your friends. In addition to making your body look sexy and sculpted, they burn calories *all the time*, even when you're asleep.

TRY: eggs, beans, tofu, edamame, turkey, roast beef, pork tenderloin, 0% Greek yogurt, low-fat milk, nuts and nut butters, seeds, and fish

high-fiber carbohydrates
Fiber is a type of indigestible carbohydrate that slows carbohydrate digestion, blunting the rise in blood sugar and keeping hunger at bay. It's also linked to reduced risk of heart disease and diabetes.

TRY: oatmeal, nuts and seeds, fruit, beans, peas, whole wheat bread, whole wheat pasta, whole grains (like brown rice, quinoa, and popcorn), and vegetables

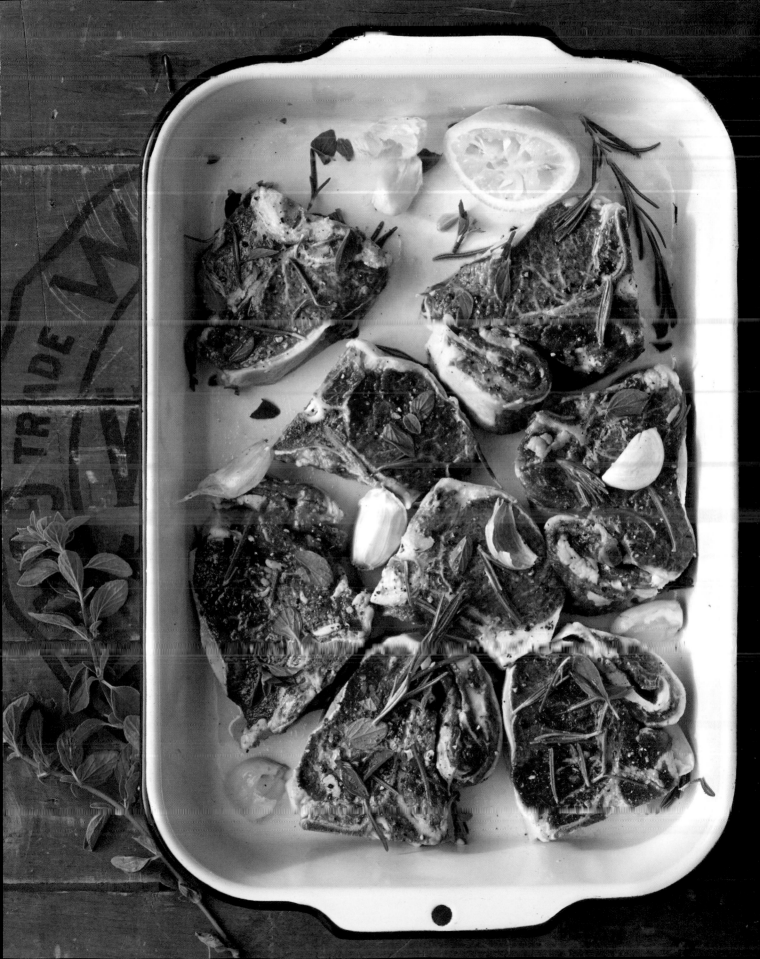

PASS ON PERFECTION

Theodore Roosevelt said it best: "Comparison is the thief of joy." This is my favorite quote, and it can apply to so many facets of life. In this case, I mean the idea of that perfect body. We all come in different shapes and sizes, so try to be the best version of yourself and stop comparing yourself to those perfect magazine models. By the way, I worked for years in photo retouching, where we'd spend hours retouching the models to get that "perfect" look. You would be surprised if you saw the before and after photos. Even the prettiest of models and celebrities have flaws just like you and me.

GIVE YOURSELF A BREAK

Food is my life. I test recipes, write about food, attend food blog conferences, and go on lots of awesome food trips hosted by large brands where I get fed some pretty darn good food. If you think I'm passing up any of these delightful dishes because I'm watching my weight, you're wrong. I make good choices all week so I can still enjoy a great meal out here and there. Going out to dinner with my husband or enjoying a night out with the girls is one of my favorite things to do. I learn about new flavors and foods, and I get inspiration from those meals. But I still maintain my healthy weight because I factor that in to my life.

So shed that all-or-nothing attitude. Perfection does not equal success when it comes to losing weight or becoming comfortable in the kitchen. Allow yourself some wiggle room and be patient. Remember, you didn't put on the extra weight overnight.

Also keep in mind that no food is considered off-limits or "bad" when eating the Skinnytaste way. The more you deprive yourself of certain foods, the more you're going to crave them. Enjoy your favorite foods in moderation from time to time, be it a planned indulgence once in a while or a spontaneous bite of a favorite dessert. This is a realistic way of eating that you can keep up for the rest of your life.

EXERCISE, STRESS LESS, AND GET PLENTY OF SLEEP

As irresistible as my healthy recipes are, eating a nutritious diet alone is not enough to get your best body—you have to consider the big picture. It involves all the components of a healthy life: a healthy balance of exercise, plenty of sleep, stress relief, and fun.

Exercise is an important part of life, as staying fit and being active on a regular basis will not only help you lose weight and decrease your risk for a variety of diseases, but it will also boost your energy levels and improve your mood. It is also a great way to relieve stress. High levels of stress can wreak havoc on your body, so it's also important to manage your stress levels. Unwind by doing some yoga, treating yourself to a massage or other spa treatment, playing with your kids, or even just listening to music. And don't forget sleep!

Don't Forget to Hydrate

Even mild dehydration can bring on fatigue and snack attacks. Aim for a daily goal of at least eight 8-ounce glasses of fluid, with most of that coming from water. Be wary of calorie-dense high-sugar teas, energy drinks, and juice. It takes just a few minutes to drink a few hundred calories, and you'll still feel hungry when you're done because your body doesn't feel as full from drinking liquid as it does from eating food.

I function best after seven to nine hours a night, though everyone is different. When I'm well rested, I'm alert and ready to take on the new day. Figure out the amount of sleep you need to function at your best, and then make sure you get that amount each night.

Lastly, don't forget about the fun factor. You're creating this amazing, healthy Skinny life for yourself—make sure you take full advantage of it. Take some time to think about what you enjoy, and then make a point to do one or more of those things each day.

A SKINNY KITCHEN MAKEOVER

Ready to get on the path to a healthier, leaner new you? Your first step is to give your fridge, freezer, and pantry a healthy makeover. Some of you might think you already have this all figured out, but I'm sure if I sneaked a peek at your pantry, I'd find at least a few hidden obstacles just waiting to trip you up. Use the strategies below to set up your kitchen for healthy eating success.

THE FRIDGE

keep it real

Your focus should be on health before weight. To accomplish this goal, stock your fridge with real ingredients—that means whole, unprocessed foods and no substituting eggs with liquid egg replacements or real bacon with turkey bacon. A little real and flavorful food goes a long way, so I keep it in moderation.

be choosy with cheese

Cheese is a stellar source of calcium and protein. For certain varieties—like mozzarella, Swiss, or cheddar—I don't mind opting for reduced-fat. But for stronger flavored cheeses,

such as sharp cheddar, Gorgonzola, and Romano, I stick with the real thing because I can use smaller quantities to get the same flavor hit. And I always have naturally lower-in-fat cheeses, such as Pecorino Romano or Parmigiano-Reggiano, in my fridge to boost the flavor in a variety of dishes.

toss light butters and vegetable spreads

You're better off going for a dab of real or whipped butter instead of those highly processed spreads. I usually cook with healthy oils, but once in a while, butter is necessary. Cookies, crusts, and scones, for instance, often require butter; and for those occasions, I go for the real thing and simply use smaller amounts.

replace artificially sweetened yogurt

Stock up instead on plain, nonfat, or low-fat yogurt or Greek yogurt. You'd be surprised by how many low-calorie yogurts use artificial sweeteners to keep the calories down. Plain Greek yogurt doesn't have any added sweeteners and it's higher in protein. Sweeten it yourself with fresh fruit or a drizzle of honey.

give up nondairy creamers

Instead, use real dairy milk or soy- or nut-based milks. You might think you're saving calories by using creamer in your coffee, but do you really need it? Most nondairy fat-free creamers are made with partially hydrogenated oils and a whole list of artificial ingredients. Stick to the real thing. If I want to flavor my coffee, I sprinkle in some ground cinnamon, cocoa powder, pumpkin spice, or vanilla extract.

dispose of store-bought salad dressings

Toss those bottled salad dressings (yes, even the low-fat ones) and make your own from scratch.

It's easy, tastes better, will save you money, and will put you in control over what you add to your recipe. (See Fabulous Main-Dish Salads on page 123 for dressing recipes.)

toss the soda

Don't drink your calories away! You can save hundreds of calories by simply swapping out soda and other sugar-sweetened beverages for water, seltzer, or sparkling water. Need a little flavor? Toss in some fruit, such as watermelon slices, berries, or lemon, lime, or orange wedges; or add some slices of cucumbers or fresh mint.

THE FREEZER

forgo frozen entrées

How about real home cooking instead of all those preservatives? Sure, it takes some extra time to prepare, but the health benefits are worth the effort—look for all my recipes with the FF tag and make your own healthier, freezer-friendly meals!

stock up on frozen fruits and vegetables

The problem with canned vegetables is that they tend to lose a lot of nutrients during the preservation process (notable exceptions include tomatoes and pumpkin). Frozen vegetables, on the other hand, may be even more healthful than some of the fresh produce sold in supermarkets because they are flash-frozen when they're at their peak. Choose packages marked with a USDA "U.S. Fancy" shield, which designates produce of the best size, shape, and color. Vegetables of this standard also tend to be more nutrient-rich than the lower grades "U.S. No. 1" or "U.S. No. 2."

opt for better ice cream alternatives

Don't break the calorie bank on full-fat ice creams. Instead, opt for nonfat frozen yogurt or sorbet. I love Stonyfield Organic Nonfat Frozen Yogurt. Or you can make your own healthier frozen treats: Try freezing ripe bananas to make a quick and healthy one-ingredient frozen treat in your food processor, or make your own popsicles with fresh fruit purees, or create a granita (see recipe on page 310).

THE PANTRY

replace white with whole grains

This one simple swap—replacing refined white bread, pasta, and rice with whole grains—will increase the amount of fiber and antioxidants you get each day. Plus, whole grains take longer to digest so they keep you feeling fuller, longer. Experiment with different varieties of rice and pastas or try some new grains, such as quinoa, farro, barley, bulgur, wheatberries, spelt, and more.

opt for healthy oils

Say hello to a variety of heart-healthy oils: Canola, olive, and peanut oils are all high in monounsaturated fats, while sunflower, soybean, and sesame oils are high in healthy polyunsaturated fats.

stock up on whole-grain cereals

Skip the sugary cereals and instead load up on a variety of fiber-rich whole-grain cereals. Go for oats and granola, or try using quinoa in place of your porridge.

buy beans and legumes

Dried or canned beans and legumes are not only economical, they're also a perfect pantry staple because they keep for a while and can be used in a variety of dishes. They're a smart buy for health: They're high in fiber and protein as well as B vitamins and iron.

sweeten smartly

Less refined sweeteners, like raw sugar, raw honey, and pure maple syrup, contain more antioxidants and give your blood sugar a gentler rise. Still, you'll want to sweeten smartly because these more natural sweeteners are high in calories, so use them sparingly.

be prepared for a snack attack

Toss all those salty fried snacks and instead opt for raw or dry-roasted nuts, like almonds, peanuts, cashews, and walnuts. A handful of nuts is a fiber-rich snack that's high in healthy fats. Combine them with dried fruit and whole-grain cereal to make your own trail mix. You can also stock up on nut butters, baked tortilla chips, whole-grain crackers, air-popped popcorn, dark chocolate, and fresh fruit (on the counter or in the fridge) so you always have healthier snack alternatives on hand.

Bottom line: Having a properly stocked kitchen can help set you up for success. In fact, when your pantry, fridge, and freezer are loaded with the right ingredients and products, healthy eating becomes a breeze.

Stay Motivated

Everyone gets in a slump once in a while, and sometimes it's hard to find your way out. But don't throw in the towel! Instead, find a way to get back in control. Here some tricks that work for me:

- **SURROUND YOURSELF WITH PEOPLE WHO INSPIRE YOU.** I like to be around fit people because they inspire me to work out more. Finding a workout buddy can also help give you that push to keep you on track.

- **PENCIL YOURSELF IN.** We are all busy, and finding time for exercise can be hard. I schedule my workouts in my calendar, as I would a business meeting or doctor's appointment.

- **GO PUBLIC.** Committing yourself publicly, whether it's to friends in person or on social media or even via a blog, can help you stay on track. We don't like to let others down, so this public proclamation can keep us from breaking our commitment to ourselves.

- **THINK SMALL.** Sure, you may want to lose 20, 30, or 40 pounds, or maybe even more. But think of it this way: Every pound lost brings you a pound closer to your goal. So celebrate every small accomplishment, whether it's simply hitting the gym instead of the snooze button or passing on seconds of your favorite dessert.

- **MAKE A LIST AND CHECK IT OFTEN.** Jot down a list of all the reasons you want to eat healthfully, get in better shape, and lose weight. Maybe it's for your family or an upcoming vacation; maybe you're sick and tired of feeling sick and tired. Keep the list handy and refer to it whenever your motivation starts to flag.

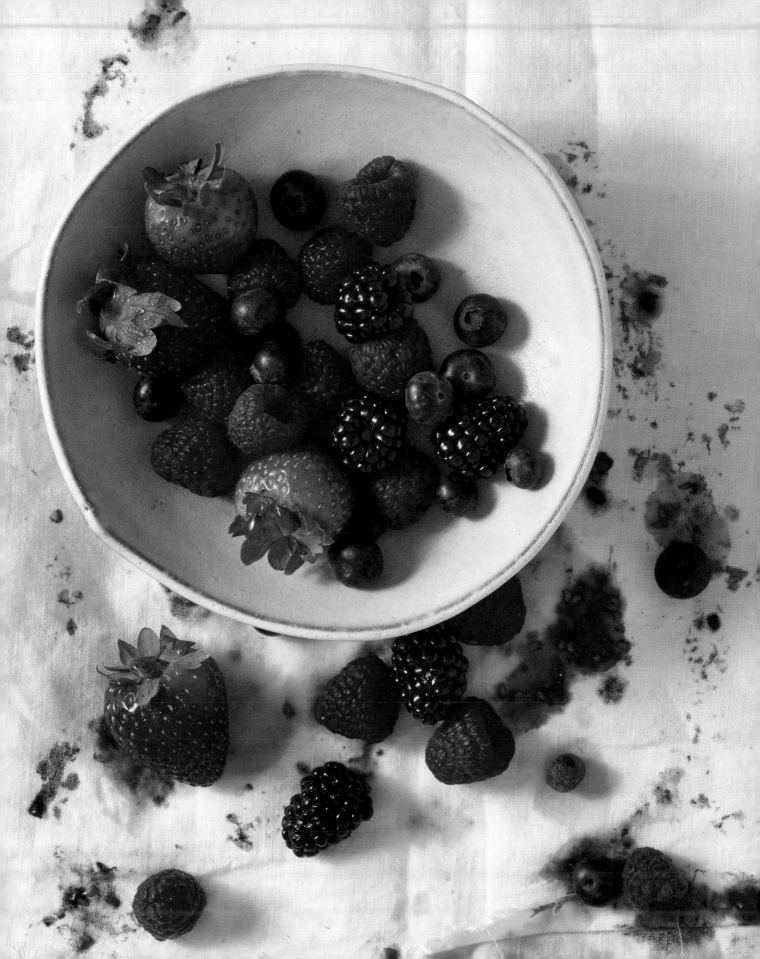

SUNNY MORNINGS

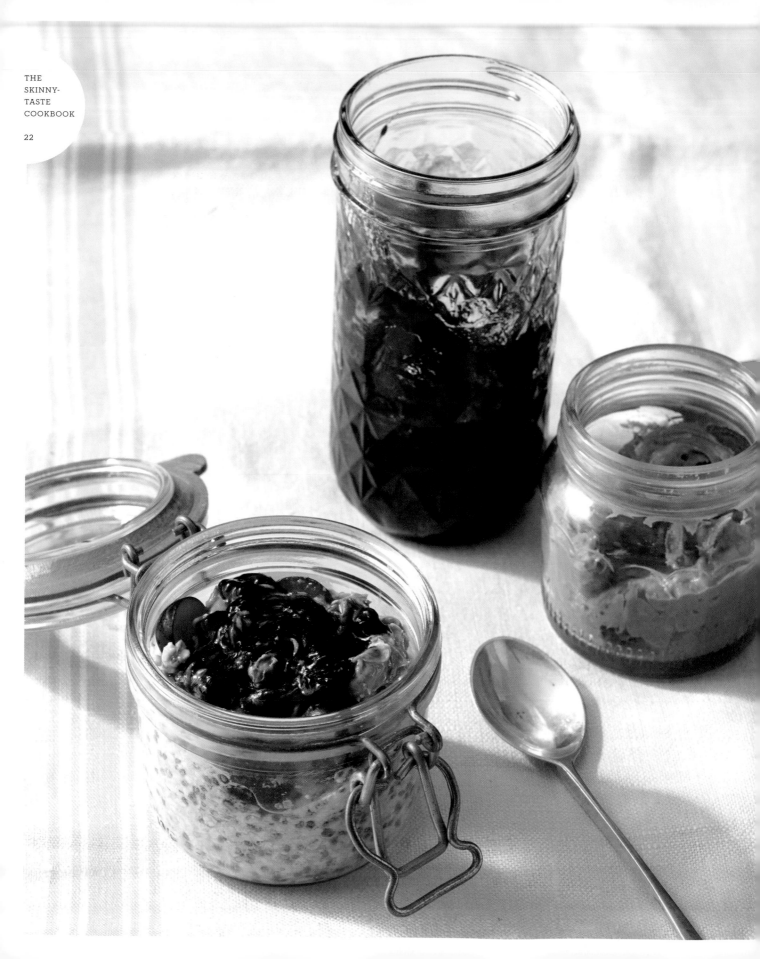

PB & J Overnight Oats in a Jar

SERVES 1

I always found comfort in those mornings when my mom made us warm oatmeal for breakfast. I've never liked the instant stuff, and so I've always made my oatmeal from scratch, just like my mom did. But recently, I discovered overnight oats, which makes a made-from-scratch version possible on those busy weekdays. Plus, it's packed with protein, fiber, vitamins, and nutrients—score!

OATS

½ cup unsweetened almond milk (or skim, or soy)

¼ cup quick-cooking oats*

¼ cup red seedless grapes, halved

½ tablespoon chia seeds

1 teaspoon sugar (I prefer raw cane sugar)

TOPPINGS

1 tablespoon crunchy peanut butter

1 tablespoon reduced-sugar grape jelly

Read the label to be sure this product is gluten-free.

For the oats: In an 8-ounce mason jar, combine the milk, oats, grapes, chia seeds, and sugar. Close the jar with the lid, shake the mixture, and refrigerate overnight.

For the toppings: The next day, take the jar out of the refrigerator, stir in the peanut butter and jelly, and serve.

FOOD FACTS fill up with oats

If you're looking for an easy and satisfying morning meal that can keep hunger in check until lunchtime, oats are the answer. Oats are loaded with soluble fiber, which slows digestion and can keep you feeling fuller longer. They also contain a good amount of protein, which is more satiating than fat or carbs. And studies show the soluble fiber in oats can help reduce LDL ("bad") cholesterol, which can cut your risk for heart disease.

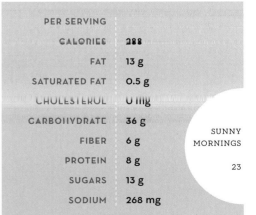

PER SERVING	
CALORIES	288
FAT	13 g
SATURATED FAT	0.5 g
CHOLESTEROL	0 mg
CARBOHYDRATE	36 g
FIBER	6 g
PROTEIN	8 g
SUGARS	13 g
SODIUM	268 mg

Coco-Loco Mango Green Smoothie

SERVES 1

(V) (GF) (Q)

The first time I made a green smoothie, I was a little scared to taste it. But after my first sip, I was hooked. In fact, I start my morning with a green smoothie three or four days each week. Even my toddler loves them, and I like knowing that she's getting a healthy serving of greens. You can use any combination of fruit you like, but I'm wild about the pairing of coconut and sweet ripe mango. I like adding chia seeds to my smoothies, but I also play around with other superfoods, such as flaxseed, hemp seeds, and berries. And I also experiment with different greens, like baby kale and baby chard.

1 cup So Delicious original coconut milk beverage

½ cup chopped ripe mango

1 cup baby spinach

1 tablespoon sweetened coconut flakes*

1 teaspoon chia seeds

1 medium dried pitted date (or 1 teaspoon sugar)

1 cup ice

*Read the label to be sure this product is gluten-free.

In a blender, combine the coconut milk, mango, spinach, coconut flakes, chia seeds, and the date and blend until smooth. Add the ice and blend again until smooth.

FOOD FACTS little seed, big nutrition
Indigenous to Central America, chia seeds have been a staple energy source for centuries and are high in omega-3 fatty acids, which have been shown to improve cardiovascular health. They have incredible satiating effects, a high fiber content, and a good amount of healthy fats and antioxidants.

PER SERVING	
CALORIES	240
FAT	8 g
SATURATED FAT	5.5 g
CHOLESTEROL	0 mg
CARBOHYDRATE	36 g
FIBER	8 g
PROTEIN	3 g
SUGARS	30 g
SODIUM	56 mg

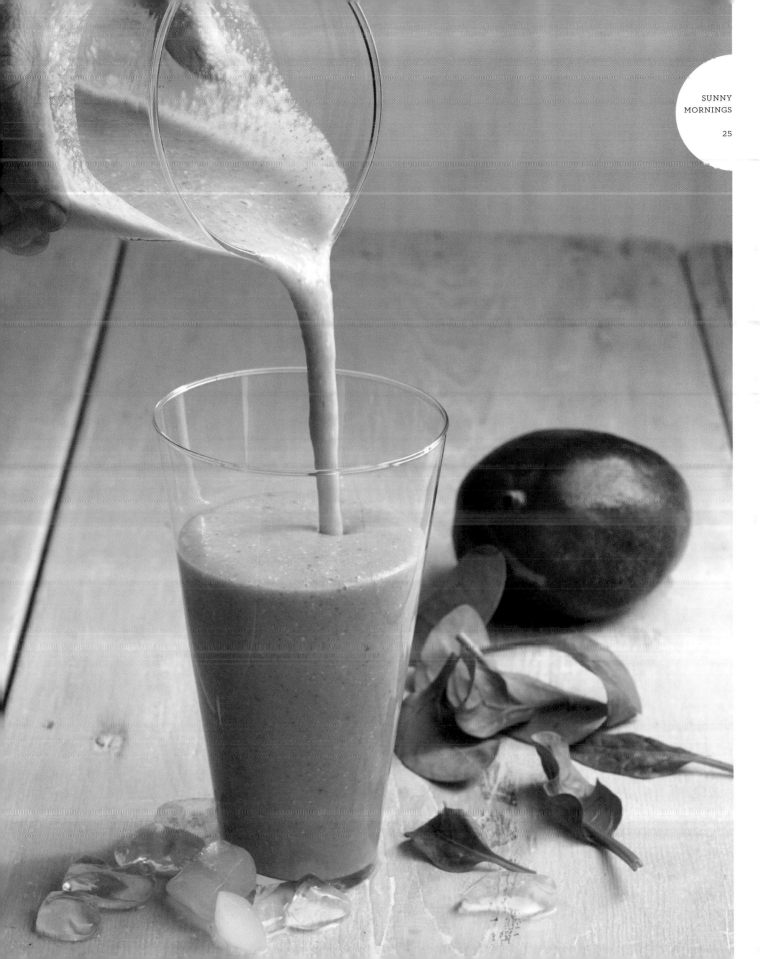

Good-for-You Granola

MAKES 3¾ CUPS • SERVES 11

Here's how I like my cereal: Fill a bowl with a cup of whatever fruit is on hand, top it with ⅓ cup homemade granola, and pour in some unsweetened almond milk. This is my basic granola recipe—you can add any combination of dried fruit, nuts, or other ingredients that you like. Whatever you use, you'll feel good knowing that this recipe is lower in fat than store-bought granola.

¼ cup quinoa

1½ cups rolled oats*

¼ cup unsweetened shredded coconut

¼ cup ground flaxseeds

¼ cup slivered almonds

¼ cup chopped walnuts

¼ cup dried blueberries

¼ cup dried cherries

¼ cup honey

1 teaspoon virgin coconut oil (or canola)

½ teaspoon pure vanilla extract

¼ teaspoon ground cinnamon

Kosher salt

skinny**scoop**

I make a batch of granola on weekends when I have free time. Kept in an airtight jar, it can last a month or longer.

*Read the label to be sure this product is gluten-free.

Preheat the oven to 325°F. Line a baking sheet with parchment paper.

Rinse the quinoa thoroughly under cold water in a fine-mesh sieve. Drain well and pat dry with paper towels.

Spread the quinoa, oats, and coconut out on the baking sheet. Toast in the oven, stirring once, until golden, about 10 minutes. Transfer the oat mixture to a medium bowl and add the ground flaxseeds, almonds, walnuts, and dried fruit. (Leave the oven on.)

In a separate medium bowl, combine the honey, oil, vanilla, cinnamon, and a pinch of salt. Pour the mixture over the oats and stir together with a spatula.

Spread the mixture out on the lined baking sheet. Bake until golden brown, 10 to 12 minutes.

PER SERVING	(⅓ CUP)
CALORIES	173
FAT	6.5 g
SATURATED FAT	2 g
CHOLESTEROL	0 mg
CARBOHYDRATE	27 g
FIBER	3.5 g
PROTEIN	4 g
SUGARS	13 g
SODIUM	8 mg

Paradise Parfait

SERVES 2

When I make a parfait, there are no rules—I use whatever I have on hand. However, the one guideline I try to follow is to make it as colorful as possible. We eat with our eyes, so I often consider how something will look when I make it. Layering is one way to make a dish more visually appealing. The mango and coconut give it a tropical flair and offer up one-and-a-half fruit servings, as well as protein and fiber.

1¼ cups (10 ounces) 0% plain Greek yogurt

½ cup chopped strawberries

¼ cup chopped pineapple

½ cup chopped mango

¼ cup sweetened coconut flakes*

2 teaspoons honey

Read the label to be sure this product is gluten-free.

Layer the yogurt, strawberries, pineapple, and mango in clear parfait cups or champagne glasses. Top with sweetened coconut flakes, drizzle with honey, and serve.

A DIY Parfait Party Bar

Start with nonfat Greek yogurt and let your guests pick their favorite mix-ins. Choose a variety for maximum flavor, color, and crunch:

FRUITY: fresh berries, cherries, bananas, peaches, kiwi, pomegranate seeds, pineapple, mango, fresh figs, dried fruit

CRUNCHY: granola, toasted nuts (chopped pecans, walnuts, pistachios, and almonds), coconut flakes (toasted, optional)

SWEET: cacao nibs, dark chocolate, honey, peanut butter, honey, maple syrup

"SPICE-Y:" cinnamon, cocoa powder, nutmeg, pumpkin pie spice

NUTRITION BOOSTERS: chia seeds, hemp seeds, ground flaxseeds, goji berries, toasted quinoa

PER SERVING	(1 PARFAIT)
CALORIES	220
FAT	3 g
SATURATED FAT	3 g
CHOLESTEROL	0 mg
CARBOHYDRATE	32 g
FIBER	3 g
PROTEIN	18 g
SUGARS	26 g
SODIUM	85 mg

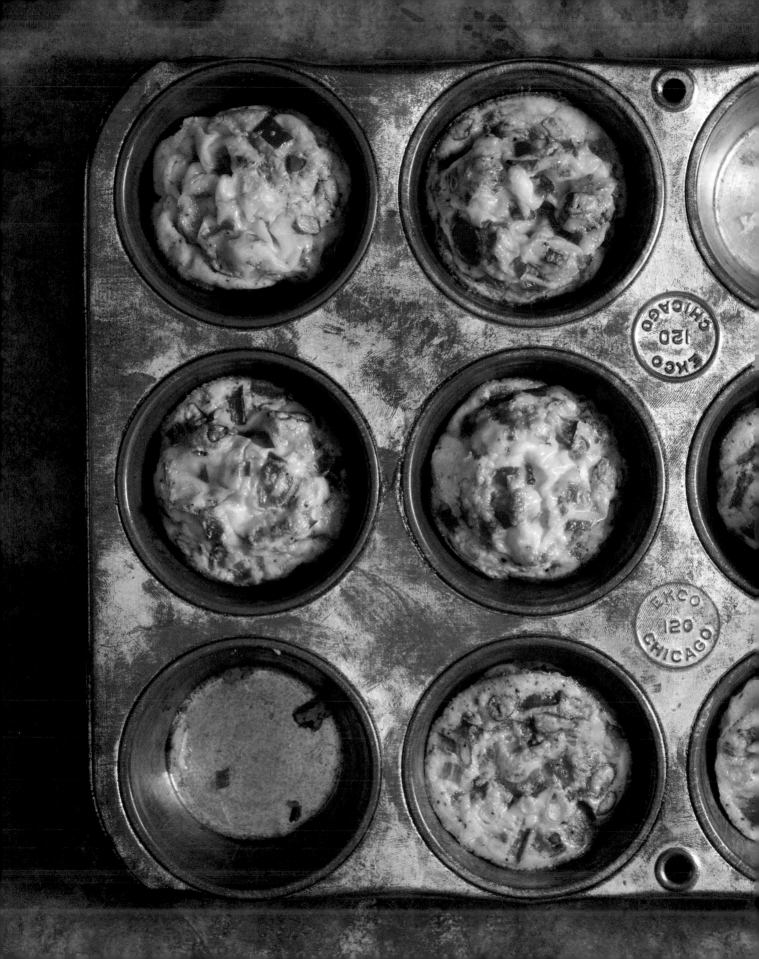

Make-Ahead Western Omelet "Muffins"

MAKES 12 MUFFIN-SIZE OMELETS • SERVES 6

GF **Q** **FF**

These make-ahead muffin-size omelets are the perfect solution for breakfasts on the run. Bake them up and you'll have breakfast ready for the next few days. Just keep them refrigerated and portioned in zip-top plastic bags. Simply reheat right before heading to work or the gym, or getting your kids off to school. To make these light, I swap half the egg yolks with egg whites. That way, you still get the nutrients of the egg yolk, but with half the fat.

Olive oil cooking spray or oil mister

6 large eggs

6 large egg whites

¼ teaspoon kosher salt

Freshly cracked black pepper

3 ounces sliced ham (about 4 slices), finely chopped

2 ounces reduced fat Swiss cheese, chopped

½ cup finely chopped red or orange bell pepper

¼ cup chopped scallions

Preheat the oven to 350°F. Lightly spray a standard 12-cup nonstick or silicone muffin tin with oil.

In a medium bowl, beat the whole eggs and egg whites with a fork. Season them with the salt and a pinch of black pepper. Mix in the ham, Swiss cheese, bell pepper, and scallions. Pour about ¼ cup of egg mixture into each muffin cup and carefully place the pan in the oven.

Bake until the eggs set, 20 to 24 minutes.

skinny**scoop**

You can freeze leftovers or make a double batch. To freeze, wrap cooled egg muffins in plastic wrap. To reheat, unwrap frozen egg muffins and microwave about 1 minute or place on a cookie sheet and bake at 350°F until heated through, about 25 minutes.

PER SERVING	(2 MUFFIN-SIZE OMELETS)
CALORIES	119
FAT	6 g
SATURATED FAT	2 g
CHOLESTEROL	195 mg
CARBOHYDRATE	2 g
FIBER	0.5 g
PROTEIN	14 g
SUGARS	1 g
SODIUM	329 mg

Apple 'n' Spice Baked Oatmeal

SERVES 6

Apples and spice and everything nice! I love baked oatmeal. It's almost like having dessert for breakfast—without the guilt. Whenever I make it, I can trick my toddler, Madison, into eating it cold because she thinks it's cake. I personally prefer eating it warm, right out of the oven, and I make this anytime I need something delish for brunch or a breakfast potluck.

APPLE FILLING

2 tablespoons honey

2 cups peeled and chopped Gala apples

¾ cup golden raisins

1 tablespoon cornstarch

¾ teaspoon ground cinnamon

¼ teaspoon ground nutmeg

Cooking spray or oil mister

OATMEAL

1 cup quick-cooking oats*

⅓ cup chopped walnuts or pecans

½ teaspoon baking powder

Kosher salt

1 cup fat-free milk

1 large egg

2 tablespoons raw honey

1 teaspoon pure vanilla extract

FOOD FACTS fill up on fiber! Studies show that people lose more weight when they fill up on high-fiber foods, such as fruit, oats, and other whole grains. Your goal: at least 25 grams of fiber a day for women, 38 grams for men.

Read the label to be sure this product is gluten-free.

For the apple filling: In a large heavy pot, combine ⅓ cup water, the honey, apples, raisins, cornstarch, cinnamon, and nutmeg. Bring to a simmer over low heat and cook, stirring occasionally, until the apples are soft, about 25 minutes.

Preheat the oven to 375°F. Lightly spray an 8 × 8-inch or 9 × 9-inch ceramic baking dish with oil. Put the apples into the bottom of the prepared baking dish.

For the oatmeal: In a bowl, combine the oats, half of the walnuts, baking powder, and a pinch of salt. Pour over the apples.

In a separate bowl, whisk together the milk, egg, honey, and vanilla. Pour the milk mixture over the oats, making sure to distribute the mixture as evenly as possible.

Sprinkle the remaining walnuts over the top. Bake until the top is golden brown and the oatmeal is set, about 30 minutes. Cut into 6 rectangles and serve warm from the oven.

PER SERVING	(1 RECTANGLE)
CALORIES	250
FAT	6 g
SATURATED FAT	1 g
CHOLESTEROL	32 mg
CARBOHYDRATE	47 g
FIBER	3 g
PROTEIN	6 g
SUGARS	30 g
SODIUM	89 mg

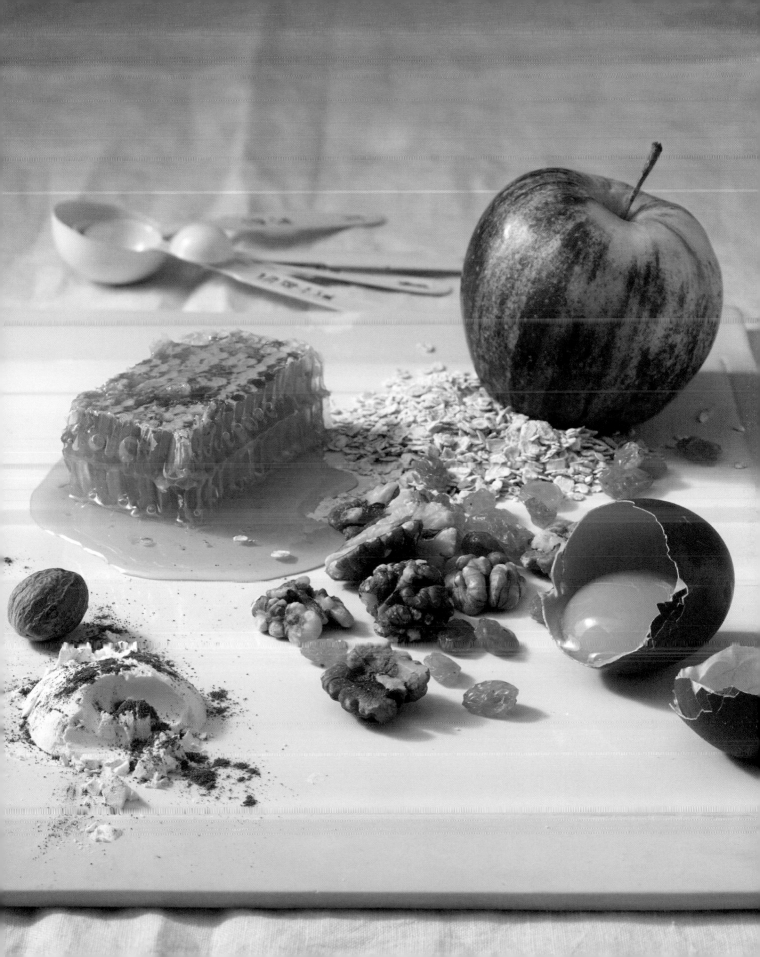

Naked Eggs Benedict

SERVES 4

When I was a teenager, my mom owned a luncheonette eponymously named Marlene's Kitchen. She worked behind the counter cooking breakfast for all her customers and I helped out, working as a waitress on weekends. It was a quaint little place, where everyone knew one another and felt at home. Of all the breakfast options there, poached eggs topped with cheese were my favorite. I'm also fond of another popular poached pick: Eggs Benedict. But the Hollandaise sauce is all butter, and just a few tablespoons contain a whopping 200 calories. No thanks! My "skinny" solution is simple: Use whole-grain English muffins, add some greens, and skip the Hollandaise sauce. Then I don't feel bad splurging with a little light Havarti cheese on top.

4 slices Canadian bacon

4 large eggs

2 light multigrain English muffins, split and toasted

1 cup loosely packed baby spinach

Kosher salt and freshly cracked black pepper

2 ounces light Havarti cheese, grated

1 tablespoon minced fresh chives, for garnish

Heat a large skillet over medium-high heat. Add the Canadian bacon and cook until lightly browned on each side, about 1 minute.

Fill a large deep skillet with about 2 inches of water and bring to a boil. Reduce the heat to low to maintain a simmer. Crack the eggs into individual bowls. Gently slide the eggs one at a time into the simmering water. Using a spoon, gently nudge the egg whites in toward the yolk. Cook for 2 to 3 minutes for a semi-soft yolk or 3 to 4 minutes for a firmer-set yolk. Using a slotted spoon or spatula, transfer the eggs one at a time to a plate lined with paper towels to drain.

Divide the toasted muffin halves among 4 serving plates. Top each muffin half with a piece of Canadian bacon, ¼ cup baby spinach, and a poached egg. Season each with a pinch of salt and black pepper to taste. Sprinkle with shredded cheese and minced chives, and serve hot.

PER SERVING	(1 SANDWICH)
CALORIES	206
FAT	7 g
SATURATED FAT	3.5 g
CHOLESTEROL	230 mg
PROTEIN	19 g
CARBOHYDRATE	14 g
FIBER	4 g
SUGARS	1 g
SODIUM	609 mg

Greek-a-licious Egg White Omelet

SERVES 4

V GF Q

Egg white omelets can be boring, but not when you fill them with flavor! This savory omelet is packed with spinach, tomatoes, feta, and dill, reminiscent of the popular Greek pie *spanakopita*. Greek food holds a special place in my heart because I was born in Astoria, New York, which has a large Greek population. Years later, I landed one of my first jobs there, and I used to eat at a little Greek hole-in-the-wall that made the best spanakopita—I ordered it nearly every day. This dish has a lot fewer calories than the original since it skips the flaky pastry, calls for egg whites, and uses reduced-fat feta cheese.

1 tablespoon extra-virgin olive oil

½ cup finely chopped scallions

1 garlic clove, minced

2 plum tomatoes, finely chopped (about 1 cup)

1 (10-ounce) package frozen chopped spinach, thawed and excess liquid squeezed out

1 tablespoon chopped fresh dill

2 tablespoons chopped fresh parsley

Kosher salt

½ cup crumbled reduced-fat feta cheese (2½ ounces)

2 tablespoons grated Parmesan cheese

12 large egg whites

Freshly cracked black pepper

Cooking spray or oil mister

In a medium skillet, heat the oil over medium heat. Add the scallions and garlic and cook until soft, about 2 minutes. Add the tomatoes, spinach, dill, parsley, and a pinch of salt. Cook until the tomatoes soften and everything is heated through, 3 to 5 minutes. Season with ¼ teaspoon salt and cook for 1 more minute. Remove the pan from the heat, stir in the feta and Parmesan, and cover the pan to keep warm.

In a medium bowl, whisk the egg whites with 2 tablespoons water, ⅛ teaspoon salt, and a pinch of black pepper. Lightly spray a large nonstick skillet with oil and heat the skillet over medium-low heat. When hot add one-fourth of the egg mixture (about ½ cup), swirling to evenly cover the bottom of the pan. Cook until set, about 2 minutes. Spoon one-fourth of the spinach mixture (about ½ cup) onto half of the omelet, fold the omelet over, and slide it onto a serving plate. Repeat with the remaining ingredients.

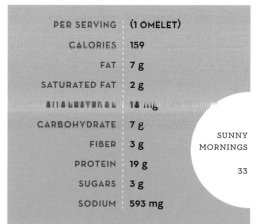

PER SERVING	(1 OMELET)
CALORIES	159
FAT	7 g
SATURATED FAT	2 g
CHOLESTEROL	18 mg
CARBOHYDRATE	7 g
FIBER	3 g
PROTEIN	19 g
SUGARS	3 g
SODIUM	593 mg

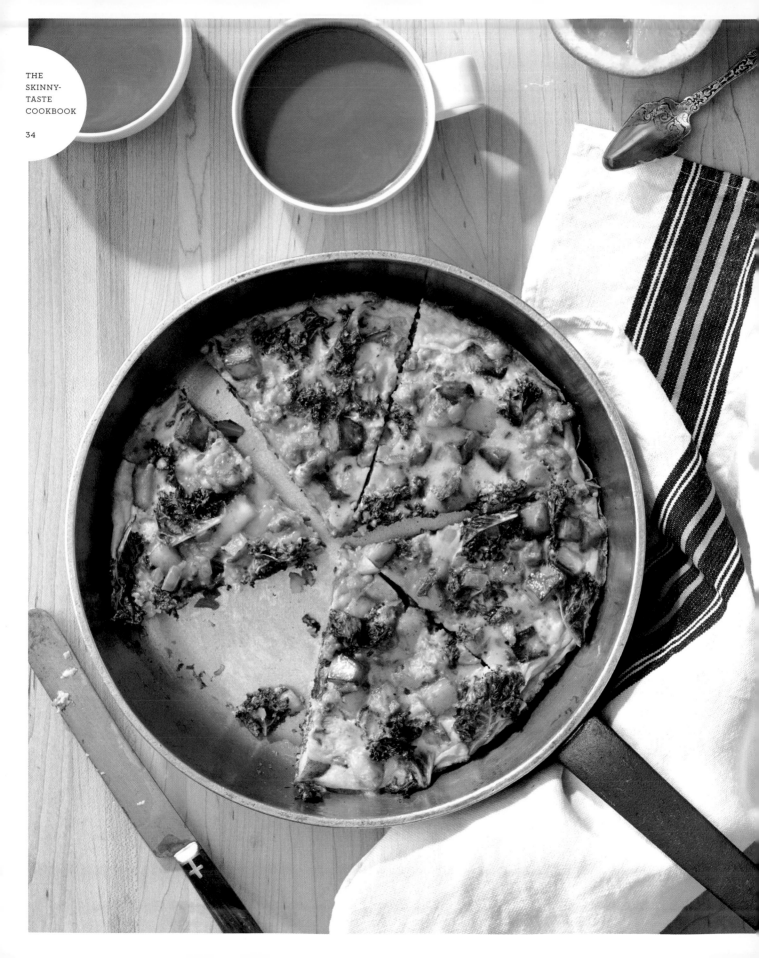

Winter Potato, Kale, and Sausage Frittata

SERVES 6

(GF) (Q) (FF)

With sausage, potatoes, eggs, and kale, this frittata is a meal in one! Frittatas are so versatile, both in what you can put in them and for the fact that they're delicious for breakfast, lunch, *or* dinner. You can literally clean out your refrigerator to come up with countless ways to whip one up. This dish starts out on the stovetop and finishes in the oven, so you'll need to use an ovenproof skillet. If you don't own one, you can also slide the half-cooked frittata onto a large plate, then carefully flip it back into the skillet and finish cooking the other side over low heat on the stovetop.

5 large eggs

3 large egg whites

2 tablespoons grated Pecorino Romano cheese

Kosher salt

Freshly cracked black pepper

2 teaspoons olive oil

6 ounces fresh sweet Italian chicken or turkey sausage,* casings removed

1 small onion, chopped

12 ounces (2 medium) peeled Yukon Gold potatoes, diced into ½-inch pieces

⅛ teaspoon garlic powder

⅛ teaspoon paprika

1 cup chopped kale, stems and ribs removed

*Read the label to be sure this product is gluten-free.

Preheat the oven to 400°F.

Crack the eggs and egg whites into a large bowl. Add grated Pecorino Romano, ⅛ teaspoon of the salt, and a pinch of black pepper and beat until blended.

Heat a 10-inch nonstick oven-safe skillet over medium heat. Add 1 teaspoon of the oil, the sausage meat, and the onions to the pan and cook, breaking the meat up with a wooden spoon, until it's cooked through and the onions are golden, 5 to 6 minutes. Transfer the sausage and onions to a plate.

Add the remaining 1 teaspoon of oil to the pan, then add the potatoes. Season with ½ teaspoon salt, garlic powder, paprika, and a pinch of black pepper. Cover and cook the potatoes over medium-low heat, stirring occasionally, until crisp and tender,

(recipe continues)

PER SERVING	(1 WEDGE)
CALORIES	184
FAT	8.5 g
SATURATED FAT	2.5 g
CHOLESTEROL	175 mg
CARBOHYDRATE	13 g
FIBER	2 g
PROTEIN	14 g
SUGARS	1 g
SODIUM	383 mg

skinny**scoop**

Any dark leafy green can be swapped out for the kale—try spinach or Swiss chard. You can freeze leftovers to reheat for another day. To freeze, cut the cooked, cooled frittata in wedges, wrap each wedge in plastic wrap, wrap in foil, and freeze until hard. To reheat, unwrap frozen frittata and microwave it, or bake at 350°F until heated through, about 35 minutes.

10 to 12 minutes. Add the kale, cover, and cook until wilted, 2 to 3 minutes.

Add the cooked sausage and onions to the skillet and stir to combine. Pour the egg mixture into the skillet. Reduce the heat to low and cook until the edges are set, 6 to 8 minutes.

Transfer the skillet to the oven and bake until the frittata is completely set and cooked through, 8 to 10 minutes. Remove from the oven, place a plate over the pan, and turn the frittata out onto the plate. Cut into 6 wedges and serve.

Breakfast Excuse Buster

Research shows that skipping meals—breakfast in particular—can lead to weight gain. The fact is breakfast should be a morning must! But it doesn't have to be time-consuming—it could be something as simple as a slice of whole-wheat toast with nut butter and bananas (five minutes, tops!), yogurt, or some hard-boiled eggs with fruit.

For an egg-streamly easy breakfast, I boil a dozen eggs in advance and keep them in the refrigerator for a handy, hunger-busting breakfast. A piece of fruit plus one large egg are only 200 calories, and the mix of protein, fat, and fiber will keep you satisfied until lunch. For a more substantial start to the day, you can whip up my favorite Egg, Tomato, and Scallion Sandwich (page 90) in minutes, because the eggs are already cooked. (Bonus: no sticky skillet to clean!)

Cali Avocado Egg Sandwich

SERVES 4

Ⓥ Ⓠ

I'm always impressed with how health-conscious people in California are, and it excites me to see that they put avocados on everything. (If you haven't noticed yet, I'm a bit avocado-obsessed myself. I always have three or four avocados in my kitchen at any given time.) You can find healthy food options everywhere in the Golden State—even the airport, which is where I actually got the inspiration for this sandwich.

8 large egg whites
(about 1 cup)

Kosher salt

Freshly cracked black pepper

Cooking spray or oil mister

¼ cup chopped scallions

¼ cup seeded and chopped tomatoes

¼ cup chopped red bell pepper

8 slices whole wheat bread, toasted

1 medium (4 ounces) Hass avocado, thinly sliced

In a medium bowl, beat together the egg whites, ¼ teaspoon salt, and black pepper to taste.

Heat a 9-inch nonstick skillet over medium heat. When hot, lightly spray the pan with oil. Add 1 tablespoon each of the scallions, tomatoes, and bell pepper, and season with a pinch of salt. Cook, stirring, for 1 minute. Pour in ¼ cup of the egg whites and rotate the pan. Reduce the heat to medium-low and cook until the eggs are set, 1 to 1½ minutes. Fold the eggs in half so they look like a half moon and cook for 30 more seconds. Fold the eggs in half again.

Transfer the eggs to a piece of toasted bread. Top each with one-quarter of the avocado, a pinch more of salt and black pepper, and a second slice of bread. Cut in half and serve. Repeat with the remaining ingredients to make 3 more sandwiches.

skinny scoop

After I get back from shopping, I leave one avocado out on the counter to ripen, and put the rest in the refrigerator so they last longer. If I don't use a whole avocado, I keep the pit in the remaining avocado, cover it tightly with plastic wrap, and refrigerate it.

PER SERVING	(1 SANDWICH)
CALORIES	170
FAT	6 g
SATURATED FAT	0.5 g
CHOLESTEROL	0 mg
CARBOHYDRATE	23 g
FIBER	7.5 g
PROTEIN	13 g
SUGARS	3 g
SODIUM	431 mg

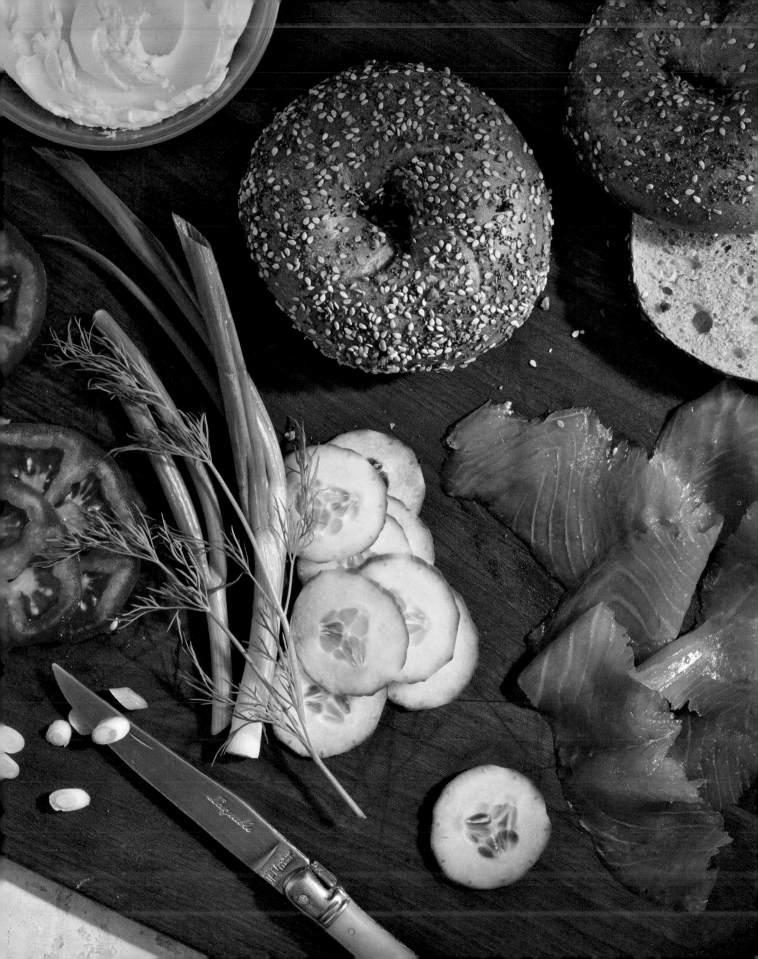

Open-Face Bagels
with Scallion-Lox Cream Cheese

SERVES 4

Q

Bagels and lox is a New York City classic. The dish—which is perfect for breakfast, lunch, or brunch—takes just minutes to whip up and is delicious, especially when topped with a few slices of fresh tomatoes and cucumbers. The bagels they sell here in New York are pretty large, so I find half a bagel, which is roughly 2½ ounces, to be the perfect size. My favorite bagel is whole wheat "everything," but pumpernickel or any whole-grain type is a great option.

4 ounces ⅓-less-fat cream cheese, at room temperature

2 ounces Nova lox or smoked salmon, finely chopped

¼ cup finely chopped scallions

1 tablespoon finely chopped fresh dill

2 large whole wheat "everything" bagels, sliced in half (5 ounces each)

1 medium tomato, thinly sliced

½ medium cucumber, thinly sliced

Kosher salt

Freshly ground black pepper

In a medium bowl, combine the cream cheese, salmon, scallions, and dill. Spread 3 tablespoons of the cream cheese mixture onto each bagel half. Top each half with tomatoes and cucumber slices, and finish with a pinch of salt and black pepper.

skinny**scoop**

Although smoked salmon and lox can be refrigerated for about a week (make sure they're tightly wrapped), they're best eaten as soon as possible because the intensity of flavor and firmness of texture will diminish as the days go by.

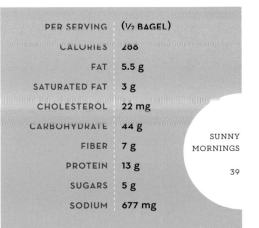

PER SERVING	(½ BAGEL)
CALORIES	288
FAT	5.5 g
SATURATED FAT	3 g
CHOLESTEROL	22 mg
CARBOHYDRATE	44 g
FIBER	7 g
PROTEIN	13 g
SUGARS	5 g
SODIUM	677 mg

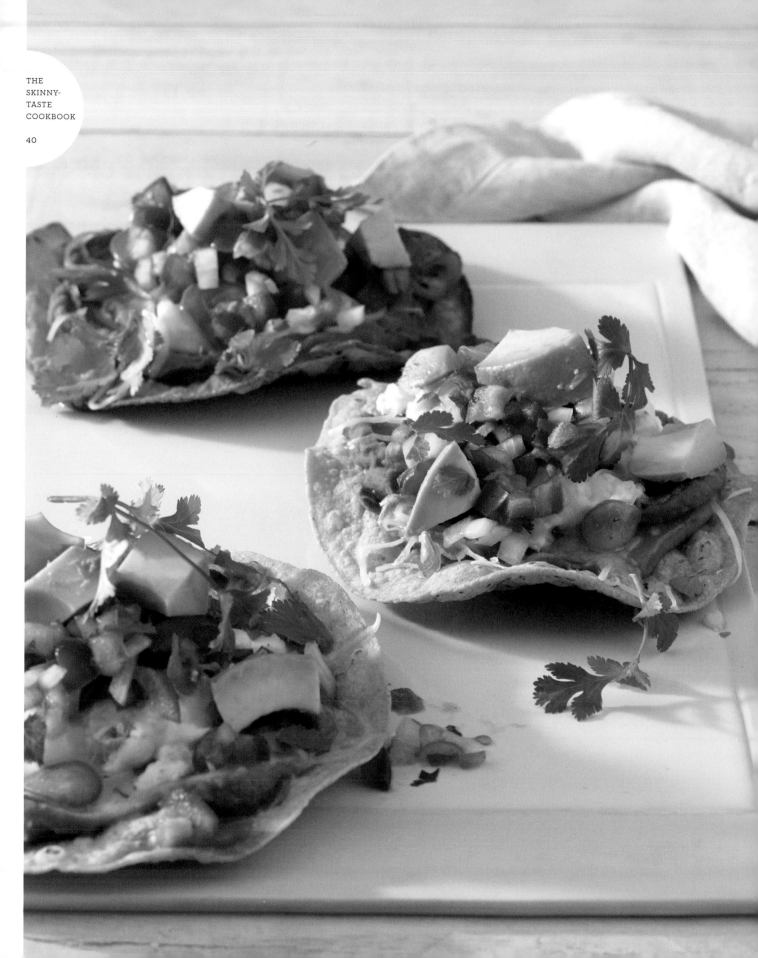

"Que Rico" Breakfast Tostada

SERVES 4

Scrambled egg whites with scallions piled high on a crispy tostada with refried beans, melted cheese, pico de gallo, jalapeño, and diced avocado—can I get an "Olé!" Whenever I'm craving a bit of spice to start my day, I love making these Mexican-inspired breakfast tostadas. (No worries if you don't care for spicy food—you can easily leave out the jalapeño.)

8 large egg whites

Kosher salt

Freshly cracked black pepper

3 tablespoons chopped scallions

Cooking spray or oil mister

1 cup fat-free refried beans* (I recommend Trader Joe's)

1 teaspoon ground cumin

4 corn tostadas*

1 cup reduced-fat Mexican cheese blend (I recommend Sargento)

1 fresh jalapeño pepper, thinly sliced

¼ cup pico de gallo, homemade (page 120) or store-bought

½ medium (2 ounces) Hass avocado, cut into ½-inch chunks

4 sprigs of fresh cilantro, for garnish (optional)

*Read the label to be sure this product is gluten-free.

Preheat the oven to 350°F.

In a medium bowl, beat together the egg whites, ¼ teaspoon salt, and a pinch of black pepper. Add the scallions and mix well.

Heat a medium nonstick skillet over medium heat. When hot, lightly spray the pan with oil and add the eggs. Cook, stirring occasionally, until set, about 3 minutes. Remove the pan from the heat.

In a medium bowl, combine the refried beans, cumin, and ⅛ teaspoon salt. Arrange the tostadas on a baking sheet and spread ¼ cup of the bean mixture over each tostada. Top each with ⅓ cup of the scrambled egg whites, ¼ cup of the cheese, and a few slices of jalapeño.

Bake the tostadas until the cheese melts, 4 to 5 minutes. Transfer the tostadas to serving plates. Top with pico de gallo and avocado, and garnish with cilantro, if desired.

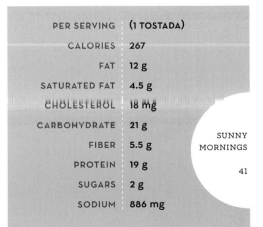

PER SERVING	(1 TOSTADA)
CALORIES	267
FAT	12 g
SATURATED FAT	4.5 g
CHOLESTEROL	18 mg
CARBOHYDRATE	21 g
FIBER	5.5 g
PROTEIN	19 g
SUGARS	2 g
SODIUM	886 mg

SUNNY MORNINGS

41

Pumpkin-Obsessed Vanilla-Glazed Scones

MAKES 12 SCONES

V

These light and fluffy buttermilk scones—made with pumpkin puree, fall spices, and a vanilla bean glaze—will warm up your home and fill it with an intoxicating scent that no fancy candle can come close to replicating. I've lightened these up substantially by using low-fat buttermilk instead of cream and replacing some butter with pumpkin puree. They taste just as good as any scone you would buy in a fancy coffee shop with half the calories.

SCONES

Cooking spray or oil mister

½ cup cold lowfat 1% buttermilk

1 large egg

1 teaspoon pure vanilla extract

5 tablespoons canned unsweetened pumpkin puree

¼ cup packed dark brown sugar

1 vanilla bean

1 cup white whole wheat flour (I recommend King Arthur)

1 cup unbleached all-purpose flour, plus more for the work surface

1 tablespoon baking powder

2 teaspoons pumpkin pie spice

¼ teaspoon ground nutmeg

¼ teaspoon ground cinnamon

½ teaspoon kosher salt

3 tablespoons very cold butter, cut into small pieces

GLAZE

2 tablespoons cold fat-free milk

1 cup powdered sugar, sifted

Preheat the oven to 375°F. Spray a baking sheet with oil.

For the scones: In a medium bowl, whisk together the buttermilk, egg, vanilla, pumpkin puree, and brown sugar. Using the tip of a sharp knife, cut along the length of the vanilla bean to split it open. Scrape half of the seeds into the bowl and whisk well; reserve the remaining seeds for the glaze.

In a large bowl, whisk together the flours, baking powder, pumpkin pie spice, nutmeg, cinnamon, and salt. Using a pastry blender or 2 knives, cut in the chilled butter until the mixture resembles coarse meal. Add the buttermilk mixture and stir until just moist.

(recipe continues)

PER SERVING	(1 SCONE)
CALORIES	172
FAT	4 g
SATURATED FAT	2 g
CHOLESTEROL	24 mg
CARBOHYDRATE	32 g
FIBER	2 g
PROTEIN	4 g
SUGARS	15 g
SODIUM	214 mg

skinny**scoop**

For perfect scones, be
careful not to overwork
the dough and be sure
your butter is well chilled.
I always keep a stick of
butter in the freezer just
for making scones.

Turn the dough out onto a floured work surface and knead lightly four times with floured hands. Transfer the dough to the baking sheet and shape it into a 9-inch round about ¾ inch thick. Using a knife, cut the dough all the way through into 12 wedges.

Bake until golden brown, 18 to 20 minutes. Transfer to a wire rack and let cool for about 10 minutes before glazing.

For the glaze: Meanwhile, in a medium bowl, whisk together the remaining seeds from the vanilla bean and the milk. In another medium bowl add the powdered sugar. Using a spatula mix in the milk and combine well until it is mixed through and forms a thick glaze.

Put the scones on parchment or wax paper and drizzle the vanilla glaze over the scones using a spoon. Alternatively you can dip the tops of the scones into the glaze, and then let them sit on the paper to harden.

Serve warm. Leftovers can be stored in airtight containers for up to 2 days.

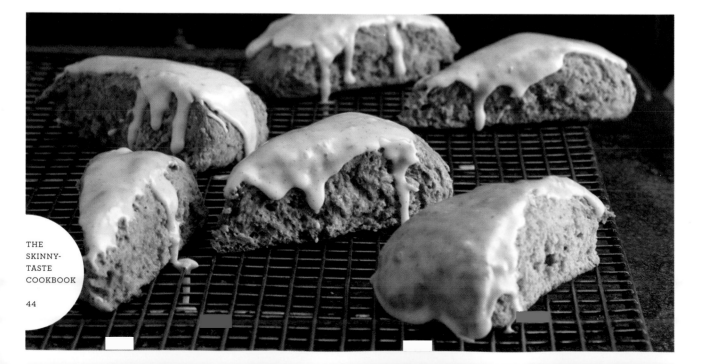

Heavenly Banana-Nut Oat Muffins

MAKES 12 MUFFINS

(V) (FF)

This recipe is like a cross between banana bread and baked oatmeal—two of my favorite breakfast foods! They are so delicious, you won't believe that the recipe calls for just a single tablespoon of oil. They get their moisture instead from very ripe mashed bananas, which also add a natural sweetness, allowing you to use less sugar. Aside from the fact that these just taste pretty darn good, you'll also score some filling fiber and satiating protein from the oatmeal.

Cooking spray or oil mister

1½ cups quick-cooking oats

1¼ cups unsweetened almond milk

½ cup packed dark brown sugar

1 cup mashed ripe bananas

2 large egg whites

2 tablespoons honey

1 tablespoon canola oil

1 teaspoon pure vanilla extract

½ cup white whole wheat flour (I recommend King Arthur)

1 teaspoon baking powder

½ teaspoon baking soda

½ teaspoon kosher salt

¾ cup chopped walnuts

Preheat the oven to 400°F. Line a standard muffin tin with 12 liners and lightly spray the liners with oil.

Pour the oats into a large bowl, add the almond milk and mix well; soak for about 30 minutes.

Add the brown sugar, mashed bananas, egg whites, honey, oil, and vanilla to the oats and mix well.

In a medium bowl, whisk together the flour, baking powder, baking soda, and salt. Slowly add the flour mixture ingredients to the liquid ingredients and mix with a spatula until just incorporated. Fold in the walnuts. Pour the batter into the prepared muffin tin.

Bake until a toothpick inserted comes out clean, 24 to 28 minutes. Let cool before serving.

skinny scoop

Make a batch of these muffins and freeze what you don't eat in a freezer-safe zip-top plastic bag. Pop frozen muffins In the microwave for a few seconds and you'll have a quick breakfast ready for when you're on the go.

PER SERVING	(1 MUFFIN)
CALORIES	162
FAT	6.5 g
SATURATED FAT	0.5 g
CHOLESTEROL	0 mg
CARBOHYDRATE	24 g
FIBER	2.5 g
PROTEIN	4 g
SUGARS	12 g
SODIUM	167 mg

SUNNY MORNINGS

45

skinnyscoop

Make a double batch of pancakes, and then freeze what you don't eat. Leftover pancakes can be refrigerated for up to 3 days or kept frozen for at least 1 month. To freeze, stack cooled pancakes on a freezer-safe dish with a sheet of wax paper between each one. Cover with plastic wrap or foil and freeze. Reheat them in the toaster or microwave.

Guiltless Chocolate Chip Pancakes

MAKES 10 PANCAKES • SERVES 5

(V) (Q) (FF)

These fluffy pancakes are lighter than a standard flapjack because I've replaced most of the fat with applesauce and egg whites—but no one would know. I make these on the weekends for my daughter Madison—she just loves them. Sometimes for fun, I make a smiley face, using fruit for eyes and chocolate chips as the mouth. She usually gets a big chuckle out of that. Personally, I prefer topping my pancakes with fresh strawberries and honey, because they complement the flavor of the chocolate.

½ cup white whole wheat flour (I recommend King Arthur)

½ cup unbleached all-purpose flour

2 teaspoons baking powder

¼ teaspoon kosher salt

½ cup unsweetened applesauce

1 cup unsweetened almond milk (or soy or low-fat dairy milk)

3 large egg whites

2 teaspoons canola oil

1 teaspoon pure vanilla extract

Cooking spray or oil mister

¼ cup mini chocolate chips

5 large strawberries, sliced

Honey or pure maple syrup, for serving (optional)

In a large bowl, whisk together the flours, baking powder, and salt.

In a separate bowl, combine the applesauce, almond milk, egg whites, oil, and vanilla. Stir the flour mixture into the applesauce mixture until just moist, being careful not to overmix.

Heat a large nonstick griddle over medium-low heat. When hot, lightly spray the pan with oil. Scoop out ¼ cup of pancake batter for each pancake, then sprinkle 1 teaspoon of chocolate chips on top. Cook until the pancakes start to bubble and the edges begin to set, 1½ minutes. Flip the pancakes over and cook the second side until golden, 1½ minutes. Repeat with the remaining batter.

To serve, put 2 pancakes on each of 5 serving plates and then top with strawberry slices and honey or maple syrup (if using).

PER SERVING	(2 PANCAKES)
CALORIES	192
FAT	6 g
SATURATED FAT	1.5 g
CHOLESTEROL	0 mg
CARBOHYDRATE	30 g
FIBER	3.5 g
PROTEIN	6 g
SUGARS	8 g
SODIUM	368 mg

Corny Banana-Blueberry Pancakes

MAKES 10 PANCAKES · SERVES 5

(V) (Q) (FF)

I love cornbread and corn muffins, so I thought, Why not add some cornmeal to my pancakes? The result: naturally sweet, fluffy, whole-grain pancakes with a corn muffin–like texture. A single serving—2 pancakes—provides almost 3 grams of fiber, which can help control your appetite until lunch. I often swap out all-purpose flour for 100% white whole wheat flour, which is milled from hard white spring wheat rather than traditional red wheat. It's just as nutritious as darker whole wheat flour, but it has a milder flavor and a lighter color, which makes it ideal for pancakes and muffins.

¾ cup white whole wheat flour (I recommend King Arthur)

½ cup fine-grind cornmeal

2 teaspoons baking powder

¼ teaspoon kosher salt

1 large ripe banana, mashed well

1 cup plus 2 tablespoons low-fat buttermilk

3 large egg whites

2 teaspoons canola oil

1 teaspoon pure vanilla extract

1 cup plus 2 tablespoons blueberries

Cooking spray or oil mister

5 tablespoons pure maple syrup, for serving

FOOD FACTS beware of maple syrup substitutes
Be careful what you pour over your pancakes. You might be topping your stack with "pancake syrup," which is a mix of different types of sugar, flavorings, and other ingredients. Real maple syrup has just one ingredient: maple syrup. Be sure to check the ingredients list.

In a large bowl, whisk together the flour, cornmeal, baking powder, and salt.

In a separate bowl, combine the mashed banana, buttermilk, egg whites, oil, and vanilla.

Add the flour mixture to the banana mixture and stir until just moist, making sure not to overmix. Gently fold in the blueberries.

Heat a large nonstick griddle pan over medium-low heat. When hot, lightly spray with oil.

Scoop out ⅓ cup of batter for each pancake. Cook until it starts to set and the bottom is golden brown, about 3 minutes. Flip the pancake and cook the second side until golden brown, about 2 minutes. Repeat with the remaining batter.

Arrange 2 pancakes on each of 5 plates and serve topped with 1 tablespoon of maple syrup.

PER SERVING	(2 PANCAKES)
CALORIES	259
FAT	3 g
SATURATED FAT	0.5 g
CHOLESTEROL	2 mg
CARBOHYDRATE	51 g
FIBER	3 g
PROTEIN	7 g
SUGARS	22 g
SODIUM	349 mg

skinny**scoop**

If you have only medium-grind or coarse-grind cornmeal on hand, you can grind it in a clean spice mill to a fine grind.

skinnyscoop

Crêpes can be refrigerated for up to 3 days or kept frozen for 2 to 3 months. To freeze, stack cooled crêpes on a freezer-safe dish with a sheet of wax paper between each one. Cover tightly with plastic wrap and freeze. Defrost in the refrigerator a day ahead, and then warm them gently in a skillet or in the microwave 4 at a time covered with a damp paper towel for 40 to 60 seconds before serving.

Dad's Jammin' Crêpes

MAKES 12 CRÊPES • SERVES 6

(V) (Q) (FF)

Crêpes are pretty easy to make once you get the hang of them. My father is originally from the Czech Republic, and crêpes, known there as *palacinky*, were a staple in our home for breakfast or dessert. I've played around with my dad's recipe, swapping out the white flour for white whole wheat and the whole milk with fat-free for nearly identical results that would make Dad proud. This is the perfect breakfast when you have guests you want to impress. I buy a variety of fancy fruit preserves, set out different bowls of fruit and fillings, and let everyone compose their own.

CRÊPES

1¾ cups fat-free milk

2 large egg whites

1 large egg

1 teaspoon canola oil

1 teaspoon pure vanilla extract

1 cup white whole wheat flour

1 teaspoon ground cinnamon

Cooking spray or oil mister

FILLING AND TOPPINGS

¼ cup of your favorite fruit preserves (I like Whole Foods 365 Organic)

3 bananas, sliced

¾ cup sliced strawberries

¾ cup blueberries

¾ cup raspberries

1 tablespoon powdered sugar, for dusting

For the crêpes: In a blender, combine the milk, egg whites and egg, oil, and vanilla. Add the flour and cinnamon and blend until smooth. At this point, the batter may be refrigerated for up to 2 days.

Heat a 10 inch nonstick skillet over medium low heat. When hot, lightly spray with oil. Pour ¼ cup of batter into the skillet, swirling the pan slightly to form a thin, even coating on the bottom of the skillet. Cook until the bottom of the crêpe sets and is golden in color, 1 to 2 minutes. Gently flip with a spatula and cook the second side for about 1 minute. Repeat with the remaining batter, stacking the finished crêpes on a plate. You should have 12 crêpes.

For the filling and toppings: To serve, spread 1 teaspoon of the fruit preserves in the center of each crêpe, fold the edge of the crêpe over the filling, and roll it into a tube shape. Place the rolled crêpe on a plate, seam side down. Top with fresh fruit, lightly dust with powdered sugar, and serve immediately.

PER SERVING	(2 CRÊPES)
CALORIES	235
FAT	2.5 g
SATURATED FAT	0.5 g
CHOLESTEROL	32 mg
CARBOHYDRATE	48 g
FIBER	6 g
PROTEIN	9 g
SUGARS	22 g
SODIUM	67 mg

SKINNY-LICIOUS SOUPS & CHILIS

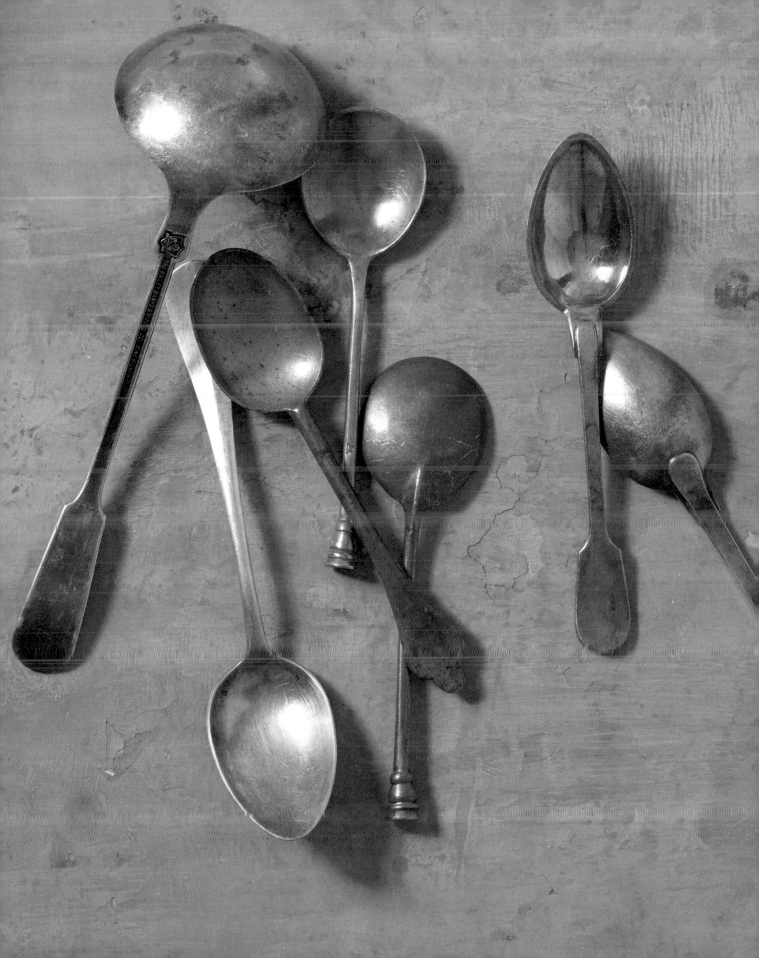

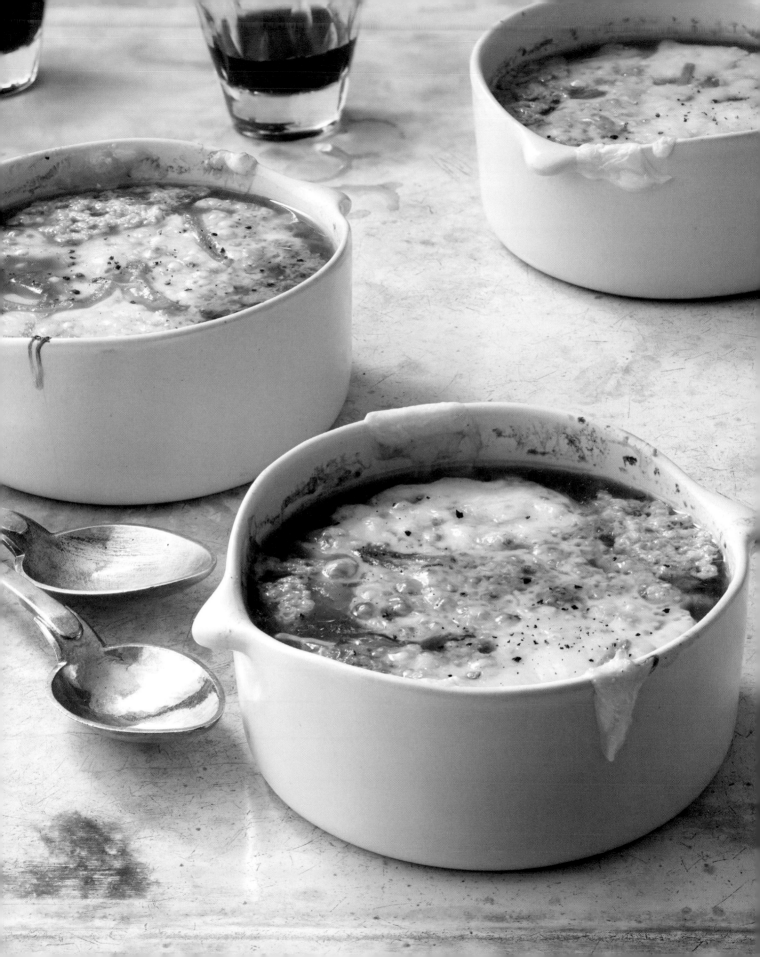

Breadless French Onion Soup with Parmesan-Asiago Crisps

SERVES 6

GF FF

What's the best part of French onion soup? The melted cheese on top of the savory broth that's loaded with sweet caramelized onions. Personally, I've never cared for the soggy bread—I'd rather save my carbs for something I really enjoy. So, instead I make a cheese crisp to float on top. Not only is it easy, but the combination of the two cheeses is also absolutely heavenly.

SOUP

1 tablespoon olive oil

1 tablespoon unsalted butter

2 pounds sweet yellow onions, cut into ⅛-inch slices

¼ cup dry sherry

¼ cup dry white or red wine

2 tablespoons all-purpose flour (use sweet rice flour* for gluten free)

8 cups Swanson beef stock (from 2½ containers)

1 sprig of fresh thyme

1 bay leaf

Freshly cracked black pepper

6 (1-ounce) slices reduced-fat low-sodium Swiss cheese

PARMESAN-ASIAGO CRISPS

½ cup freshly grated Parmigiano-Reggiano cheese

¼ cup freshly grated Asiago cheese

Read the label to be sure this product is gluten-free.

For the soup: In a Dutch oven or large nonstick pot, heat the oil and butter over medium-low heat until the butter melts, add the onions, and slowly cook until the onions become soft, stirring from time to time, about 30 minutes. Increase the heat to medium and cook until the onions begin to caramelize, about 20 to 25 minutes, stirring every few minutes. Add the sherry and wine and reduce the heat to low, stirring any brown bits stuck to the pot. Simmer until the liquid cooks down and evaporates, 2 to 3 minutes. Add the flour and cook, stirring, for 3 to 4 minutes. Add the stock, thyme, and bay leaf, increase heat to high, and bring to a boil. Cover, reduce heat to moderately low heat, and simmer until the onions are tender, about 30 minutes. Remove and discard the herbs, and then season with black pepper to taste.

(recipe continues)

PER SERVING	(1⅓ CUPS SOUP)
CALORIES	264
FAT	11 g
SATURATED FAT	5.5 g
CHOLESTEROL	15 mg
CARBOHYDRATE	19 g
FIBER	2.5 g
PROTEIN	19 g
SUGARS	9 g
SODIUM	984 mg

For the Parmesan-Asiago crisps: Meanwhile, preheat the oven to 400°F. Line a baking sheet with a silicone baking mat or parchment paper.

In a small bowl, combine the Parmesan and Asiago. Put 2 tablespoons of the cheese mixture onto the baking sheet and lightly pat it with your fingers into a 4-inch round. Repeat with the remaining cheese to make 6 rounds, leaving ½ inch space in between each. Bake until golden and crisp, 6 to 8 minutes. Set aside to cool.

When ready to serve, adjust an oven rack 4 to 6 inches from the heating element and preheat the broiler.

Ladle the soup into 6 ovenproof onion soup bowls, lay one cheese crisp on top of each (it should float), and then lay 1 slice of Swiss cheese over each crisp. Put the bowls on a baking sheet.

Broil until the cheese melts, watching closely so that it doesn't burn, 3 to 4 minutes. Serve hot.

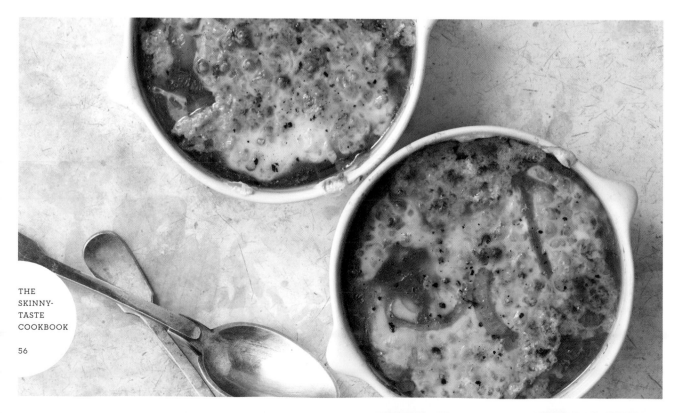

Italian Escarole and White Bean Soup

SERVES 6

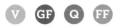

I love the old-world, rustic flavors of this hearty soup. Credit for this recipe goes to my friend Julia. Her parents emigrated from Sicily to America, and cooking is in her veins. Italians are known for feeding large families on tight budgets with peasant dishes such as this, and beans were often used because they are inexpensive, filling, and nutritious. This dish takes about 20 minutes to make, start to finish. Leftovers are great for lunch.

10 ounces ditalini pasta (use brown rice pasta for gluten-free)

Kosher salt

1 teaspoon olive oil

1 medium onion, chopped

8 cups (64 ounces) Swanson 33% less sodium chicken or vegetable broth*

1 (15-ounce) can cannellini beans,* rinsed and drained

Freshly cracked black pepper

1 head escarole, leaves washed and torn into a few pieces

Freshly grated Parmigiano-Reggiano cheese, for serving (optional)

*Read the label to be sure this product is gluten free.

Cook the pasta to al dente in a pot of salted boiling water according to package directions. Drain and set aside.

Heat a large nonstick pot over medium heat. When hot, add the oil and onion and cook, stirring, until golden, 3 to 4 minutes. Add the broth and beans and bring to a boil. Season with black pepper to taste, and then add the escarole. Cook until the escarole wilts, about 15 minutes.

To serve, divide the cooked pasta among 6 serving bowls. Ladle the soup over the pasta, sprinkle with Parmesan, if desired, and serve.

FOOD FACTS meet escarole

Escarole (pronounced ESS-ka-roll) is a variety of endive whose leaves are broader, paler, and less bitter. It contains a number of nutrients, including folate, fiber, and vitamins C and K. If you can't find it, you can substitute Swiss chard or any other leafy green vegetable.

skinny scoop

Nothing can ruin a dish like mushy pasta. To avoid that situation, cook the pasta in a separate pot. Then when you're ready to serve, divide the pasta among serving bowls, ladle in the soup, and top with cheese.

PER SERVING	(2 GENEROUS CUPS NOT INCLUDING PARMESAN)
CALORIES	300
FAT	2 g
SATURATED FAT	0.5 g
CHOLESTEROL	0 mg
CARBOHYDRATE	55 g
FIBER	7 g
PROTEIN	15 g
SUGARS	2 g
SODIUM	779 mg

SKINNY-LICIOUS SOUPS & CHILIS

Too-Good-to-Be-True Baked Potato Soup

SERVES 5

GF **Q**

This soup is one of my most popular recipes on Skinnytaste. It offers everything you love about a baked potato in soup form! In fact, a fan once described it as a "warm bowl of awesomeness." You can totally enjoy it without the guilt because it's soooo much lighter than a baked potato. That's because I hide some cauliflower in there, which gives the great taste and texture for fewer calories.

2 medium russet (baking) potatoes, about 6 ounces each

3½ cups (16 ounces) cauliflower florets (from 1 small head)

1½ cups Swanson 33% less sodium chicken broth*

1½ cups 1% reduced-fat milk

½ cup light sour cream

6 tablespoons chopped fresh chives

¾ teaspoon kosher salt

Freshly cracked black pepper

10 tablespoons shredded reduced-fat sharp cheddar cheese

3 slices center-cut bacon, cooked and crumbled

Read the label to be sure this product is gluten-free.

Pierce the potatoes all over with a fork and microwave on high for 5 minutes. Turn them over and microwave until tender, 3 to 5 minutes longer. (Alternatively, bake at 400°F for 1 hour or until tender.) Let cool. When cool enough to handle, peel and coarsely chop the potatoes.

Set a steamer basket in a large pot and fill with about 1 inch of water. Bring the water to a boil over high heat. Add the cauliflower, cover, and steam until tender, 5 to 6 minutes. Drain, remove the steamer basket, and return the cauliflower to the pot.

Set the pot over medium heat and add the broth, milk, and potatoes. Bring to a boil. Use an immersion blender to puree the soup until smooth. Add the sour cream, 3 tablespoons of the chives, and season with the salt and black pepper to taste. Reduce the heat to low and cook, stirring occasionally, until thick and creamy, 8 to 10 minutes.

Remove the pot from the heat. Ladle the soup into 5 soup bowls. Top each with 2 tablespoons of cheese, and divide the remaining chives and the bacon among them. Serve hot.

PER SERVING	(1 GENEROUS CUP)
CALORIES	200
FAT	7 g
SATURATED FAT	3 g
CHOLESTEROL	17 mg
CARBOHYDRATE	23 g
FIBER	3.5 g
PROTEIN	14 g
SUGARS	6 g
SODIUM	323 mg

FOOD FACTS another cruciferous standout
Cruciferous vegetables are one of the most potent disease-fighting groups of foods out there. You've likely heard all about broccoli's benefits, but cauliflower offers some health perks, too. The veggie contains glucosinolates, compounds that may have anticancer properties, according to some studies.

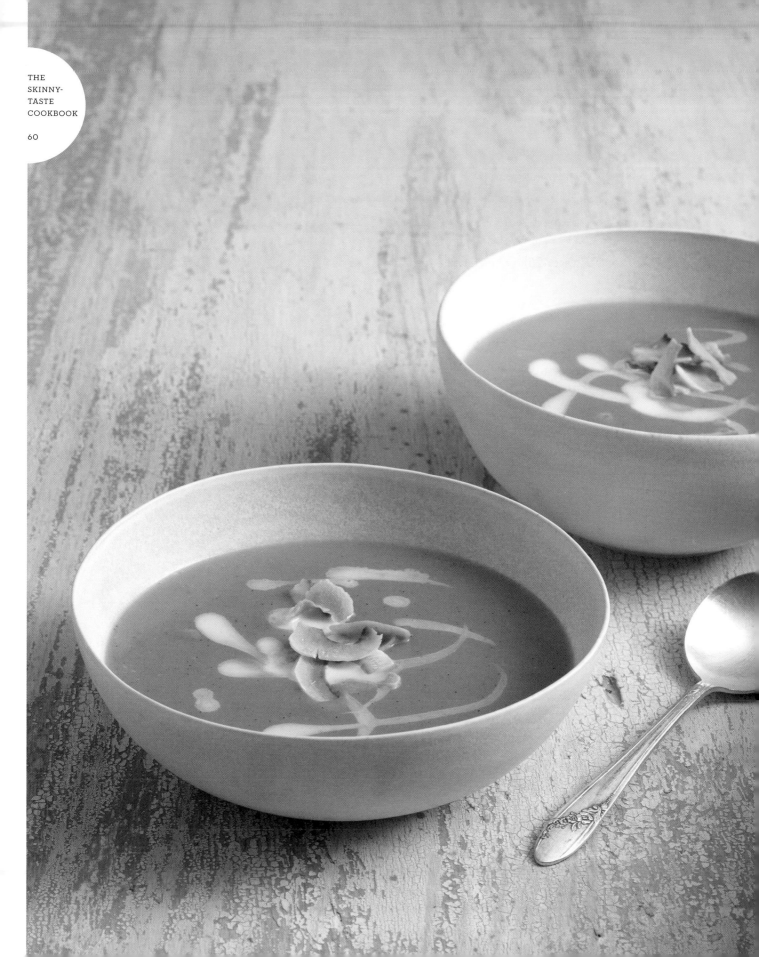

Cinnamon-Roasted Butternut Squash Soup

SERVES 6

I get my inspiration for my soups from the fresh produce available as the seasons change. Butternut squash is wonderful when roasted with nutmeg and cinnamon. I then balance out the sweetness with sautéed shallots and puree the whole thing until it's creamy and velvety. I had an "aha" moment when I was trying to think of a good garnish for the soup. I just happened to be making Coconut Chicken Salad (page 126) for lunch while testing this recipe when it hit me: toasted coconut!

40 ounces peeled and seeded butternut squash, cut into 1½-inch cubes, from 1 whole

¾ teaspoon ground cinnamon

¼ teaspoon ground nutmeg

6 tablespoons sweetened coconut flakes*

1 tablespoon coconut oil

¼ cup minced shallots

2¼ cups Pacific organic vegetable broth,* plus more as needed

1 cup plus 2 tablespoons light canned coconut milk

¾ teaspoon kosher salt

Freshly cracked black pepper

Read the label to be sure this product is gluten-free.

Preheat the oven to 375°F.

Put the squash on a large baking sheet. Toss with the cinnamon and nutmeg, cover with foil, and roast until tender, 40 to 50 minutes. Let cool. (Reduce the oven temperature to 350°F.)

Spread the coconut on a baking sheet and toast in the oven, stirring every 2 minutes, until golden, 6 to 8 minutes. Let cool.

Heat a large nonstick pot over medium heat. Add the coconut oil and shallots and cook, stirring, until tender, 5 minutes.

Add the roasted squash to the pot with shallots. Add the broth and 1 cup of the coconut milk and simmer about 5 minutes. Using an immersion blender or a regular blender in batches, puree the soup until smooth. Add more broth if needed and simmer for 2 to 3 more minutes. Season with salt and pepper.

To serve, ladle the soup into 6 serving bowls and top each with 1 tablespoon toasted coconut and 1 teaspoon coconut milk.

PER SERVING	(1 CUP)
CALORIES	186
FAT	8 g
SATURATED FAT	5.5 g
CHOLESTEROL	0 mg
CARBOHYDRATE	30 g
FIBER	5 g
PROTEIN	3 g
SUGARS	7 g
SODIUM	370 mg

Silky Edamame Soup

SERVES 4

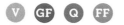

I often get inspiration from great restaurants when I go out to eat, and this soup is the perfect example. While dining with my husband at a new Asian-fusion restaurant in my area, I felt as if the edamame soup on the menu was calling my name. It was a silky soup made of pureed edamame (soybeans), baby spinach, shallots, and broth, topped with a dollop of crème fraîche. I loved it so much, I ran straight to the store afterward to re-create it myself. Here's the result!

SOUP

1 teaspoon sesame oil

¼ cup chopped shallots

2 garlic cloves, chopped

4 cups Swanson 33% less sodium chicken broth* (or vegetable broth can be used)

1 tablespoon reduced-sodium soy sauce (use tamari for gluten-free)

12 ounces fresh or frozen shelled edamame

3 cups baby spinach

TOPPINGS

Freshly cracked black pepper

1 tablespoon sliced scallions

¼ cup crème fraîche or light sour cream

Roasted Edamame with Sea Salt (page 107; optional)

PERFECT PAIRINGS
Enjoy this soup as a main course with a salad on the side or as a starter to your own Asian-fusion entrée. Need a suggestion? Try the **Sweet 'n' Spicy Sriracha-Glazed Salmon (page 215).**

Read the label to be sure this product is gluten-free.

For the soup: In a medium saucepan, heat the sesame oil over medium heat. Add the shallots and garlic and cook, stirring, until lightly golden and fragrant, 1 to 2 minutes. Add the broth, soy sauce, and edamame and bring to a boil. Cover, reduce the heat to medium-low, and simmer until the edamame are tender, 15 to 20 minutes. Add the spinach and cook 1 more minute.

Working in batches, puree the soup in a blender. Return it to the saucepan to keep warm.

For the toppings: To serve, ladle the soup into 4 serving bowls, top each with some black pepper, scallions, and a touch of crème fraîche and roasted edamame.

FOOD FACTS the skinny on soybeans
Soybeans are a super source of protein, with more than 8 grams per 1/2 cup. In fact, soybeans are considered a complete protein, meaning they contain all of the essential amino acids that our bodies cannot make on their own.

PER SERVING	(1½ CUPS SOUP NOT INCLUDING OPTIONAL GARNISH)
CALORIES	173
FAT	10 g
SATURATED FAT	3.5 g
CHOLESTEROL	20 mg
CARBOHYDRATE	11 g
FIBER	4.5 g
PROTEIN	11 g
SUGARS	3 g
SODIUM	732 mg

THE SKINNY-TASTE COOKBOOK

"Un"Stuffed Cabbage Soup

SERVES 8

GF FF

Stuffed cabbage is one of my favorite comfort dishes that my mom used to make, but it can take quite a bit of time to make. These days, time is not something I have a lot of with a toddler running around and a full-time career. So when I'm in a rush, I rely on this shortcut: I throw all the ingredients into a big pot and make this soup instead. Most of the cooking time is unattended, so I can spend more time with my family and less time in the kitchen. Bonus: Leftovers are even better the next day.

1 pound 95% lean ground beef

1⅛ teaspoons kosher salt

1 large white onion, finely chopped

3 garlic cloves, minced

1¼ teaspoons sweet paprika

½ teaspoon dried thyme

2 (14.5-ounce) cans petite diced tomatoes

1 (8-ounce) can tomato sauce

5 cups Swanson unsalted cooking beef stock*

4 cups chopped green cabbage

Freshly cracked black pepper

1 cup cooked brown rice

*Read the label to be sure this product is gluten-free.

In a large pot or Dutch oven set over high heat, season the ground beef with ¼ teaspoon of the salt and cook, using a wooden spoon to break the meat into small pieces as it browns. Drain any fat from the pot and reduce the heat to medium-low. Add the onion, garlic, paprika, and thyme and cook until the onions are soft, 5 to 7 minutes. Add the tomatoes, tomato sauce, beef stock, and cabbage, and season with the remaining salt and black pepper to taste. Bring to a boil, reduce the heat to low, cover, and simmer until the cabbage is soft, about 35 minutes.

Add the cooked brown rice and simmer 5 more minutes before ladling the soup into 8 serving bowls to serve.

skinny**scoop**

Soups and stews like this are perfect for freezing. Freeze leftovers in labeled, portion-size containers so you'll have quick meals to reheat when you're pressed for time.

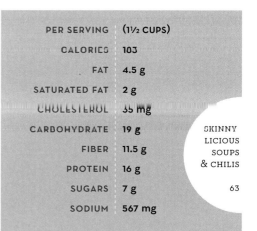

PER SERVING	(1½ CUPS)
CALORIES	103
FAT	4.5 g
SATURATED FAT	2 g
CHOLESTEROL	35 mg
CARBOHYDRATE	19 g
FIBER	11.5 g
PROTEIN	16 g
SUGARS	7 g
SODIUM	567 mg

SKINNY LICIOUS SOUPS & CHILIS

63

Slow-Cooker Chicken Enchilada Soup

SERVES 6

Call me lazy, but I love a meal that can pretty much cook itself. I also love turning classic meals into a hearty bowl of soup, and the slow cooker allows me to do both. For this dish, I took my standard chicken enchilada recipe and threw the ingredients into a slow cooker. What emerged a few hours later was this delicious, chunky soup that I topped with cheese, scallions, cilantro, and avocado. If I don't have avocado, I add a touch of light sour cream or crushed chips on top. It's everything I love about enchiladas in one neat bowl!

SOUP

2 teaspoons olive oil

½ cup chopped onion

3 garlic cloves, minced

3 cups Swanson 33% less sodium chicken broth*

1 (8-ounce) can tomato sauce

1 to 2 teaspoons chipotle chile in adobo sauce, chopped

¼ cup chopped fresh cilantro

1 (15-ounce) can low-sodium black beans, rinsed and drained

1 (14.5-ounce) can petite diced tomatoes

2 cups frozen corn kernels

1 teaspoon ground cumin, plus more to taste

½ teaspoon dried oregano

1 pound boneless, skinless chicken breasts

TOPPINGS

¾ cup shredded reduced-fat cheddar cheese

¼ cup chopped scallions

¼ cup chopped fresh cilantro

1 medium (4 ounces) Hass avocado, sliced

6 tablespoons reduced-fat sour cream (optional)

Read the label to be sure this product is gluten-free.

For the soup: In a medium nonstick skillet, heat the oil over medium heat. Add the onion and garlic and cook, stirring, until soft, about 3 minutes. Add to the slow-cooker along with the broth, tomato sauce, chipotle in adobo, cilantro, beans, tomatoes, corn, cumin, and oregano. Add the chicken breasts. Cover and cook on low for 4 to 6 hours.

Remove the chicken, shred it with two forks, and return it to the slow cooker.

For the toppings: To serve, ladle into 6 serving bowls and dividing evenly, top each with 2 tablespoons of cheddar, scallions, cilantro, avocado, and sour cream (if using).

PER SERVING	(1½ CUPS PLUS TOPPINGS)
CALORIES	368
FAT	12 g
SATURATED FAT	3 g
CHOLESTEROL	58 mg
CARBOHYDRATE	28 g
FIBER	8.5 g
PROTEIN	31 g
SUGARS	6 g
SODIUM	821 mg

skinny**scoop**

If you're not a fan of the
smoky taste of chipotle
peppers, you can replace
them with other spicy
chiles, such as jalapeños or
serranos.

Aztec Chicken, Quinoa, and Avocado Soup

SERVES 6

GF **FF**

Never seen avocado used in soup before? My mom is from Colombia, where it's quite common to add fresh avocado to soup just before eating. It adds a cool, sweet, creamy texture to a warm, hearty bowl of soup. As a kid, I didn't really care for it, but as an adult, I just love it. And luckily, so does my family. To brighten and round out the flavors of this soup, I like to finish it with a squeeze of fresh lime juice just before serving.

2 teaspoons olive oil

7 scallions, chopped

2 garlic cloves, minced

1 cup chopped tomato

6 tablespoons chopped fresh cilantro

1 teaspoon ground cumin

½ teaspoon ground annatto or sweet paprika

5 cups Swanson 33% less sodium chicken broth*

1 cup sliced carrots

½ cup chopped yellow bell pepper

Kosher salt

Freshly ground black pepper

1 pound boneless, skinless chicken breasts

1 medium jalapeño, diced (optional)

½ cup quinoa, rinsed well

1½ cups fresh or frozen corn kernels

1 medium (4 ounces) Hass avocado, chopped, for garnish

6 lime wedges, for serving

Read the label to be sure this product is gluten-free.

In a large pot or Dutch oven, heat the oil over medium-low heat. Add the scallions and garlic and cook, stirring, until soft, about 3 minutes. Add the tomato, ¼ cup of the cilantro, the cumin, and the annatto and cook 2 more minutes. Add the broth, carrots, bell pepper, ½ teaspoon of salt, and black pepper to taste, and bring to a boil. Reduce to a simmer, cover, and cook until the vegetables are tender, about 30 minutes.

Add the chicken and jalapeño (if using) and cook until the chicken is cooked through, about 15 to 18 minutes. Remove the chicken, shred it using two forks, and set it aside.

Meanwhile, in a medium saucepan, cook the quinoa according to package directions.

PER SERVING	(GENEROUS 1½ CUPS)
CALORIES	230
FAT	8 g
SATURATED FAT	1 g
CHOLESTEROL	48 mg
CARBOHYDRATE	21 g
FIBER	4.5 g
PROTEIN	21 g
SUGARS	4 g
SODIUM	702 mg

Add the cooked quinoa and corn to the soup, increase the heat to medium, and cook for 5 more minutes. Remove the pot from the heat. Return the shredded chicken to the pot, season with ⅛ teaspoon salt and black pepper to taste, and stir in the remaining 2 tablespoons cilantro.

To serve, ladle the soup into 6 serving bowls, garnish with the avocado, and serve with lime wedges on the side for squeezing.

FOOD FACTS crazy for quinoa
This grain is a hunger-curbing, power-packed nutritional all-star. Loaded with protein, fiber, calcium, iron, and vitamins, this superfood is digested slowly, which keeps blood sugar and insulin levels (and, therefore, energy and appetite) steady.

skinny**scoop**

Annatto is a staple in Latin American cooking, imparting flavor as well as color. It can be found in Spanish and Latin American markets. Sweet paprika can be used in its place if annatto is not available.

4 Tips for Making a Better Bowl of Soup

There's nothing better than a one-pot meal (easy cleanup!), and making soup is the easiest way to achieve this. Sure you could pop open a can, but believe it or not, making soups from scratch is a cinch once you master these simple, basic techniques.

SIMMER SEASONAL
You can capture the essence of each season and come up with endless varieties of soups by simmering seasonal vegetables—it's a smart and healthy way to cook.

START WITH DELICIOUS BROTH
I often make my own homemade stocks when it's time to clean out the refrigerator. But there is no mistaking the convenience of using packaged broth. Adding fresh herbs and aromatics, such as onions, garlic, leeks, and shallots, to your store-bought broth will make them taste like you were simmering them for hours.

SAY CHEESE!
Add a Parmesan rind to your pot—this is simple, but it works like a charm. They are like magic flavor boosters and add a rich, savory, umami character to your soup. I always save my Parmigiano-Reggiano or Pecorino Romano rinds and keep them in my freezer just for this.

BE FRESH
Flavoring your soup at the very end with something fresh and uncooked, such as fresh herbs, avocado, or a squeeze of lime juice, will brighten the deep, delicious, melded tastes of the rest of the soup and add a much needed touch of freshness.

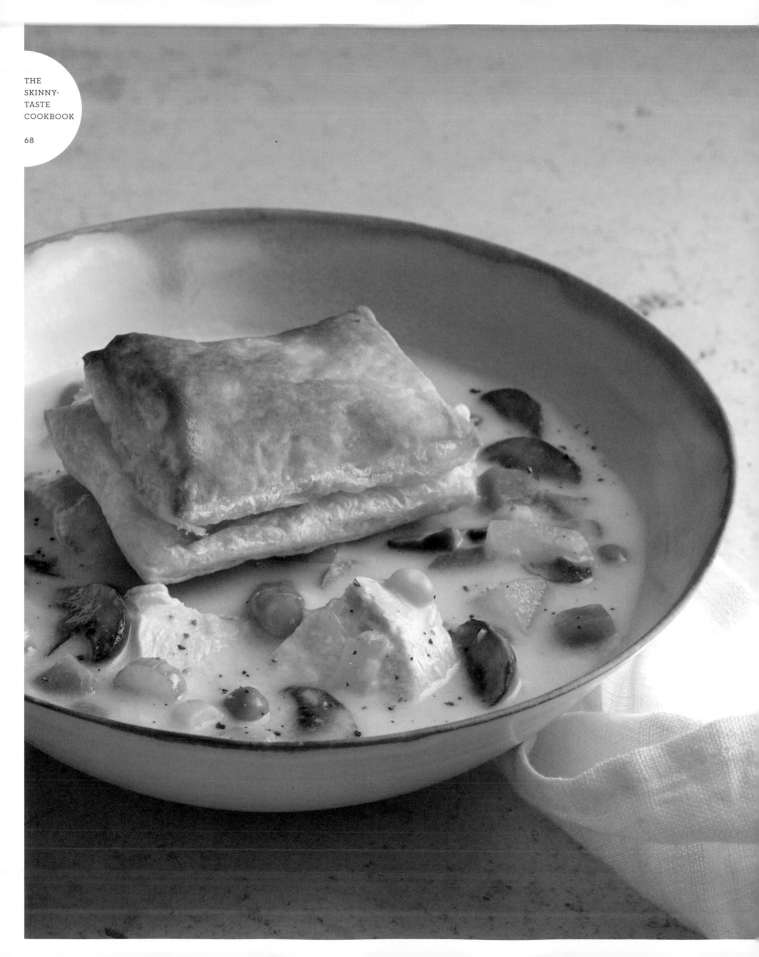

Chicken Pot Pie Soup

SERVES 6

GF

Why not take a classic comfort food and put a new spin on it? Chicken pot pie—one of my childhood favorites—is every bit as delightful when served as a soup. On the nights I want to get extra fancy, I cut out "croutons" from frozen pie crust or puff pastry into half-ounce shapes, bake them until golden, and serve on top.

¼ cup unbleached all-purpose flour (or 2 tablespoons cornstarch for gluten-free)

4 cups fat-free milk

1¼ pounds boneless, skinless chicken breasts

1 (10-ounce) package frozen classic mixed vegetables (peas, carrots, green beans, corn)

1 large celery stalk, chopped

½ medium onion, chopped

8 ounces sliced cremini mushrooms

2 tablespoons chicken Better Than Bouillon*

Pinch of dried thyme

Freshly cracked black pepper

2 medium Yukon Gold potatoes, peeled and diced

Kosher salt, if needed

*Read the label to be sure this product is gluten-free.

In a small bowl, make a slurry by whisking together ½ cup cold water and the flour or cornstarch if making this gluten-free. Set aside.

In a large pot, combine 1½ cups water and the milk and slowly bring to a boil over medium-low heat. Add the chicken, frozen vegetables, celery, onion, mushrooms, bouillon, thyme, and black pepper to taste and bring to a boil. Partially cover, reduce the heat to low, and simmer 15 minutes. Remove the chicken and set it aside. Continue to cook the soup until the vegetables are soft, about 5 more minutes. Add the potatoes and cook until soft, about 5 minutes.

Meanwhile, chop or shred the chicken into small pieces. Add the chicken to the soup, and slowly stir in the slurry. Cook until the soup thickens, 2 to 3 minutes. Adjust salt and black pepper to taste and serve.

PER SERVING	(1½ CUPS NOT INCLUDING CROUTON)
CALORIES	269
FAT	3.5 g
SATURATED FAT	0.5 g
CHOLESTEROL	11 mg
CARBOHYDRATE	32 g
FIBER	4 g
PROTEIN	30 g
SUGARS	12 g
SODIUM	983 mg

Rustic Italian Gnocchi Soup

SERVES 8

Let's test your memory. Think back to fourth-grade science: How many different tastes are there? If you remember that there were four (bitter, sweet, salty, and sour), you'd be wrong today. There's actually a fifth flavor called *umami*, a Japanese word used to describe something savory. This hearty bowl of soup is bursting with umami. Using a Parmesan rind is a must when I want to add the subtle umami flavor to soups. I always save my rinds when I'm done with my cheese, keeping them in the freezer until I need them.

3 tablespoons all-purpose flour

14 ounces fresh sweet Italian chicken sausage, casings removed

4½ cups Swanson 33% less sodium chicken broth

1 cup fat-free milk

1 small onion, chopped

1 celery stalk, chopped

1 carrot, chopped

4 garlic cloves, minced

Rind from Parmigiano-Reggiano (optional)

2 large roasted red bell peppers, jarred or homemade (see page 233)

½ teaspoon freshly ground black pepper, plus more as needed

1 (16-ounce) package gnocchi

3 cups baby spinach, chopped

2 tablespoons chopped fresh basil

Freshly grated Parmigiano-Reggiano, for serving (optional)

skinny scoop

To save time, I buy fresh gnocchi at a nearby Italian store in my neighborhood. You can even find refrigerated, dried, or frozen gnocchi in the supermarket. And if you really want to speed this up, you can also use jarred roasted peppers.

In a small bowl, make a slurry by whisking together ½ cup cold water and the flour.

Heat a large nonstick pot over medium heat. Add the sausage and cook, using a wooden spoon to break the meat into small pieces, until cooked through and slightly browned, 4 minutes.

Add ½ cup water, broth, and milk and bring to a boil. Add the onion, celery, carrot, garlic, Parmesan rind (if using), roasted peppers, and black pepper and return to a boil. Partially cover the pot, reduce the heat to low, and simmer until the vegetables are soft, 15 to 20 minutes. Uncover, slowly stir in the slurry, and continue stirring while the soup returns to a boil.

Add the gnocchi, spinach, and basil. Cook until the gnocchi start to float to the top and become puffy (or according to the gnocchi package directions) and the soup thickens. Season with black pepper to taste. Discard the Parmesan cheese rind. To serve, ladle the soup into 8 serving bowls and sprinkle evenly with grated Parmesan, if desired.

PER SERVING	(1¼ CUPS, NOT INCLUDING PARMESAN)
CALORIES	203
FAT	8 g
SATURATED FAT	3.5 g
CHOLESTEROL	49 mg
CARBOHYDRATE	20 g
FIBER	2 g
PROTEIN	13 g
SUGARS	5 g
SODIUM	860 mg

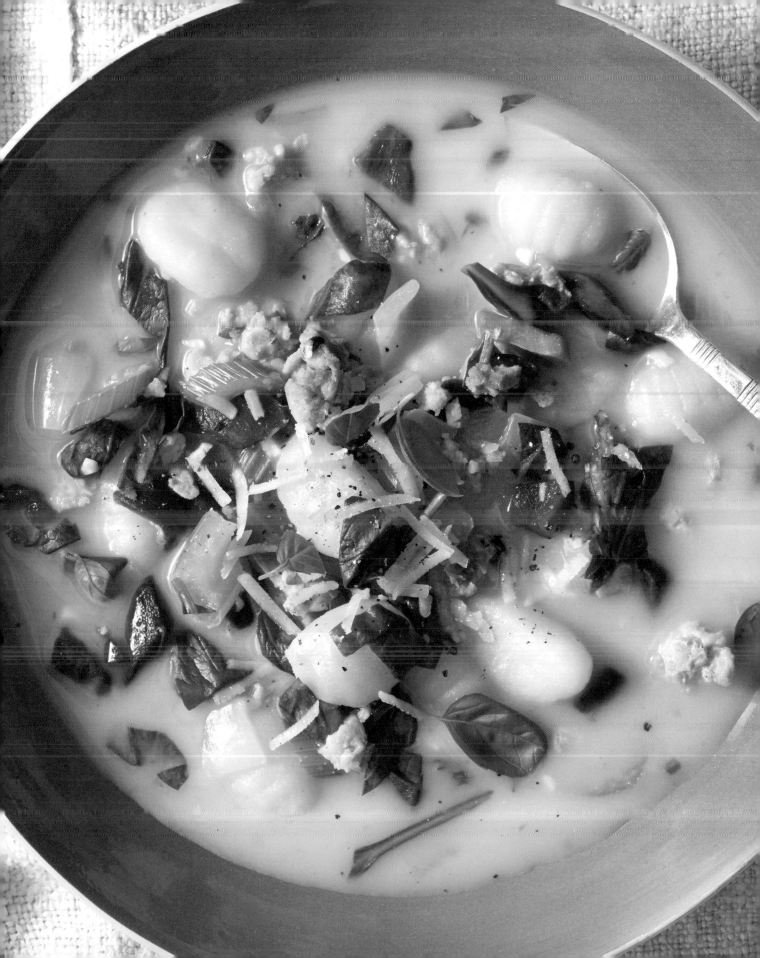

Katia's Caldo Gallego

SERVES 8

GF **FF**

A magnificent hearty soup, *caldo gallego* is from the Galician region of Spain. It's the kind of soup that will stick to your bones on chilly winter nights. This recipe comes from my cousin Katia, who is a terrific cook. I asked Katia to share her recipe, and together we brainstormed ways to slim down the already healthy dish, including replacing fatty cuts of meat with leaner ones. We were able to re-create the same great taste without losing the integrity of her original.

3 medium russet (baking) potatoes, peeled

3.5 ounces dry chorizo sausage, cut crosswise into ¼-inch-thick slices

14 ounces boneless, skinless chicken thighs, trimmed of all fat, cut into 1-inch chunks

1 beef marrow bone, about 4 inches long

½ large head green cabbage, cored and roughly chopped

1 medium yellow onion, finely chopped

2 garlic cloves, minced

1 (15.5-ounce) can small white beans,* rinsed and drained

1 bunch collard greens, stemmed and cut into ½-inch strips

1 teaspoon smoked paprika

2 teaspoons kosher salt

Freshly cracked black pepper

Read the label to be sure this product is gluten-free.

Cut one of the potatoes in half, put it into a large pot, and add the chorizo, chicken thighs, and beef bone. Add 8½ cups water and bring to a boil over medium-high heat. Reduce the heat to medium. Cut the remaining potatoes into cubes (to help thicken the soup) and add to the pot. Add the cabbage, onion, and garlic. Cover and cook for 15 minutes. Add the beans, collard greens, paprika, salt, and black pepper to taste. Reduce the heat to low, cover, and simmer until the collards are tender, about 20 minutes. Discard the bone and serve.

PER SERVING	(SCANT 2 CUPS)
CALORIES	263
FAT	7.5 g
SATURATED FAT	2.5 g
CHOLESTEROL	58 mg
CARBOHYDRATE	30 g
FIBER	9.5 g
PROTEIN	20 g
SUGARS	3 g
SODIUM	500 mg

Slow-Cooker Santa Fe Chicken

SERVES 8

This recipe is one of the most popular recipes on Skinnytaste, and probably because it has everything you could want in a slow-cooker dish: It requires no prep or precooking; it's inexpensive, healthy, kid-friendly; and it's delicious. I use lots of fresh herbs and spices to boost the flavors without adding extra fat or sodium. Plus, some herbs contain antioxidants, which help fight off a variety of diseases.

STEW

1 (14.4-ounce) can Swanson 99% fat-free chicken broth*

1 (15-ounce) can low-sodium black beans,* rinsed and drained

2 cups (8 ounces) frozen corn kernels

1 (14.5-ounce) can diced tomatoes with mild green chiles

¼ cup chopped fresh cilantro

3 scallions, chopped

1 teaspoon garlic powder

1 teaspoon onion powder

1¼ teaspoons ground cumin

1 teaspoon cayenne pepper

¼ teaspoon kosher salt

1½ pounds boneless, skinless chicken breasts

TOPPINGS

½ cup chopped scallions

¼ cup chopped fresh cilantro

Read the label to be sure this product is gluten-free.

For the stew: In a slow cooker, combine the broth, beans, corn, tomatoes, cilantro, scallions, garlic powder, onion powder, cumin, and cayenne. Season the chicken with salt and lay it on top. Cover and cook on low for 10 hours or high for 6 hours.

Thirty minutes before serving, remove the chicken, shred it with two forks, and return it to the slow cooker.

For the toppings: To serve, divide the soup among 8 serving bowls and top with the scallions and cilantro.

PERFECT PAIRINGS

Top this dish with a little sour cream and reduced-fat cheddar; spoon it over cilantro-lime rice (combine ¾ cup cooked brown rice with a squeeze of lime juice and a tablespoon chopped fresh cilantro); sprinkle it over baked tortilla chips and top with reduced-fat cheese and jalapeños; or serve it over greens as a salad. (Psst! It's also great as a filling for enchiladas: see page 171 for my awesome enchilada sauce recipe.)

skinny scoop

Beat the morning rush by preparing all the ingredients the night before. Then, all you have to do is add them to the slow cooker in the morning and turn it on!

PER SERVING	(1 CUP)
CALORIES	181
FAT	2.5 g
SATURATED FAT	0.5 g
CHOLESTEROL	70 mg
CARBOHYDRATE	18 g
FIBER	4.5 g
PROTEIN	23 g
SUGARS	1 g
SODIUM	736 mg

SKINNY LICIOUS SOUPS & CHILIS

Slow-Cooker White Bean Chicken Chili Verde

SERVES 6

GF FF SC

In this lighter twist on the classic Mexican chili verde, chicken is used in place of pork along with white beans simmered in a rich, spicy sauce. Cubanelle peppers are sweet banana-shaped peppers, and I like using them for their milder flavor, which doesn't overpower the other flavors in this dish. Since slow cookers mellow out the flavors of spices, it's always best to taste your dishes at the very end and adjust the spices as needed. Leftovers are even better the next day, so don't worry if you think you've made too much. You can even freeze whatever you don't plan to eat right away.

1 teaspoon olive oil

1 small onion, chopped

1 cup chopped cubanelle pepper

3 medium tomatillos, chopped

3 garlic cloves, minced

2¾ teaspoons ground cumin

2 (15.5-ounce) cans Great Northern or navy beans,* rinsed and drained

1 (7-ounce) can fire-roasted chopped green chiles

¼ cup chopped jalapeño pepper, fresh or pickled (remove seeds if you prefer mild heat)

2½ cups Swanson 33% less sodium chicken broth*

1½ pounds boneless, skinless chicken breasts

¼ cup chopped fresh cilantro

1 teaspoon dried oregano

¼ teaspoon chili powder*

2 bay leaves

¼ teaspoon kosher salt

¼ cup finely chopped scallions or red onion, for serving

Read the label to be sure this product is gluten-free

Heat a medium nonstick skillet over medium heat. Add the oil, then the onions and cubanelle pepper. Cook, stirring, until golden and soft, about 5 minutes. Add the tomatillos, garlic, and 2½ teaspoons of the cumin and cook for 2 more minutes. Transfer the mixture to the slow cooker and add the beans, green chiles, jalapeño, broth, chicken breasts, cilantro, oregano, chili powder, and bay leaves.

Cover and cook on low for 8 hours or high for 4 hours. Remove the chicken from the broth, shred with 2 forks, and return it to the slow cooker.

Season with the salt and the remaining ¼ teaspoon cumin, or to taste, and discard the bay leaves. To serve, ladle the chili into 6 serving bowls and top with the scallions.

PERFECT PAIRINGS

My favorite combination of toppings for this chili is chopped scallions and shredded Colby-Jack cheese. Sometimes, though, I keep it simple and add just a few slices of avocado. My husband prefers his with light sour cream, shredded Jack cheese, and tortilla chips on the side.

PER SERVING	(1½ CUPS)
CALORIES	382
FAT	5 g
SATURATED FAT	1 g
CHOLESTEROL	55 mg
CARBOHYDRATE	46 g
FIBER	18 g
PROTEIN	38 g
SUGARS	4 g
SODIUM	532 mg

SKINNY-LICIOUS SOUPS & CHILIS

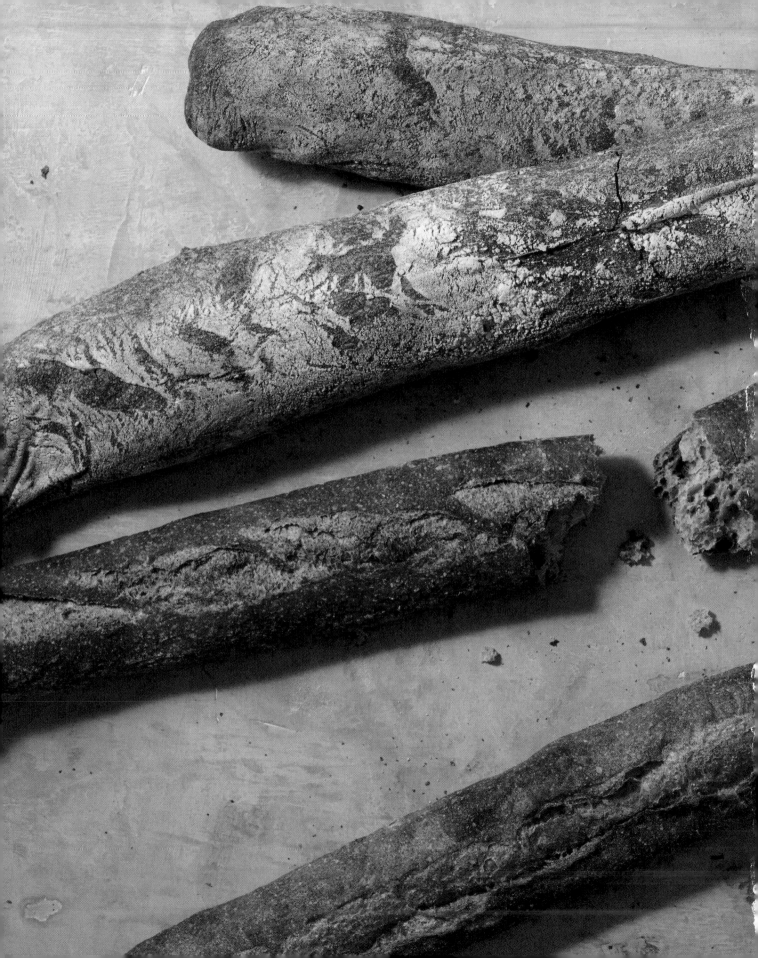

SANDWICHES
ON THE LIGHTER SIDE

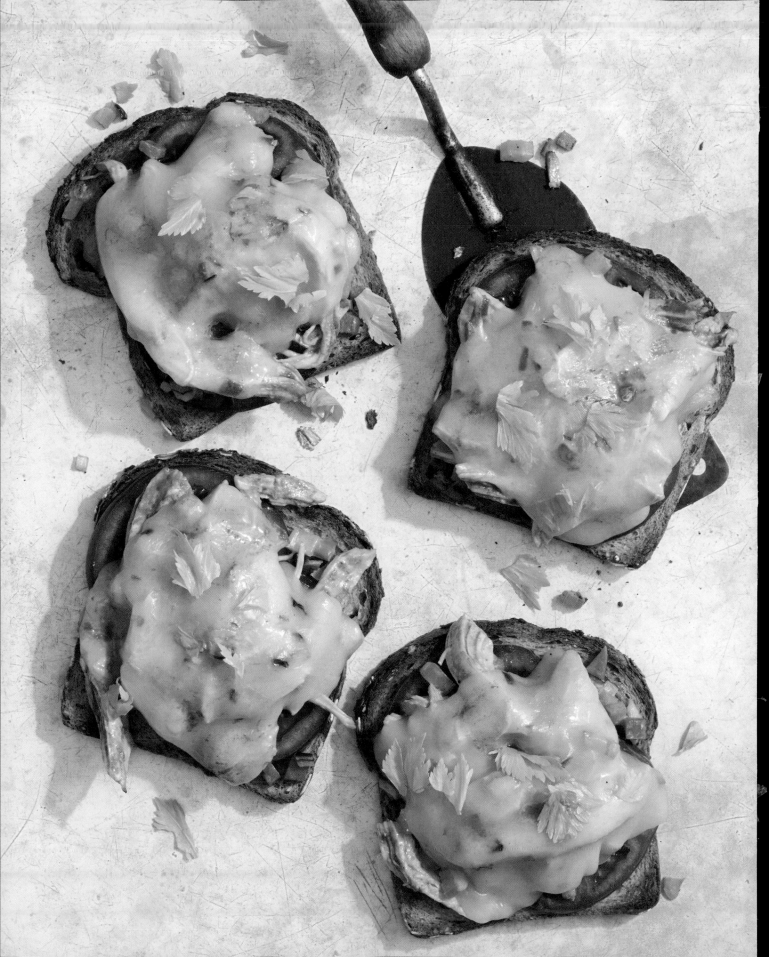

Buffalo Chicken Melts

SERVES 4

Q

I grew up on tuna melts, and now I often make them for my kids. I love this spicier twist on the classic: In place of tuna I use chicken salad made with a Louisiana-style hot sauce and minced carrots, celery, and onions. It's served open-face on toasted whole-grain bread and topped with thin slices of tomatoes and melted pepper Jack cheese, which adds just the right amount of heat.

1½ cups (7 ounces) Convenient Slow-Cooker Shredded Chicken (recipe follows) or breast meat from a store-bought rotisserie chicken

¼ cup finely chopped carrots

¼ cup finely chopped celery

1 tablespoon finely chopped red onion

1 tablespoon light mayonnaise such as Hellmann's

2½ tablespoons Frank's RedHot sauce

Pinch of cayenne pepper (optional)

4 slices multigrain bread, lightly toasted (such as Arnold)

8 thin slices tomato

4 slices (2.6 ounces total) reduced-fat pepper Jack cheese (such as Sargento)

Adjust an oven rack in the top third of the oven and preheat the broiler.

In a medium bowl, combine the chicken, carrots, celery, red onion, mayonnaise, hot sauce, and cayenne (if using).

Arrange the toast on a baking sheet and put 2 slices of tomato on each. Divide the chicken salad evenly among the slices and top with 1 slice of pepper Jack. Broil until the cheese is golden and bubbling, about 2 minutes, keeping a close eye on it to avoid burning. Serve hot.

(recipe continues)

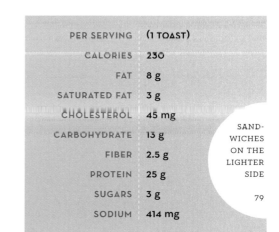

PER SERVING	(1 TOAST)
CALORIES	230
FAT	8 g
SATURATED FAT	3 g
CHOLESTEROL	45 mg
CARBOHYDRATE	13 g
FIBER	2.5 g
PROTEIN	25 g
SUGARS	3 g
SODIUM	414 mg

SAND-
WICHES
ON THE
LIGHTER
SIDE

Convenient Slow-Cooker Shredded Chicken

MAKES 18 OUNCES · SERVES 6

GF

Wanna know my secret to making quick weeknight meals? I use my slow cooker to make shredded chicken. It's my favorite technique because the chicken gets so tender that it just falls apart and it requires almost no attention whatsoever.

I opt for organic chicken and buy it in bulk to save money. I throw 3 pieces in my slow cooker and wrap the rest in plastic to freeze for another day. A few hours later, the chicken easily shreds into pieces. You can use chicken broth to add more flavor, or just use water with salt instead. If I have some herbs, celery, or parsley in my refrigerator, I may even throw them in. There are really no rules—use whatever you have on hand.

3 boneless, skinless chicken breasts, trimmed of all fat (1½ pounds total)

3 cups Swanson 33% less sodium chicken broth* (or water)

1 onion, quartered (optional)

1 celery stalk (optional)

1 sprig of fresh parsley (optional)

*Read the label to be sure this product is gluten-free.

In a slow cooker, combine the chicken breast, just enough broth (or water) to cover the chicken, and onion, celery, and parsley, if using. Cover and cook on high for 4 hours.

Remove the chicken and shred it with two forks. Discard the remaining liquid and vegetables. Use the shredded chicken in any recipe that calls for it, or refrigerate it for up to 3 days.

PER SERVING	(3 OUNCES)
CALORIES	66
FAT	1.5 g
SATURATED FAT	0.5 g
CHOLESTEROL	31 mg
CARBOHYDRATE	2 g
FIBER	0 g
PROTEIN	11 g
SUGARS	1 g
SODIUM	300 mg

Roast Beef Sandwiches with Creamy Horseradish Spread

SERVES 4

Q

I distinctly remember the first time I tried a roast beef sandwich with watercress and cucumbers. From my very first bite, I thought it was a magical combination. I've been making roast beef sandwiches this way ever since. The horseradish spread really gives this an extra punch of flavor!

HORSERADISH CREAM

3 tablespoons light sour cream

1 tablespoon prepared horseradish

1 tablespoon Dijon mustard

1 tablespoon finely chopped fresh chives

Kosher salt and freshly cracked black pepper

SANDWICHES

8 ounces whole wheat baguette, cut into 4 pieces

8 ounces thinly sliced lean roast beef

1 cup watercress or baby arugula

20 thin slices English cucumbers (2 ounces)

Kosher salt and freshly cracked black pepper

For the horseradish cream: In a small bowl, combine the sour cream, horseradish, mustard, and chives. Season with a pinch of salt and black pepper.

For the sandwiches: Split each piece of baguette in half lengthwise and spread the horseradish cream onto the bread. Layer each sandwich with 2 ounces roast beef, ¼ cup watercress, and 5 slices cucumber. Season each with a pinch each of salt and black pepper and serve.

FOOD FACTS say "yes" to watercress!
This tiny vegetable has big time cancer fighting compounds. One cup of these peppery leaves is loaded with antioxidants: 25% of your recommended daily intake of vitamin C, 20% of your recommended intake of vitamin A, and carotenoids, the same glaucoma-fighting plant pigments found in carrots.

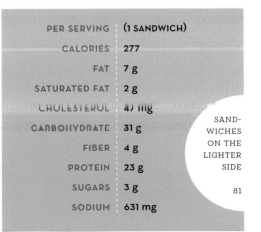

PER SERVING	(1 SANDWICH)
CALORIES	277
FAT	7 g
SATURATED FAT	2 g
CHOLESTEROL	47 mg
CARBOHYDRATE	31 g
FIBER	4 g
PROTEIN	23 g
SUGARS	3 g
SODIUM	631 mg

SAND-WICHES ON THE LIGHTER SIDE

Greek Salad Pita Pizzas

SERVES 4

V Q

Greek goodness—that's what I call these personal salad pita pizzas. I came up with the idea after tasting a savory Greek tart at the farmers' market. The flavors were so fresh and tasty that I wanted to come up with a quick, lighter way anyone could enjoy it. This is so easy to make and takes less than 5 minutes to put together!

2 teaspoons red wine vinegar

1 teaspoon extra-virgin olive oil

3 tablespoons chopped Kalamata olives

1 tablespoon chopped red onion

¾ cup hummus, homemade (see page 111) or store-bought

4 (1-ounce) whole wheat pitas, unsplit and toasted

4 thin slices beefsteak tomato

⅓ cup seeded and chopped cucumber

⅓ cup chopped orange bell pepper

2 tablespoons crumbled feta cheese

skinny**scoop**

Trader Joe's carries organic whole wheat pita breads that are 100 percent whole grain and have no artificial ingredients. If you don't live near a TJ's, look for small whole wheat pitas that are about 1 ounce each, or cut a larger one in half.

In a small bowl, whisk together the vinegar and olive oil. Stir in the olives and onion.

Spread 2 tablespoons hummus on the top of each toasted pita. Top each with a slice of tomato, spread with 1 more tablespoon hummus in the center of the tomato, and top with the cucumber, bell pepper, onion-olive mixture, and feta.

PER SERVING	(1 PITA)
CALORIES	194
FAT	7.5 g
SATURATED FAT	1.5 g
CARBOHYDRATE	4 mg
CHOLESTEROL	27 g
FIBER	4.5 g
PROTEIN	6 g
SUGARS	2 g
SODIUM	370 mg

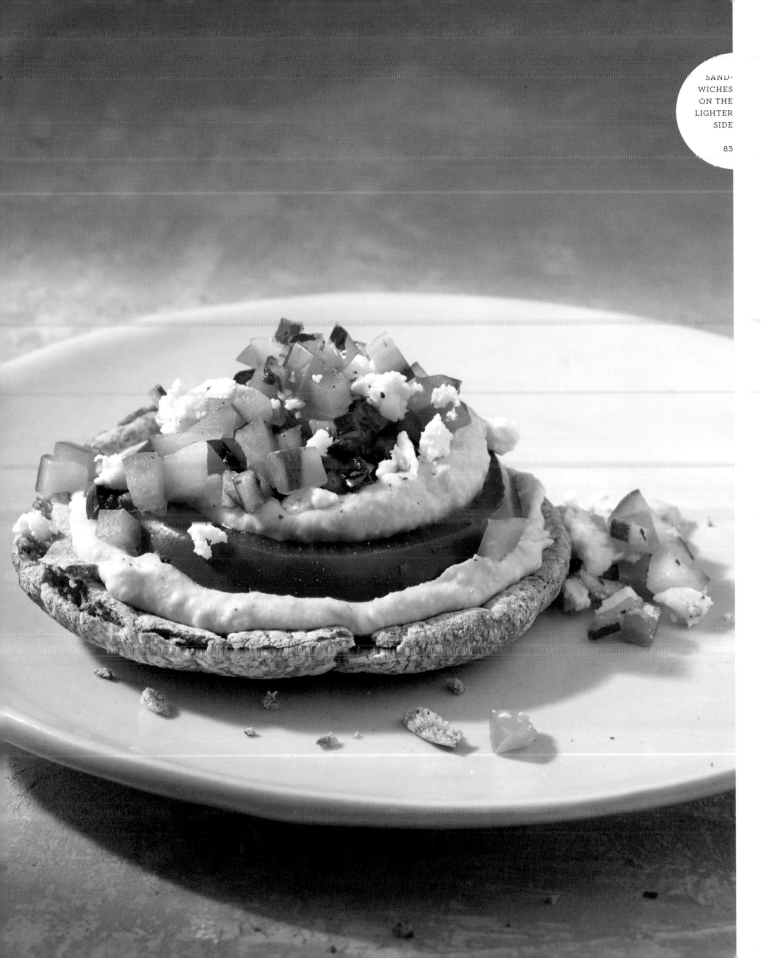

Chicken Philly Cheesesteaks

SERVES 4

Q

I must confess, I have a real weakness for cheesesteaks. I used to work near a sandwich shop that made a pretty decent Philly chicken sub. Whenever I'd walk by during my lunch break, I'd have a hard time passing one up. But at more than 500 calories and 15 grams of fat per sub (yikes!), I always felt guilty if I ordered one. So I made up my own leaner version. It's so good and only about 350 calories!

10 ounces boneless, skinless thin chicken breast cutlets

½ teaspoon garlic powder

Kosher salt

Freshly cracked black pepper

Cooking spray or oil mister

1 teaspoon olive oil

½ medium green bell pepper, thinly sliced

½ large onion, halved and thinly sliced

8 ounces sliced mushrooms

8 ounces whole wheat French or Italian bread, split horizontally and cut crosswise into 4 pieces

4 (1-ounce) slices reduced-fat provolone cheese

Preheat the oven to 425°F or the broiler to low.

Season the chicken with the garlic powder, ¼ teaspoon salt, and black pepper to taste. Heat a large nonstick skillet over high heat. When hot, spray the skillet with oil and add half of the chicken, making sure you don't overcrowd the pan. Cook until browned, about 1 minute, turn the chicken over, and cook the second side for 1 additional minute. Transfer to a large dish. Repeat with the remaining chicken.

Add ½ teaspoon of the oil to the hot skillet. Add the bell pepper and onion and season with a pinch of salt and black pepper. Cook 1 minute, stir, and then cook until the onions are golden and slightly browned, 4 to 5 minutes. Transfer to the plate of chicken.

Reduce the heat to medium and add the remaining ½ teaspoon olive oil to the skillet. Add the mushrooms, season with ⅛ teaspoon salt and a pinch of black pepper, and cook until the mushrooms are slightly browned on one side, 1 to 2 minutes.

PER SERVING	(1 SANDWICH)
CALORIES	356
FAT	9 g
SATURATED FAT	4 g
CHOLESTEROL	61 mg
CARBOHYDRATE	38 g
FIBER	2.5 g
PROTEIN	31 g
SUGARS	4 g
SODIUM	730 mg

Turn the mushrooms over and cook until soft, 1 to 2 more minutes. Transfer to the plate of chicken, onions, and peppers.

Divide the chicken and vegetables evenly among the bottom halves of the bread, and top each with a slice of cheese. Place the sandwiches on a baking sheet.

Heat the sandwiches in the oven or broiler until the cheese melts, 2 to 3 minutes, being careful not to burn the cheese if using the broiler. Remove from the oven, close the sandwiches, and serve.

skinny**scoop**

I love making sandwiches using a good-quality whole wheat crusty bread from my local bakery. However, a 2- or 3-ounce slice of French bread is pretty small and leaves little room for whatever you want to fill your sandwich with. My solution: Cut a larger piece of bread and scoop out some of the guts. This allows me to enjoy a larger sandwich without the extra calories. I usually cut a 3- or 4-ounce piece of bread and scoop out about an ounce, saving me about 65 calories.

Go Topless

EMBRACING THE OPEN-FACE SANDWICH

A tartine is an open-face sandwich that's often made with a rich spread. Leaving the top piece of bread off cuts calories, making a slimmer sandwich. And topping it with fruit, veggies, healthy fats, and more good-for-you ingredients allows you to create a truly healthy bite. Try one of these deliciously skinny, quick tartines, each of which is 300 calories or less.

Top a 2-ounce slice of crusty whole-grain bread with . . .

- 2 sliced heirloom tomatoes, chiffonade-cut fresh basil, and 1 teaspoon olive oil drizzled on top (211 CALORIES)

- 3 ounces (about ½ cup) mashed avocado and a sprinkle of salt and freshly ground black pepper (276 CALORIES)

- 2 tablespoons ⅓-less-fat cream cheese, diced scallions, and sliced tomatoes and cucumbers (221 CALORIES)

- 1 chopped hard-boiled egg, thinly sliced red onion, capers, and 1 teaspoon olive oil drizzled on top (261 CALORIES)

- 2 ounces flaked tuna (packed in water), ¼ medium sliced Hass avocado, chopped tomatoes, and a handful of sprouts (300 CALORIES)

Turkey Panini with Avocado, Spinach, and Roasted Peppers

SERVES 4

Ⓠ

Looking for a fresh way to dress your sandwich? Try mashed avocado seasoned with a touch of salt and black pepper. The spread adds a nice flavor to this crisp, warm panini made with lean turkey breast, sweet roasted peppers, and wilted baby spinach pressed between two slices of ciabatta bread.

½ cup mashed avocado

4 pieces (2.75 ounces each) ciabatta bread, sliced open

Kosher salt and freshly cracked black pepper

2 cups baby spinach

8 ounces thinly sliced turkey breast

8 thin slices roasted red bell peppers, jarred (not oil-packed) or homemade (see page 233)

Olive oil spray or oil mister

skinny**scoop**

No panini press? No problem. Place the sandwich onto a heated skillet or griddle, top with a weight, such as another heavy pan, and push down on the weight to press and crisp the sandwich. When the bread is toasted, flip the sandwich and toast the other side.

Preheat a panini press.

Spread 2 tablespoons of the avocado on the top of each piece of ciabatta bread. Season the avocado with a pinch of salt and black pepper. Place ½ cup spinach on the bottom of each sandwich and top each with 2 ounces of turkey and 2 slices roasted pepper. Close the sandwiches and lightly spray the tops with a little olive oil.

Place the sandwiches one at a time on the hot panini press and close. Cook until the bread is toasted and crisp, about 5 minutes. Cut the sandwiches in half diagonally and serve immediately.

PER SERVING	(1 PANINI)
CALORIES	300
FAT	6 g
SATURATED FAT	1 g
CHOLESTEROL	25 mg
CARBOHYDRATE	41 g
FIBER	3.5 g
PROTEIN	21 g
SUGARS	5 g
SODIUM	864 mg

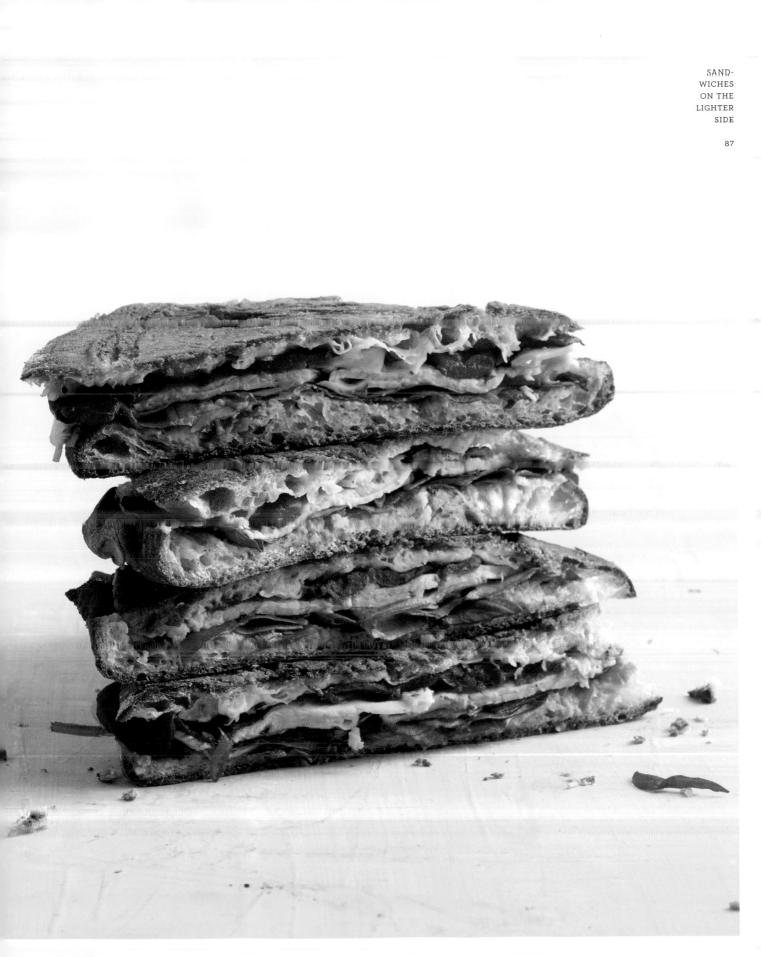

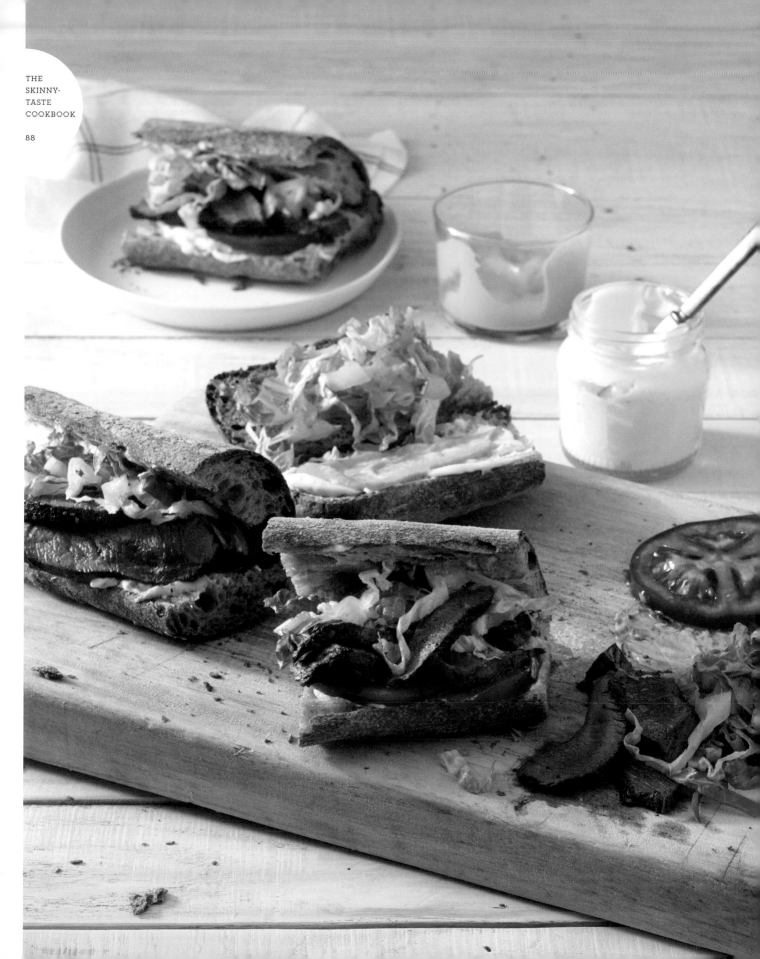

Grilled Steak Sandwiches

SERVES 4

Q

These steak sandwiches are simple—you probably already have most of the ingredients in your pantry—but put them all together and you have yourself a pretty darn good sandwich. Cook lean sirloin steaks on the grill, top with juicy tomatoes and crisp lettuce, and serve on a whole wheat baguette. Dinner is ready in less than 15 minutes and it's absolutely delicious!

STEAK

14 ounces sirloin steak, trimmed of fat

½ teaspoon garlic powder

¼ teaspoon kosher salt

Freshly cracked black pepper

Cooking spray or oil mister

SANDWICHES

8 ounces whole wheat baguette, cut into 4 pieces

2 tablespoons yellow mustard

¼ cup light mayonnaise

2 cups shredded romaine lettuce

1 large beefsteak tomato, sliced

For the steak: Season the sirloin with the garlic powder, salt, and black pepper to taste.

Preheat a grill to high (or preheat a grill pan over high heat). Lightly rub the grates with oil or spray a grill pan with oil and add the steaks. Grill for about 3 minutes, turn the steaks over, and grill another 3 minutes for medium (cook longer or less according to your preference). Transfer the steak to a cutting board to rest for 5 minutes.

For the sandwiches: Split open each piece of bread, then spread each with ½ tablespoon mustard and 1 tablespoon mayonnaise. Divide the lettuce and tomatoes among the sandwiches.

Thinly slice the steak and divide it among the sandwiches and serve.

skinnyscoop

Always let cooked steak rest at least 5 minutes before slicing so that you don't lose all those delicious juices. I'd rather keep them in my sandwich than let them collect on the cutting board.

PER SERVING	(1 SANDWICH)
CALORIES	350
FAT	11 g
SATURATED FAT	2.5 g
CHOLESTEROL	64 mg
CARBOHYDRATE	35 g
FIBER	4 g
PROTEIN	28 g
SUGARS	5 g
SODIUM	571 mg

SAND-
WICHES
ON THE
LIGHTER
SIDE

Egg, Tomato, and Scallion Sandwiches

SERVES 4

(V) (Q)

Prior to making Skinnytaste my full-time career, I worked in Manhattan as a digital photo retoucher. In the lobby of the building where I worked, there was a small cafe that served a simple egg sandwich. My friend Tricia and I were absolutely hooked. It calls for only a few common ingredients, but the combination is just delicious! I had to remake it at home.

4 large eggs, hard-boiled, peeled, and sliced

4 whole wheat 100-calorie potato rolls (I love Martin's)

4 thick slices tomato

¼ cup chopped scallions

Kosher salt and freshly cracked black pepper

¼ cup light mayonnaise

Assemble the sandwiches by placing one sliced egg on the bottom of each roll. Top it with a tomato slice and 1 tablespoon scallions. Season each with a pinch of salt and black pepper. Spread 1 tablespoon of mayonnaise on the top of each roll, put the tops on the sandwiches, and serve.

skinny**scoop**

Here's a foolproof way to make perfect hard-boiled eggs every time: Place eggs in a pot, cover with cold water, and bring to a rolling boil. Cover the pot, remove it from the heat, and let it sit for 20 minutes without opening the lid. Drain the hot water, quickly rinse the eggs under cold water, and peel.

PER SERVING	(1 SANDWICH)
CALORIES	220
FAT	10 g
SATURATED FAT	2 g
CHOLESTEROL	215 mg
CARBOHYDRATE	22 g
FIBER	3.5 g
PROTEIN	14 g
SUGARS	5 g
SODIUM	581 mg

Pear and Brie Grilled Cheese

SERVES 4

(V) (Q)

Have you ever had baked Brie? If not, you're totally missing out. And if you have, then you'll understand why this grilled cheese sandwich works. I love the salty-sweet combination of ripe pears and Brie. Adding a touch of fig butter—a fruit spread not to be confused with butter—to this grilled cheese sandwich enhances the sweetness of the pears and makes it a real adult treat.

8 slices multi-grain bread

¼ cup fruit butter such as fig or apple

1 pear, peeled and thinly sliced

6 ounces light Brie, rind removed and sliced

Olive oil spray or oil mister

Heat a skillet over medium-low heat.

Spread each slice of bread with ½ tablespoon fig or apple butter. Top 4 of the slices with the pear and Brie, then top with the remaining slices of bread. Spray both sides of the sandwiches with a little oil.

Place the sandwiches, one at a time, in the hot skillet and cook until the bread is golden and the cheese starts to melt, about 2 minutes on each side. (Alternatively, use a panini press.) Serve hot.

skinny scoop

Fruit butters are usually available in the jelly aisle. They're basically a fruit spread made with mostly fruit and less sugar than a preserve or marmalade.

PER SERVING	(1 SANDWICH)
CALORIES	309
FAT	9 g
SATURATED FAT	4 g
CHOLESTEROL	23 mg
CARBOHYDRATE	41 g
FIBER	6 g
PROTEIN	18 g
SUGARS	15 g
SODIUM	617 mg

SAND-
WICHES
ON THE
LIGHTER
SIDE

91

French Bread Pizza Supreme

SERVES 4

Q

French bread pizza reminds me of my high school days when I would come home from school ravenous and turn French bread into an awesome after-school meal. I still make such pizzas today, although now I sneak in some whole grains and top them with tons of veggies. It's perfect because everyone can customize their toppings to their taste. I've always liked the classic combination of pepperoni, mushrooms, bell peppers, and onions, but you can use any vegetables or leftovers you have, including broccoli, sliced turkey, meatballs, spinach—the possibilities are endless!

1 (10-ounce) loaf whole wheat French bread

1 cup marinara sauce, homemade (recipe follows) or store-bought

2 mushrooms, thinly sliced

1 thinly sliced red onion, separated into rings

8 thin slices green bell pepper

1 cup shredded part-skim mozzarella cheese (4 ounces)

¼ cup shredded Parmesan cheese (0.9 ounces)

8 turkey pepperoni slices, cut in half

Preheat the oven to 425°F.

Split the bread horizontally lengthwise, then cut each half crosswise into 2 pieces to give you 4 pieces total. Scoop out the center of the bread, keeping only the crust (each should weigh about 2 ounces).

Place the bread, cut side up, on a baking sheet. Spread each piece with ¼ cup marinara sauce. Divide the mushrooms, onion rings, pepper slices, mozzarella, and Parmesan among the pieces, then top with pepperoni.

Bake until the cheese is melted and bubbling, and the bread is crisp, about 10 minutes.

PER SERVING	(1 PIZZA)
CALORIES	310
FAT	8 g
SATURATED FAT	4 g
CHOLESTEROL	20 mg
CARBOHYDRATE	42 g
FIBER	4.5 g
PROTEIN	16 g
SUGARS	4 g
SODIUM	756 mg

(recipe continues)

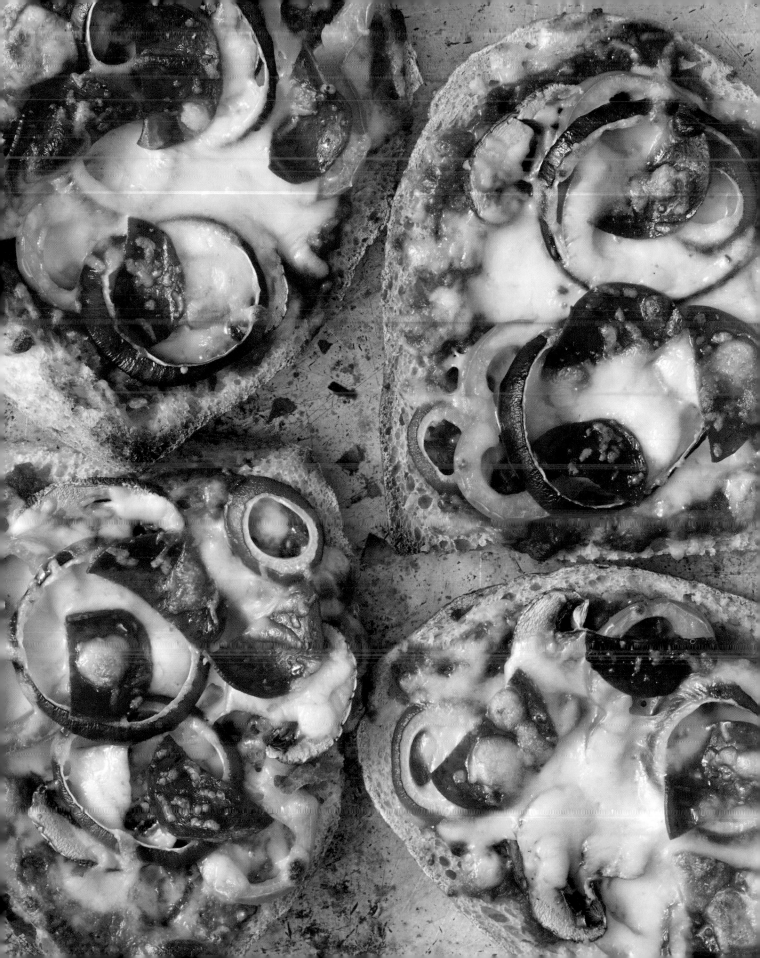

Quickest Marinara Sauce

MAKES ABOUT 6¾ CUPS

(V) (GF) (Q) (FF)

This easy-to-whip-up sauce works well for a variety of quick meals, from pizza to pasta to chicken Parm, which you can throw together on a busy weeknight. The secret to the perfect marinara is buying the right tomatoes. Not all canned tomatoes are created equal; you should look for a brand you like. I prefer Tuttorosso New World Style crushed tomatoes, which already has salt, so if you use a different brand, you may need to adjust the salt to taste.

2 teaspoons olive oil

5 garlic cloves, smashed

2 (28-ounce) cans crushed tomatoes (I recommend Tuttorosso)

¾ teaspoon kosher salt, plus more as needed

Freshly ground black pepper

¼ cup roughly chopped fresh basil

Heat a medium-large saucepan over medium heat. Add the oil and garlic and cook, stirring, until golden, about 2 minutes. (Tip: Because I don't use a lot of oil, I tilt my pan to one side so the garlic is submerged in the oil and cooks evenly.) Add ¼ cup water, the tomatoes, and salt and season with black pepper to taste. Cover the pot, bring to a boil, reduce the heat to medium-low, and simmer until the sauce is heated through, about 10 minutes. Remove the pan from the heat, stir in the basil, and adjust salt and pepper to taste if needed.

skinny**scoop**

This sauce can be stored in the refrigerator for up to 3 days, or in the freezer for up to 4 months. To freeze, let the sauce cool and transfer it to 1-quart zip-top bags (rather than gallon-size). Label the bags with the name, portion size, and date, and lay them flat in the freezer. To thaw, transfer the sauce to the refrigerator 1 to 2 days before you plan to use it, or you can heat the frozen sauce over low heat on the stovetop.

PER SERVING	(½ CUP)
CALORIES	48
FAT	0.5 g
SATURATED FAT	0 g
CHOLESTEROL	0 mg
CARBOHYDRATE	8 g
FIBER	2 g
PROTEIN	2 g
SUGARS	2 g
SODIUM	325 mg

Grilled Vegetable Sandwiches with Pesto Mayonnaise

SERVES 4

(V) (Q)

Summer is my favorite season—I love the warm weather, the beach, the long hours of daylight, and the abundance of fresh produce available at farmers' markets. This is the ideal quickie weeknight summer dinner. What really makes a sandwich is the bread it's made on—good bread is worth seeking out. For this sandwich, I like to use a crusty, whole wheat or multigrain rustic-style loaf, which you can find in any good bakery or Trader Joe's.

PESTO MAYONNAISE

1 cup fresh basil leaves

1 garlic clove

2 tablespoons grated Parmesan cheese

Freshly ground black pepper

¼ cup light mayonnaise (I prefer Hellmann's Light)

SANDWICHES

1 medium eggplant, cut lengthwise into ¼-inch-thick slabs

2 medium zucchini, sliced lengthwise ¼ inch thin

Olive oil spray or mister

2 tablespoons balsamic vinegar

¼ teaspoon dried oregano

¼ teaspoon kosher salt

Freshly ground black pepper

8 (1-ounce) slices bread from a multigrain round country loaf

1 large tomato, thinly sliced

For the pesto mayonnaise: In a food processor, combine the basil, garlic, Parmesan, and black pepper to taste and pulse until smooth. Add the mayonnaise and pulse a few times.

For the sandwiches: Preheat a grill to medium (or preheat a grill pan over medium heat).

Spray the sliced vegetables generously with olive oil and drizzle on the balsamic vinegar. Season with the oregano, salt, and black pepper to taste. Grill the vegetables until lightly browned and tender, 5 to 6 minutes on each side.

Toast the bread on the grill for about 1 minute per side. Spread the pesto mayonnaise on the bread. Divide the grilled vegetables among 4 of the bread slices, layer the sliced tomatoes on the vegetables, and then top with the remaining 4 slices of bread.

PER SERVING	(1 SANDWICH)
CALORIES	260
FAT	9 g
SATURATED FAT	2 g
CHOLESTEROL	4 mg
CARBOHYDRATE	39 g
FIBER	7 g
PROTEIN	8 g
SUGARS	9 g
SODIUM	424 mg

SAND-WICHES ON THE LIGHTER SIDE

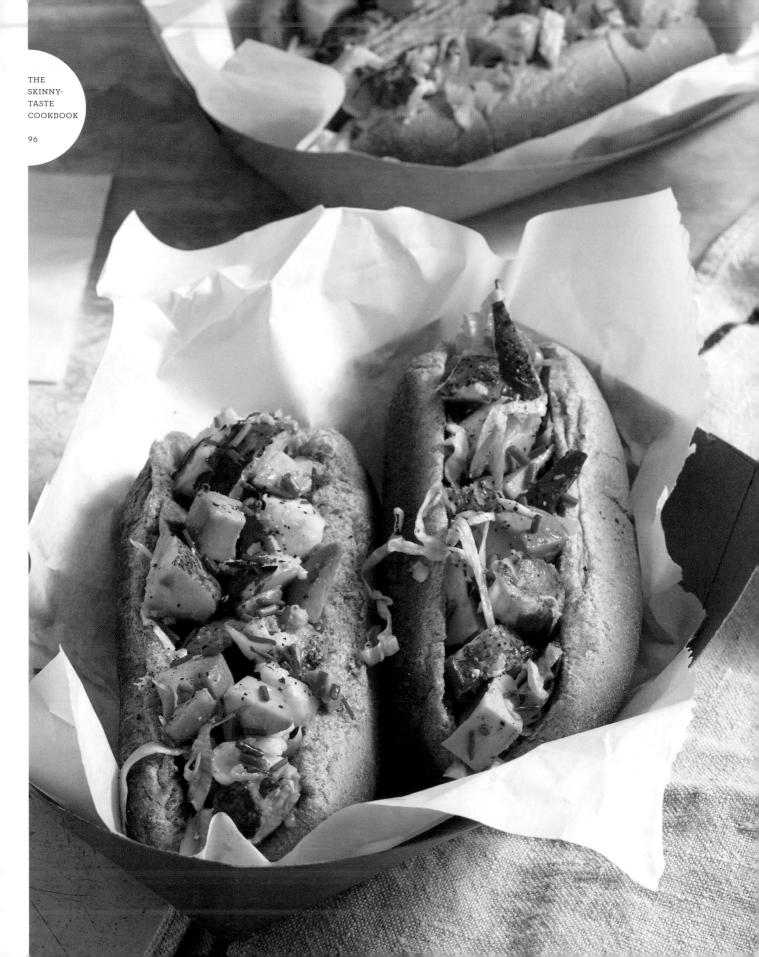

Summer Lobster Rolls

SERVES 4

Q

Lobster rolls always remind me of Fire Island, New York. In the summer I love taking day trips by ferry out to this barrier island off the south shore of Long Island and often treat myself to a lobster roll for lunch. But it's usually swimming in fatty mayonnaise, or worse, melted butter. Here, I remake this favorite summer sandwich so that it's a bit healthier. The fresh avocado gives it a creamy texture, plus a dose of heart-healthy fat.

If you want to eliminate the carbs, bypass the bread and serve this in a fancy martini glass instead. If fresh lobster isn't available to you, you can use lump crabmeat, or much less expensive imitation crab instead.

9 ounces fresh steamed lobster meat (from two 1½-pound live lobsters), chopped

1 medium (4 ounces) Hass avocado, chopped

Juice of 1 large lemon

1 teaspoon olive oil

2 teaspoons minced fresh chives

Kosher salt and freshly ground black pepper

4 whole wheat hot dog buns

1 cup shredded lettuce

In a medium bowl, combine the lobster meat, avocado, lemon juice, olive oil, and chives, and season with a pinch of salt and black pepper.

Open the hot dog buns and put the shredded lettuce inside. Top with the lobster salad and serve.

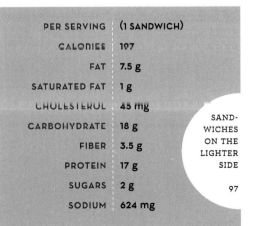

PER SERVING	(1 SANDWICH)
CALORIES	197
FAT	7.5 g
SATURATED FAT	1 g
CHOLESTEROL	45 mg
CARBOHYDRATE	18 g
FIBER	3.5 g
PROTEIN	17 g
SUGARS	2 g
SODIUM	624 mg

SAND-
WICHES
ON THE
LIGHTER
SIDE

97

SKINNY BITES

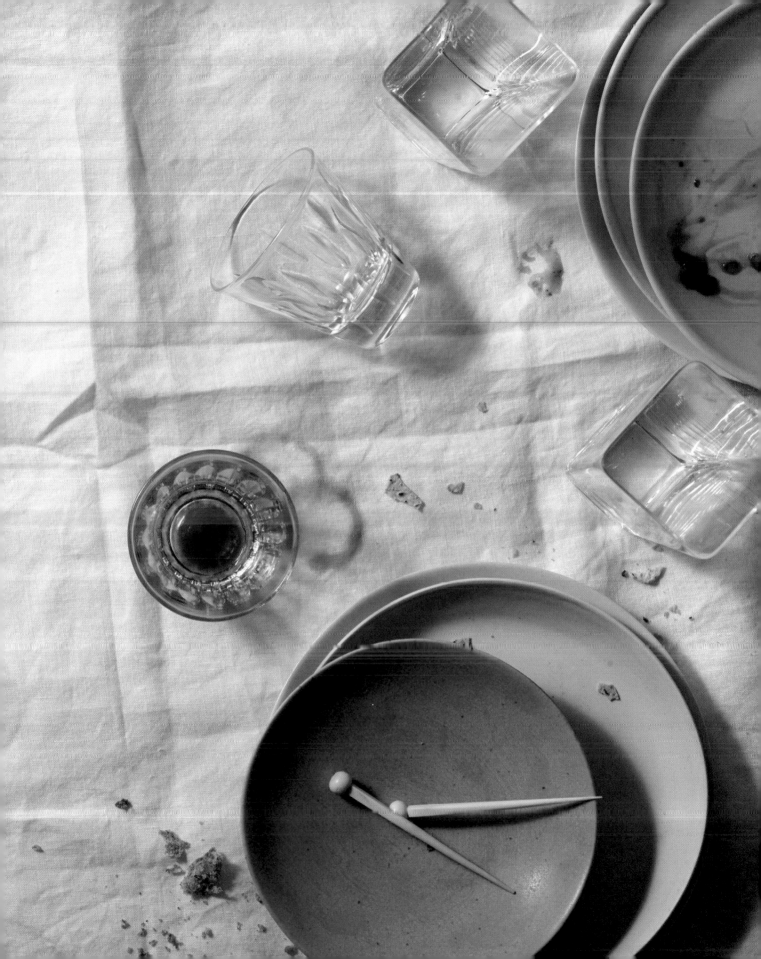

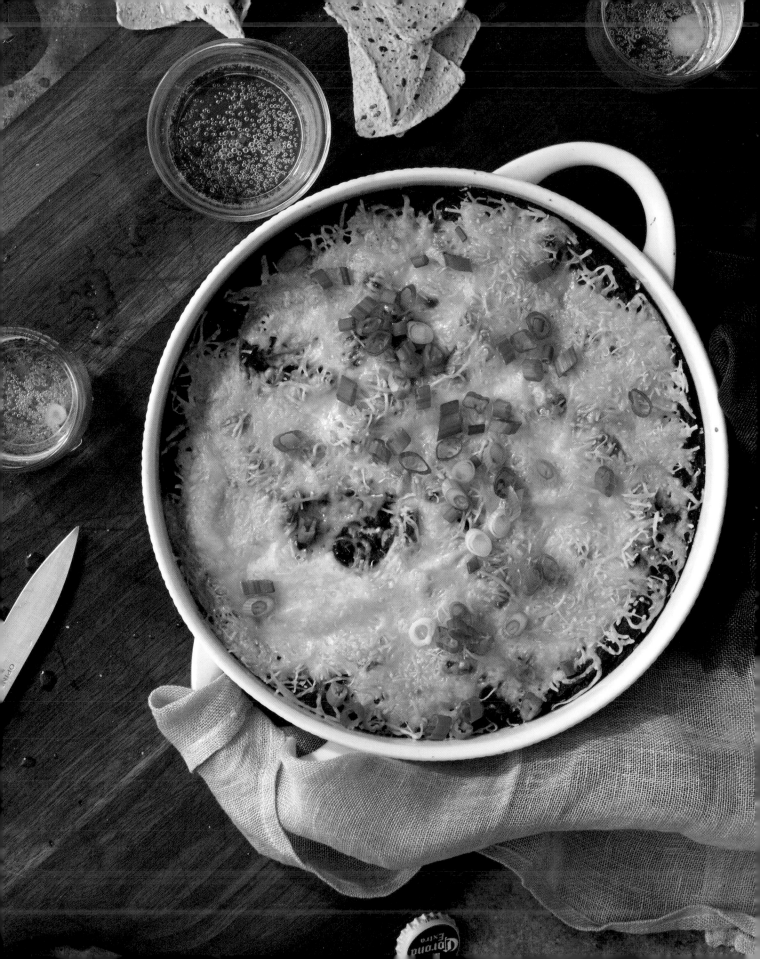

Caliente Bean and Queso Dip

MAKES 3½ CUPS • SERVES 14

(V) (GF) (Q)

Melted cheese is my weakness, but I believe in everything in moderation. Plus, there *are* some health perks associated with cheese: It's a complete protein with the right amount of amino acids to give our bodies a protein fix, and it's rich in calcium, vitamin A, and folate. Cheesy days are always happier than cheeseless days for me, so to make it work calorie-wise, I look for reduced-fat or part-skim cheese options. Sargento makes a delicious light Mexican cheese blend that melts beautifully and is perfect for making this crowd-pleasing appetizer.

Cooking spray or oil mister

1 (15-ounce) can fat-free refried beans*

1 tablespoon taco seasoning*

1¼ cups jarred medium salsa

1 (4-ounce) can diced green chiles

1½ cups shredded reduced-fat Mexican cheese blend (6 ounces)

1 teaspoon chopped fresh cilantro

Read the labels to be sure these products are gluten-free.

Preheat the oven to 350°F. Spray a 9 × 9-inch baking dish with oil.

In a small bowl, combine the refried beans and taco seasoning and spread the mixture evenly over the bottom of the baking dish. Pour the salsa and green chiles on top of the beans.

Bake until the edges begin to bubble, about 30 minutes. Remove from the oven, top with the cheese, and return to the oven. Bake just long enough to melt the cheese, 5 to 6 minutes. Remove from the oven and sprinkle with cilantro.

PERFECT PAIRING
I like to serve this dip with baked tortilla chips.

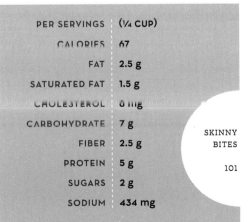

PER SERVINGS	(¼ CUP)
CALORIES	67
FAT	2.5 g
SATURATED FAT	1.5 g
CHOLESTEROL	8 mg
CARBOHYDRATE	7 g
FIBER	2.5 g
PROTEIN	5 g
SUGARS	2 g
SODIUM	434 mg

SKINNY BITES

101

Guiltless Sausage-Stuffed Mushrooms

MAKES 12 TO 14 MUSHROOMS • SERVES 6 OR 7

It's pretty hard to resist popping these bite-size sausage-stuffed mushrooms into your mouth—believe me, I know. When I was testing these out, I probably ate half of them in one sitting for lunch. Good thing these glorious snacks are made with ingredients I feel good about. But don't be fooled by their lack of fat and calories. If you serve these to company, no one would ever notice they were "light"!

14 ounces cremini or white button mushrooms

1 link fresh sweet Italian chicken sausage, casings removed (about 2.8 ounces)

1 teaspoon olive oil

⅓ cup finely chopped onion

1 celery stalk, finely chopped

¼ teaspoon kosher salt, plus more as needed

Freshly cracked black pepper

2 tablespoons whole wheat seasoned bread crumbs, homemade (see page 110) or store-bought

2 tablespoons grated Parmesan cheese

Cooking spray or oil mister

skinny**scoop**

For this recipe, I prefer the smaller mushrooms as opposed to the larger ones that are actually meant for stuffing because they taste better, they hold together better, and there's nothing better than popping those little suckers right into your mouth. If you're making these for a large party, you can prep them ahead of time and bake them in the oven when your guests arrive.

PER SERVING	(2 MUSHROOMS)
CALORIES	63
FAT	3 g
SATURATED FAT	1 g
CHOLESTEROL	13 mg
CARBOHYDRATE	5 g
FIBER	1 g
PROTEIN	5 g
SUGARS	2 g
SODIUM	162 mg

Preheat the oven to 400°F.

Stem the mushrooms, finely chop the stems, and set aside.

Heat a medium nonstick skillet over medium heat. Add the chicken sausage and cook, using a wooden spoon to break the meat into small pieces, until cooked through and browned, 3 to 4 minutes. Transfer to a plate and set aside.

Add the olive oil to the pan, then add the onion. Cook, stirring, for 1 minute, then add the celery. Reduce the heat to medium and cook, stirring, until the celery is soft, about 12 minutes. Add the chopped mushroom stems to the pan, season with the salt and a pinch of black pepper, and cook, stirring, until soft, 4 to 5 minutes. Add the cooked sausage, stir in the bread crumbs and Parmesan, then set aside.

Lightly season the inside of the mushroom caps with a pinch of salt. Fill each mushroom with about 1 heaping tablespoon sausage stuffing, rounding off the tops. It's easy to do this right over the pan one at a time. Place them in a baking dish and lightly spray the tops with oil.

Bake until golden brown, about 20 minutes. Serve hot.

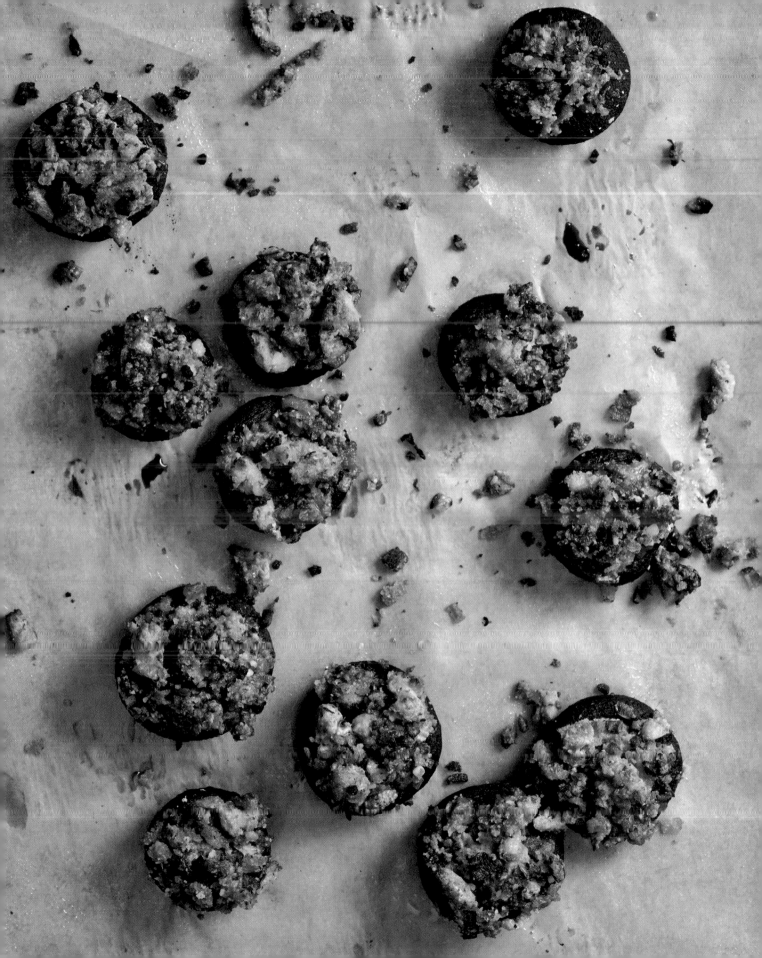

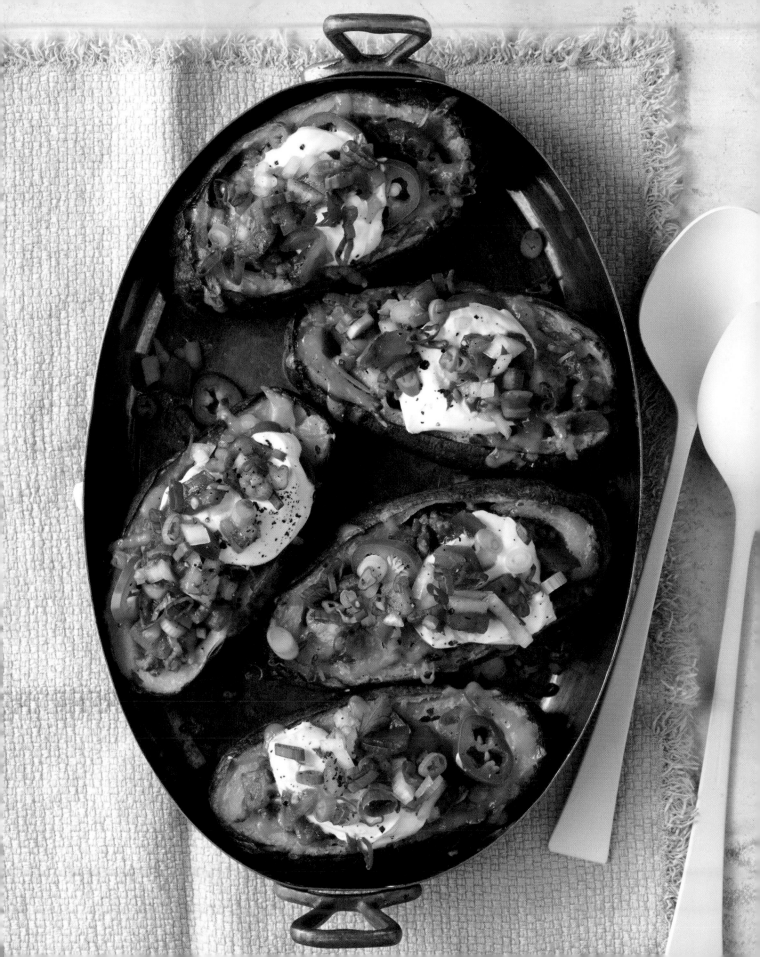

Loaded "Nacho" Potato Skins

SERVES 16

GF

I took two of my favorite party foods—loaded nachos and potato skins—and combined them into one ultimate appetizer! Thanks to the surge of low- or no-carb diets, the white potato has gotten a bad rap. But the humble spud is far from "bad." In fact, it's a nutritious whole food that's packed with nutrients, as well as fiber if the skins are left intact. Here, I even splurged and used full-fat cheddar to top them off. After all, these are potato skins, so they need to be cheesy.

8 small russet (baking) potatoes (about 2¼ pounds total)

QUICK CHILI FILLING

6 ounces 99% extra-lean ground turkey breast

¼ teaspoon kosher salt

¼ cup chopped onion

¼ cup chopped red bell pepper

1 garlic clove, minced

⅓ cup canned diced tomatoes with chiles

½ cup canned fat-free refried beans*

¾ teaspoon ground cumin

¼ teaspoon chili powder

¼ teaspoon smoked paprika

POTATO SKIN TOPPINGS

Cooking spray or oil mister

⅛ teaspoon kosher salt

Freshly ground black pepper

1 cup (4 ounces) shredded Monterey Jack or sharp cheddar cheese

¼ cup pickled jalapeño slices

½ cup light sour cream

½ cup pico de gallo, homemade (see page 120) or store-bought

¼ cup chopped scallions

Read the label to be sure this product is gluten-free.

Pierce each potato several times with a fork. Microwave on high for about 12 minutes, or until the potatoes are cooked through. (Alternatively, bake them in a 400°F oven directly on the oven rack until the skins are crisp and a knife easily pierces the potatoes, about 50 minutes.) Transfer to a wire rack and let cool until cool enough to handle, about 10 minutes.

Preheat the broiler.

(recipe continues)

PER SERVING	(1 LOADED POTATO SKIN)
CALORIES	75
FAT	3 g
SATURATED FAT	1.5 g
CHOLESTEROL	15 mg
CARBOHYDRATE	7 g
FIBER	1 g
PROTEIN	5 g
SUGARS	1 g
SODIUM	172 mg

SKINNY BITES

skinny**scoop**

For this recipe, look for potatoes in 5-pound bags; they tend to be smaller than loose potatoes sold individually. When buying potatoes, always avoid green-spotted spuds or sprouted potatoes.

For the quick chili filling: Heat a medium skillet over medium-high heat. Add the turkey and cook, using a wooden spoon to break the meat into small pieces, until no longer pink, 4 to 5 minutes. Season with the salt. Add the onion, bell pepper, and garlic and cook for 2 to 3 minutes. Add the tomatoes, refried beans, cumin, chili powder, and paprika. Reduce the heat to low, cover, and simmer for 7 to 8 minutes to blend the flavors.

For the potato skin toppings: Slice each potato in half lengthwise. Using a spoon, scoop out the flesh, leaving about ¼ inch intact. Lightly coat the insides and skin sides of the potatoes with oil, and season both sides with the salt and black pepper to taste. Arrange the potato shells on a baking sheet and broil until the skins start to crisp and brown, 2 to 3 minutes on each side. Preheat the oven to 400°F.

Divide the chili evenly among the potato skins and top with the cheese and jalapeño slices. Return to the oven and heat until the cheese is melted, 2 to 3 minutes. Remove from the oven and top with the sour cream, pico de gallo, and scallions. Serve immediately.

Roasted Edamame with Sea Salt

SERVES 4

(V) (GF)

When my daughter Madison was about one and started growing her first few teeth, one of her favorite solid foods was edamame. She would ask for it all the time, which always made me laugh—I created a foodie at the young age of one! As she got older, I would buy packages of dehydrated edamame as a snack. But a small package was so expensive that I decided to try roasting edamame myself. They turned out nutty and crunchy and, I find, a bit addicting if seasoned with a little sea salt.

12 ounces fresh or frozen shelled edamame

Cooking spray or oil mister

¼ teaspoon sea salt

If the edamame are frozen, thaw and dry them well with paper towels.

Preheat the oven to 425°F. Spray a large baking sheet with oil.

Spread the edamame out on the baking sheet, spray with a little more oil, and season with the sea salt. Bake until golden and crisp through the center, shaking the pan every 10 minutes or so to brown evenly, 28 to 38 minutes. Let cool completely.

PER SERVING	(⅓ CUP)
CALORIES	120
FAT	5.5 g
SATURATED FAT	0.5 g
CHOLESTEROL	0 mg
CARBOHYDRATE	9 g
FIBER	3.5 g
PROTEIN	11 g
SUGARS	0 g
SODIUM	353 mg

SKINNY
BITES

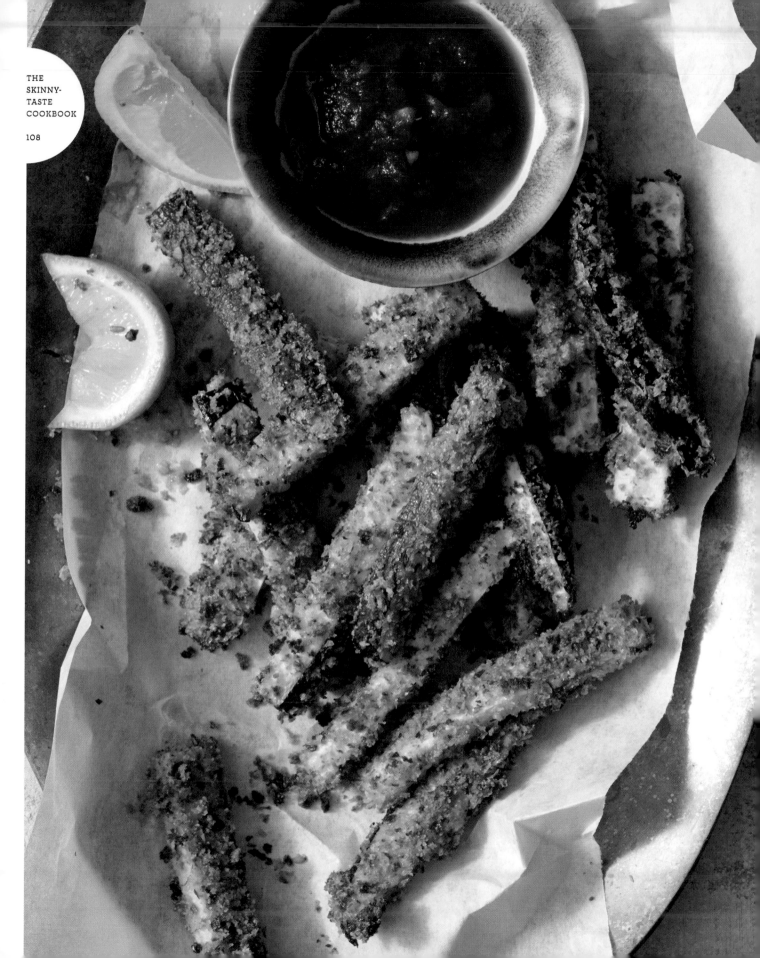

Baked Zucchini Sticks

SERWES 4

V

I guarantee that even the pickiest of eaters will love these! In fact, when my daughter Karina (a very picky eater) was younger, this was her favorite way to eat zucchini. The only complaint I used to get when I made these was that I never made enough, so if you think this is a lot for four people, keep in mind they shrink a bit when they cook.

Cooking spray or oil mister

4 medium zucchini, ends trimmed

3 large egg whites

¼ teaspoon kosher salt

Freshly ground black pepper

1 cup Seasoned Whole Wheat Bread Crumbs, homemade (recipe follows) or store-bought

2 tablespoons grated Pecorino Romano cheese

¼ teaspoon garlic powder

Preheat the oven to 425°F. Spray 2 large baking sheets with oil.

Cut each zucchini into 16 sticks about 4 inches long and about ½ inch thick for a total of 64 sticks and put them on paper towels to blot excess moisture.

In a small bowl, season the egg whites with the salt and black pepper to taste and beat well. In a medium shallow bowl, combine the bread crumbs, Romano, and garlic powder. Dip the zucchini sticks into the egg whites, and then into the bread crumbs, turning to coat well. Place the breaded zucchini sticks in a single layer on the prepared baking sheets and spray the tops with more oil.

Bake until golden brown and tender in the center, 23 to 25 minutes.

skinny**scoop**

For best results, bread the zucchini in two batches so the crumbs don't clump up. Divide the bread crumbs in half. Bread the first two zucchinis, then dump the crumbs and use the remaining crumbs to finish breading the last two.

(recipe continues)

PERFECT PAIRINGS
Serve this with warm **Quickest Marinara Sauce (page 94)** on the side for dipping.

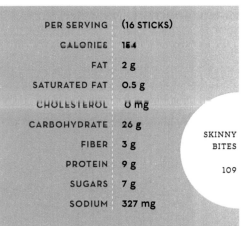

PER SERVING	(16 STICKS)
CALORIES	154
FAT	2 g
SATURATED FAT	0.5 g
CHOLESTEROL	0 mg
CARBOHYDRATE	26 g
FIBER	3 g
PROTEIN	9 g
SUGARS	7 g
SODIUM	327 mg

SKINNY BITES

Seasoned Whole Wheat Bread Crumbs

MAKES ABOUT 1¼ CUPS

Ⓥ Ⓠ

My parents are pretty old-school. I grew up in a home where nothing went to waste. For instance, stale bread in the hands of my mother usually turned into bread crumbs. Any time I have unused whole wheat French bread sitting around (especially when I make sandwiches), I turn it into these delicious seasoned bread crumbs. Mom totally rubbed off on me!

4 ounces stale whole wheat French bread, cut into bite-size pieces

3 tablespoons grated Pecorino Romano cheese

1 teaspoon dried parsley flakes

½ teaspoon Italian seasoning

½ teaspoon garlic powder

½ teaspoon onion powder

½ teaspoon kosher salt

Put the bread pieces in a blender or food processor and pulse until it turns into crumbs.

Put the crumbs in a medium bowl and add the Romano, parsley flakes, Italian seasoning, garlic powder, onion powder, and salt. Store in an airtight container for up to 3 weeks and use in any recipe calling for seasoned bread crumbs.

skinny**scoop**

This works best with very stale bread that's a few days old. If your bread is only a day old and you want to make it right away, cut the bread into cubes and toast it in the oven at 300°F for a few minutes to dry it out.

PER SERVING	(¼ CUP)
CALORIES	77
FAT	1.5 g
SATURATED FAT	0.5 g
CHOLESTEROL	3 mg
CARBOHYDRATE	12 g
FIBER	1 g
PROTEIN	3 g
SUGARS	1 g
SODIUM	270 mg

Lemony Herb Hummus

MAKES 2½ CUPS · SERVES 10

Hummus is a Middle Eastern dip made from chickpeas, tahini (sesame seed paste), and a lot of oil to make it smooth. I created a lighter version by using a lot less oil and adding Great Northern white beans to help make it extra creamy. Another trick for making extra-smooth hummus: When using canned chickpeas (or beans), bring them to a boil and blend them while they're warm. It helps soften the skin and produces a silkier texture, rather than the grainy texture you get with cold canned chickpeas. Serve this with freshly cut vegetables or baked pita chips and lavash chips.

1 (15-ounce) can chickpeas,* rinsed and drained

1 (15-ounce) can Great Northern beans,* rinsed and drained

1 garlic clove, crushed

1 tablespoon tahini

Pinch of grated lemon zest

5 tablespoons fresh lemon juice

2 tablespoons chopped fresh parsley

1½ teaspoons kosher salt

¼ teaspoon freshly cracked black pepper, plus more for garnish

1 tablespoon extra-virgin olive oil

Pinch of paprika or ground cumin, for garnish

Sprig of fresh parsley, for garnish

Read the label to be sure this product is gluten-free.

Put the chickpeas and beans in a medium pot and add just enough water to cover. Set the pot over high heat and bring the mixture to a boil. Simmer about 1 minute, then drain the beans, reserving some of the water.

Transfer the chickpeas and beans and 2 to 3 tablespoons of the reserved water to a food processor. Pulse a few times.

In a medium bowl, combine the garlic, tahini, lemon zest, lemon juice, parsley, salt, and black pepper. Add the mixture to the food processor and process until smooth and creamy, 5 to 7 minutes. If it's too thick, add more of the reserved water.

Transfer to a serving dish and smooth the top with the back of a spoon. Drizzle the olive oil over the top, sprinkle with black pepper and paprika, and put the sprig of parsley on top.

skinny scoop

This dish will stay refrigerated for up to 4 days. To serve, bring it back to room temperature.

PER SERVING	(¼ CUP)
CALORIES	131
FAT	3.5 g
SATURATED FAT	0.5 g
CHOLESTEROL	0 mg
CARBOHYDRATE	20 g
FIBER	2 g
PROTEIN	6 g
SUGARS	0 g
SODIUM	277 mg

SKINNY BITES

111

Cheesy "Fried" Mozzarella Bites

SERVES 12

FF

These fun, tasty treats are great for kids and adults alike. I mean, who doesn't love "fried" mozzarella? These bites are better for you than standard mozzarella sticks because they're made with part-skim cheese and are baked instead of fried. These actually need to be baked when they're completely frozen so they don't melt in the oven before they get golden on the outside. For this reason, I like to prep them ahead of time, and keep them ready in my freezer.

12 sticks reduced-sodium part-skim mozzarella string cheese (9 ounces; I recommend Sargento)

1 large egg

2 tablespoons all-purpose flour

5 tablespoons seasoned whole wheat bread crumbs, homemade (see page 110) or store-bought

5 tablespoons panko bread crumbs

1 tablespoon grated Parmesan cheese

1 tablespoon dried parsley flakes

Olive oil spray or oil mister

PERFECT PAIRINGS
Serve this with warm **Quickest Marinara Sauce** (page 94) for dipping.

Cut each piece of string cheese into quarters, place the pieces on a baking sheet, and freeze for at least 8 hours, or overnight.

In a small bowl, beat the egg. Put the flour in a second small bowl. In a third medium bowl, combine both the seasoned bread crumbs, panko, Parmesan, and parsley flakes.

Line a baking sheet with wax paper. Dip the frozen cheese in the flour, shaking off any excess, then into the egg, and lastly coat with the bread crumb mixture. Put the breaded cheese on the baking sheet. Freeze the breaded cheese for at least 1 hour (this is a must or they will melt in the oven before browning).

Preheat the oven to 425°F. Lightly spray a baking sheet with olive oil.

Place the frozen cheese bites on the prepared baking sheet and lightly spray the tops with a little oil. Bake for 3 minutes, turn them over, and bake until melted inside and golden on the outside, watching them closely so the cheese doesn't come out of the breading, about 2 minutes. Serve immediately as baked mozzarella hardens quicker than fried.

PER SERVING	(4 BITES)
CALORIES	107
FAT	5 g
SATURATED FAT	3 g
CHOLESTEROL	31 mg
CARBOHYDRATE	5 g
FIBER	0 g
PROTEIN	8 g
SUGARS	0 g
SODIUM	238 mg

skinny**scoop**

I like to use a combination of panko bread crumbs and seasoned bread crumbs for the topping; the panko helps give the cheese bites that extra crunch since they are baked in the oven rather than fried.

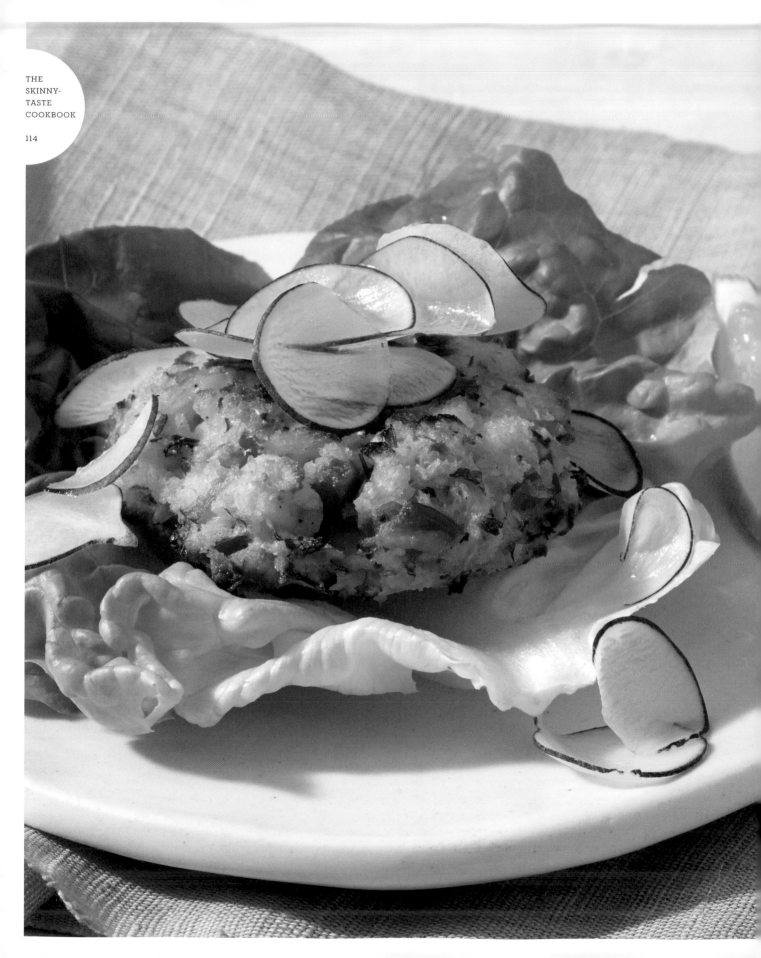

Petite Baked Crab Cakes

SERVES 8

(Q)

Fresh crab is quite plentiful here on Long Island—you can get it just about everywhere. In the warmer months, you can even see people crabbing off the side of the road. I have access to some really great fresh seafood vendors, so I usually buy lump crabmeat from a trusted source. I've had great success with everything from snow crab to king crab legs, so use whatever is freshest for you. I don't, however, recommend using crab from a can, as the taste and smell is a bit fishy and metallic, and the price is not much different. For a pretty presentation, serve the crab cakes on large leaves of lettuce, topped with thinly sliced radishes.

½ cup panko bread crumbs

1 large egg

1 large egg white

2 tablespoons finely chopped shallots

2 tablespoons finely chopped red bell pepper

1 tablespoon light mayonnaise

2 tablespoons finely chopped fresh parsley

1 tablespoon fresh lemon juice

A few dashes of Tabasco sauce

Kosher salt

⅛ teaspoon freshly ground black pepper

9 ounces lump crabmeat

Cooking spray or oil mister

8 small lemon wedges, for serving

In a large bowl, combine the panko, whole egg, egg white, shallots, bell pepper, mayonnaise, parsley, lemon juice, Tabasco, ¼ teaspoon plus ⅛ teaspoon kosher salt, and black pepper. Pick over the crabmeat to remove any bits of shell, then fold the meat into the panko mixture, being careful not to overmix. Gently shape into 8 round patties with your hands, about ¼ cup each. Refrigerate for at least 30 minutes before baking.

Preheat the oven to 425°F. Spray a nonstick baking sheet with oil and arrange the crab cakes on it. Bake until golden, turning once, 8 to 10 minutes on each side. Serve with lemon wedges for squeezing.

skinny scoop

You can form the patties ahead of time and keep them refrigerated until you're ready to bake. These are perfect as an appetizer or as a main course for four if served with a large salad.

PER SERVING	(1 CRAB CAKE)
CALORIES	69
FAT	1 g
SATURATED FAT	0.5 g
CHOLESTEROL	49 mg
CARBOHYDRATE	6 g
FIBER	0.5 g
PROTEIN	8 g
SUGARS	1 g
SODIUM	201 mg

SKINNY BITES

115

Bangin' Good Shrimp

SERVES 4

GF **Q**

I've never been to the Bonefish Grill, but fans begged me for a recipe makeover from the popular seafood chain restaurant. They would say things like, "We order Bang Bang Shrimp *every time* we go, but it's really bad for you," or "Holy Cow! We love that shrimp. Please make it lighter," and so on. Receiving *that* many e-mails, I took notice. The biggest problems with the original dish are that it's deep-fried and smothered in a fatty mayonnaise sauce. Once I made my skinny fixes, it became one of the most popular appetizers on my website. Whether you eat them as an appetizer or serve them over rice to make them a main dish, these shrimp are bangin' good!

5 tablespoons light mayonnaise (I prefer Hellmann's Light)

3 tablespoons Thai sweet chili sauce

1 to 2 teaspoons Sriracha sauce, or to taste

1 pound shelled and deveined large shrimp

2 teaspoons cornstarch

1 teaspoon canola oil

3 cups shredded iceberg lettuce

1 cup shredded red cabbage

6 or 7 cilantro leaves

¼ cup diagonally sliced scallions

In a medium bowl, combine the mayonnaise, sweet chili sauce, and Sriracha.

Toss the shrimp with the cornstarch, mixing well with your hands. Heat a large nonstick skillet or wok over high heat. Add the oil and shrimp and cook, stirring, until cooked through, about 3 minutes. Transfer the shrimp to the bowl of sauce and toss well.

In a large bowl, combine the lettuce, cabbage, and cilantro and divide among 4 serving plates. Divide the shrimp among the plates; garnish with the scallions and serve immediately.

PER SERVING	(⅔ CUP SHRIMP + 1 CUP SALAD)
CALORIES	215
FAT	7 g
SATURATED FAT	1 g
CHOLESTEROL	175 mg
CARBOHYDRATE	14 g
FIBER	1 g
PROTEIN	24 g
SUGARS	8 g
SODIUM	454 mg

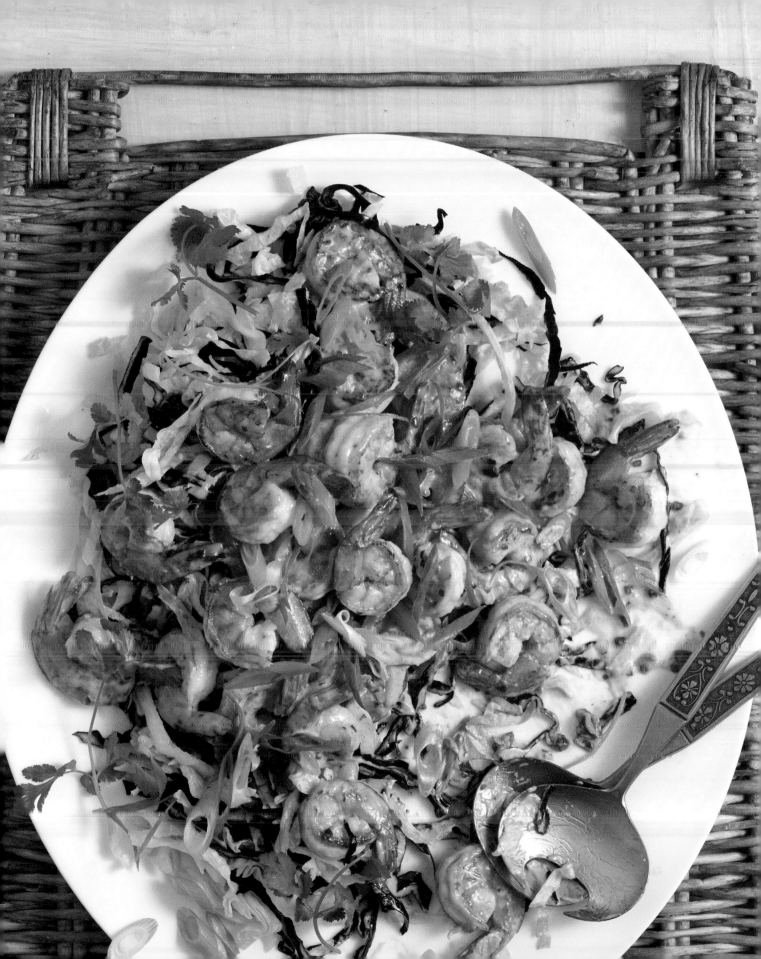

Less-Guilt Zesty Mango Guacamole

MAKES 4 CUPS · SERVES 8

(V) (GF) (Q)

My avocado obsession is so strong that I created an entire Pinterest board devoted to it. I love their taste and texture, but I also love how nutrient-rich avocados are: They're loaded with healthy fats, fiber, vitamins, and potassium. Adding mango to guacamole is brilliant; it adds a touch of sweetness which complements the savory flavors of the dip, and it gives more volume to the dish without adding any fat or a lot of calories.

2 medium (8 ounces) Hass avocados, chopped

2 large mangoes, chopped

1 small fresh jalapeño pepper, minced (include the seeds, if you want it spicy)

¼ cup chopped red onion

2 tablespoons chopped fresh cilantro

2½ tablespoons fresh lime juice

¼ teaspoon kosher salt

⅛ teaspoon freshly ground black pepper

Place the avocados in a medium bowl and mash with a fork, leaving some large chunks. Add the mango, jalapeño, onion, cilantro, lime juice, salt, and black pepper

PER SERVING	(½ CUP)
CALORIES	105
FAT	6 g
SATURATED FAT	1 g
CHOLESTEROL	0 mg
CARBOHYDRATE	15 g
FIBER	4 g
PROTEIN	1 g
SUGARS	9 g
SODIUM	44 mg

Skinny Green Goddess Dip

MAKES 1¼ CUPS • SERVES 5

This recipe is the perfect excuse to round up fresh herbs from the garden and make the most of them. I lightened it up by using Greek yogurt (in place of mayo) and some creamy mashed avocado, which adds healthy fat, makes it greener, and gives it a great texture. I've tried this with many different herbs, but as a basil lover, I like to use a big bunch of the summery ingredient. It tastes even better the next day, so it's great to make a day in advance.

½ cup 0% Greek yogurt

¼ cup light mayonnaise (I prefer Hellmann's Light)

¼ cup mashed avocado

½ cup packed chopped fresh basil

¼ cup chopped fresh chives

¼ cup chopped fresh parsley

2 anchovy fillets, rinsed and patted dry

1 garlic clove, chopped

1 tablespoon fresh lemon juice

⅛ teaspoon kosher salt

Freshly ground black pepper

In a blender, combine the yogurt, mayonnaise, avocado, basil, chives, parsley, anchovy, garlic, lemon juice, salt, and pepper to taste. Process until smooth then transfer the dip to a bowl. Keep refrigerated, covered, until ready to serve. This can be made up to a day in advance.

PERFECT PAIRING

Serve this dip with crisp, colorful vegetables cut into strips. I love using bell peppers (yellow, orange, and red), English cucumbers, baby carrots, sugar snap peas, and zucchini. You can even include some jumbo cooked shrimp.

PER SERVING	(¼ CUP)
CALORIES	68
FAT	4.5 g
SATURATED FAT	1 g
CHOLESTEROL	1 mg
CARBOHYDRATE	5 g
FIBER	1 g
PROTEIN	3 g
SUGARS	2 g
SODIUM	243 mg

SKINNY BITES

Garden Pico de Gallo

MAKES 3½ CUPS • SERVES 8

(V) (GF) (Q)

Pico de gallo is a bright, fresh salsa made from diced tomatoes, onions, cucumbers, jalapeños, cilantro, and lime juice. It's perfect served as an appetizer with baked chips, but I also love it as a condiment over tacos, tostadas, grilled meats, and salads. In the spring, I plant tomatoes, peppers, jalapeños, and fresh herbs, so that I can use them throughout the summer. This quick, fresh salsa is one way to make use of those tasty vegetables.

4 medium tomatoes, chopped

⅓ cup chopped fresh jalapeño peppers (about 2)

⅓ cup chopped cucumber

¼ cup chopped white onion

¼ cup finely chopped fresh cilantro leaves

1 garlic clove, minced

2 tablespoons fresh lime juice

¾ teaspoon kosher salt

⅛ teaspoon freshly ground black pepper

skinny**scoop**

I'm always on the prowl for a healthier alternative to chips that my picky family members will actually eat. Beanitos, which are made from beans, are a great option. They come in a few varieties, are low-glycemic, and are certified non-GMO. Plus, they're high in protein and fiber, which helps keep you feeling full longer.

In a large bowl, combine the tomatoes, jalapeños, cucumber, onion, cilantro, garlic, lime juice, salt, and black pepper. Let the salsa marinate in the refrigerator for at least 1 hour before eating.

PER SERVING	(GENEROUS ⅓ CUP)
CALORIES	16
FAT	0 g
SATURATED FAT	0 g
CHOLESTEROL	0 mg
CARBOHYDRATE	4 g
FIBER	1 g
PROTEIN	1 g
SUGARS	2 g
SODIUM	109 mg

Crave-Worthy Snacks

Slimming snacks don't have to taste like cardboard, and they shouldn't be loaded with processed junk! My real food snacks clock in at 150 calories or less and are easy to assemble at home or at the office—no cooking (or cardboard crackers) required.

- **PARMESAN POPCORN**
  2 cups air-popped popcorn topped with 2 tablespoons grated Parmesan (110 CALORIES)

- **HARD-BOILED EGG & CHIVES**
  1 large hard-boiled egg with snipped chives and a pinch of salt (80 CALORIES)

- **HUMMUS & VEGGIES**
  ¼ cup sugar snap peas and ¼ cup baby carrots dipped in ¼ cup Lemony Herb Hummus (page 111) (150 CALORIES)

- **APPLES & CHEDDAR**
  ½ sliced apple with 1 ounce cheddar (150 CALORIES)

- **PEARS & BLUE**
  ½ sliced pear with 1 ounce blue cheese (150 CALORIES)

- **GRAPES & GRUYERE**
  ½ cup grapes with 1 ounce Gruyere cheese (150 CALORIES)

- **CHIPS & GUAC**
  10 baked tortilla chips and ½ cup red bell pepper strips dipped in ¼ cup Less-Guilt Zesty Mango Guacamole (page 118) (130 CALORIES)

- **NUTTY BANANA**
  Spread 1 medium banana with ½ tablespoon almond butter (150 CALORIES)

- **CHERRIES & PISTACHIOS**
  1 cup cherries mixed with 1 tablespoon shelled pistachios (130 CALORIES)

- **ALMOND BUTTER & APPLE**
  ½ tablespoon almond butter spread on 1 apple, sliced (120 CALORIES)

- **BANANA ICE CREAM**
  Freeze 1 large ripe banana and puree in a food processor until smooth (120 CALORIES)

- **CREAMY BERRIES**
  6 ounces nonfat Greek yogurt topped with 1 cup berries (150 CALORIES)

- **SKINNY DIP**
  ¼ cup Skinny Green Goddess Dip (page 119) with 1 cup broccoli florets and 1 cup baby carrots (140 CALORIES)

- **FRESH FRUIT & NUTS**
  1 medium-size fruit (apple, pear, peach, orange, banana, etc.) with 1 tablespoon unsalted nuts (130 CALORIES)

- **FETA & WATERMELON**
  2 cups cubed watermelon with 1 tablespoon crumbled feta cheese and 1 tablespoon chopped mint (120 CALORIES)

- **GREEK TREAT**
  6 ounces nonfat Greek yogurt mixed with 1 tablespoon shaved dark chocolate and ½ tablespoon raspberry preserves (140 CALORIES)

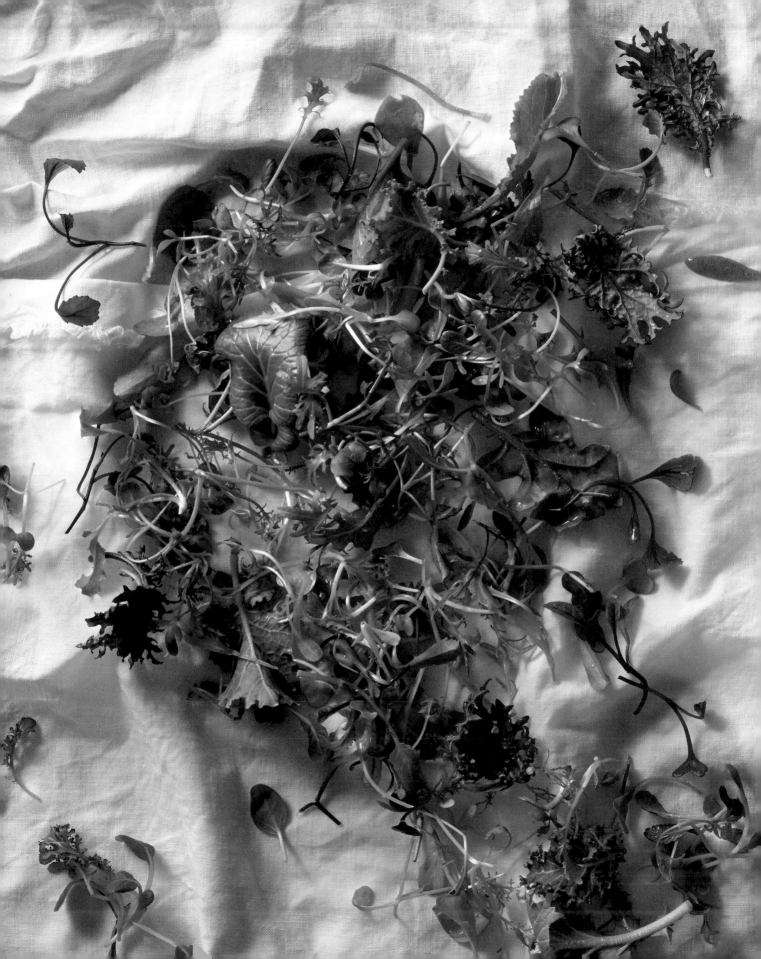

FABULOUS MAIN-DISH SALADS

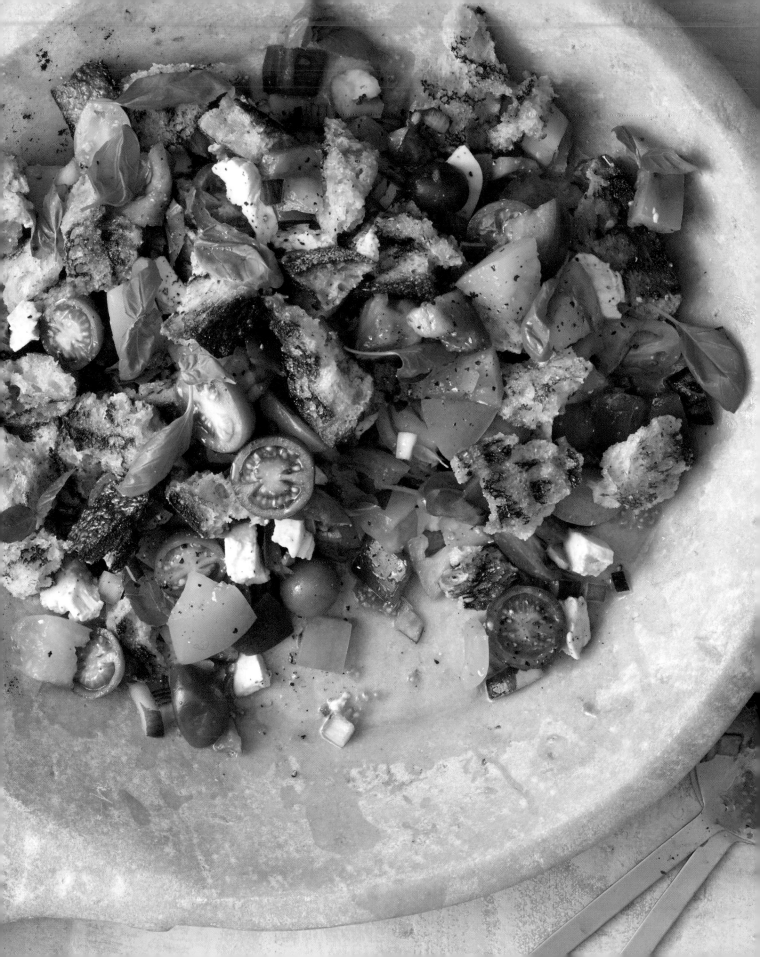

Tuscan Panzanella Salad with Grilled Garlic Bread

SERVES 4

Ⓥ Ⓠ

My husband, who's half-Italian, makes this simple salad by combining just a few quality ingredients. But here's the secret: Before adding the bread, he lets the other flavors marinate for 30 minutes at room temperature. It makes quite a difference! The bread is important, too. You'll want to look for a rustic loaf with a crunchy crust. Whole wheat Italian bread would also be great for a whole-grain option.

8 cups heirloom tomatoes, cut into 1-inch cubes

½ cup chopped red onion

8 to 10 basil leaves, cut into thin strips (chiffonade)

1 tablespoon extra-virgin olive oil

1½ teaspoons kosher salt, plus more as needed

Freshly ground black pepper

Olive oil spray or oil mister

6 ounces artisanal bread, cut into ½-inch slices

1 garlic clove, halved

4 ounces fresh mozzarella, cut into ¼-inch cubes

In a large bowl, combine the tomatoes, onion, basil, olive oil, and salt, and season with a few turns of freshly cracked black pepper. Let sit at room temperature until the flavors have blended (the juices from the tomatoes will release and create a kind of dressing), 20 to 25 minutes.

Meanwhile, preheat a grill to medium.

Lightly spray each bread slice with olive oil and season with a pinch of salt. Grill the slices until slightly toasted and golden brown on each side, about 1 minute per side. Remove the bread from the heat and rub the toasted bread all over with the garlic. Cut the bread into ½-inch cubes and set aside.

When ready to serve, toss the tomato mixture with the mozzarella and grilled bread and divide among 4 serving bowls. Eat immediately so the bread doesn't get soggy.

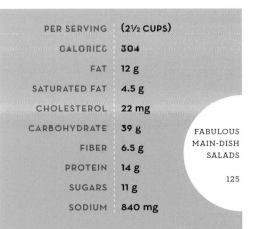

PER SERVING	(2½ CUPS)
CALORIES	304
FAT	12 g
SATURATED FAT	4.5 g
CHOLESTEROL	22 mg
CARBOHYDRATE	39 g
FIBER	6.5 g
PROTEIN	14 g
SUGARS	11 g
SODIUM	840 mg

FABULOUS
MAIN-DISH
SALADS

125

Coconut Chicken Salad
with Warm Honey-Mustard Vinaigrette
SERVES 4

I created this recipe a few years back after someone requested a makeover for a fatty deep-fried version they had on vacation. Call me loco for coco, because I love all things coconut. I happily got busy in my kitchen and played around with a faux-fried crispy coating for my chicken that is oven-baked at a high temperature to make you feel like you're eating fried.

VINAIGRETTE

1 tablespoon Dijon mustard

4 teaspoons extra-virgin olive oil

4 teaspoons honey

4 teaspoons white vinegar

CHICKEN

Olive oil spray or oil mister

½ cup sweetened shredded coconut

⅓ cup panko bread crumbs

3 tablespoons crushed cornflake crumbs

¼ teaspoon kosher salt, plus more as needed

½ cup egg whites (from about 3 large eggs)

8 chicken tenders (about 1 pound total)

SALAD

8 cups mixed baby greens

1 cup shredded carrots

1 large beefsteak tomato, thinly sliced

1 medium cucumber, sliced

For the vinaigrette: In a medium bowl, whisk together the mustard, oil, honey, vinegar, and 2 teaspoons water. Set aside.

For the chicken: Preheat the oven to 375°F. Spray a large nonstick baking sheet with olive oil.

In a medium bowl, combine the coconut, panko, cornflake crumbs, and a pinch of salt. In a second medium bowl, beat the egg whites.

Season the chicken with the remaining salt. Dip the chicken in the egg whites, then in the coconut-crumb mixture. Place the chicken on the prepared baking sheet. Lightly spray the top of the chicken with olive oil.

(recipe continues)

PER SERVING	(2 CHICKEN TENDERS + GENEROUS 2¾ CUPS SALAD)
CALORIES	340
FAT	9.5 g
SATURATED FAT	3.5 g
CHOLESTEROL	56 mg
CARBOHYDRATE	32 g
FIBER	5 g
PROTEIN	34 g
SUGARS	16 g
SODIUM	444 mg

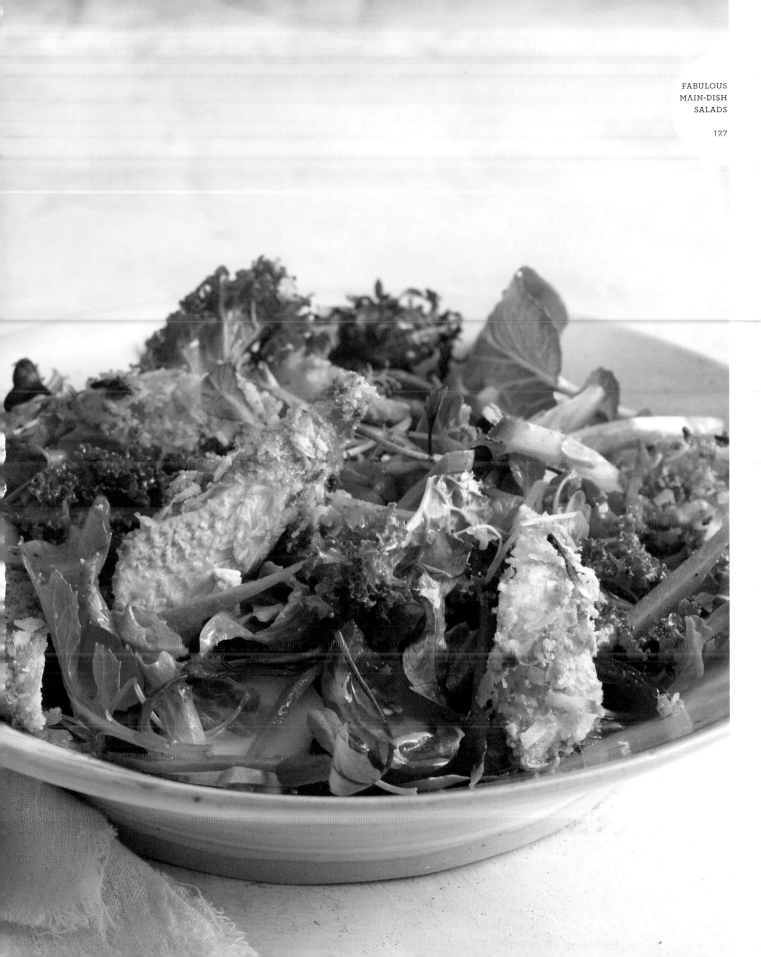

Bake for 15 minutes, flip, and cook until the chicken is cooked through, 15 more minutes.

For the salad: Place 2 cups baby greens on each of 4 serving plates. Divide the carrots, tomato slices, and cucumber slices among the plates. Slice the chicken on an angle and place on top of the greens. Heat the dressing in the microwave a few seconds and divide it among the salads.

8 Heart-Healthy Oils

Ready to give your salads and dishes a health and flavor boost? This handy primer will tell you everything you need to know about the eight healthiest oils on the shelf.

AVOCADO OIL Just like the fruit it's made from, avocado oil is rich in monounsaturated fat and antioxidants, which research suggests helps counter some of the effects of damaging free radicals that can cause diabetes and other diseases.

CANOLA OIL Canola oil is the lowest in saturated fat of all common cooking oils, and it's rich in heart-healthy omega-3s. One tablespoon of canola oil includes 16 percent of your recommended daily value for vitamin E, an antioxidant that protects your cells from damage and plays a role in immune function.

FLAXSEED OIL A delicate oil with a low smoke point, flaxseed oil is a great source of omega-3 alpha-linolenic acid (ALA). ALA appears to have anti-inflammatory properties and may also help lower blood pressure. Since flaxseed oil doesn't hold up in heat, use it in cold dishes like pesto and salads.

GRAPESEED OIL A byproduct of wine-making, this oil is high in polyunsaturated fats, which can help improve cholesterol levels and reduce your risk of heart disease. Just one tablespoon has more than a quarter of your daily recommended intake for Vitamin E.

OLIVE OIL Olive oil has earned superfood status, as it's one of the foods credited for the many health benefits associated with the Mediterranean diet. Its makeup consists mostly of monounsaturated fats, which may help lower the risk of heart disease, normalize blood clotting, and aid in blood sugar control. Extra-virgin and virgin olive oils have more antioxidants than refined olive oils.

SESAME OIL (LIGHT AND DARK) Herbalists often use sesame oil for its anti-cancer, antibacterial, and anti-inflammatory properties. Dark sesame oil has a uniquely strong, nutty flavor and should be used sparingly because a little goes a long way.

SUNFLOWER OIL Sunflower oil has more of the antioxidant vitamin E in one tablespoon than any of the other common cooking oils, delivering nearly 40 percent of your daily recommended value.

WALNUT OIL Walnut oil may reduce the risk of cardiovascular disease by improving blood vessel function, which is especially helpful for people with cardiovascular disease. Walnut oil has a strong flavor, so it's meant to be used on finished dishes.

Buffalo Chicken Salad

SERVES 4

GF **Q**

When I was in my late teens and early twenties, I loved going out to dinner with the girls to order strictly off the appetizer menu. We'd share all kinds of typical American apps, like Buffalo wings, complete with celery and blue cheese dressing. I don't think I realized—or cared—just how fattening those deep-fried wings smothered in butter actually were. Now, after having children and my metabolism has slowed a bit, I skip the fattening wings in favor of this salad, which has everything I love about Buffalo wings, but in a healthy form.

SKINNY BLUE CHEESE DRESSING

½ cup crumbled blue cheese

5 ounces 0% Greek yogurt

2 tablespoons buttermilk

1 tablespoon light mayonnaise (I prefer Hellmann's Light)

1 tablespoon white balsamic vinegar

½ tablespoon fresh lemon juice

½ teaspoon dried parsley flakes

⅛ teaspoon garlic powder

⅛ teaspoon kosher salt

Freshly ground black pepper

CHICKEN

1 pound chicken tenders

½ teaspoon chili powder*

½ teaspoon garlic powder

⅛ teaspoon freshly cracked black pepper

Cooking spray or oil mister

⅓ cup Frank's RedHot sauce

SALAD

1 medium head red leaf lettuce

1 English cucumber, sliced ¼ inch thick and halved (2 cups)

1 cup shredded carrots

2 medium celery stalks, sliced ¼ inch thick (½ cup)

1 medium tomato, chopped

¼ cup crumbled blue cheese

Read the label to be sure this product is gluten-free.

For the skinny blue cheese dressing: In a small bowl, mash the blue cheese and yogurt together with a fork. Stir in the buttermilk, mayonnaise, vinegar, lemon juice, dried parsley flakes, and garlic powder. Season with the salt and a pinch of black pepper.

For the chicken: Season the tenders with the chili powder, garlic powder, and black pepper.

(recipe continues)

PER SERVING	(2 CHICKEN STRIPS + 3 CUPS SALAD)
CALORIES	287
FAT	5 g
SATURATED FAT	4.5 g
CHOLESTEROL	93 mg
CARBOHYDRATE	11 g
FIBER	2.5 g
PROTEIN	35 g
SUGARS	6 g
SODIUM	805 mg

FABULOUS MAIN-DISH SALADS

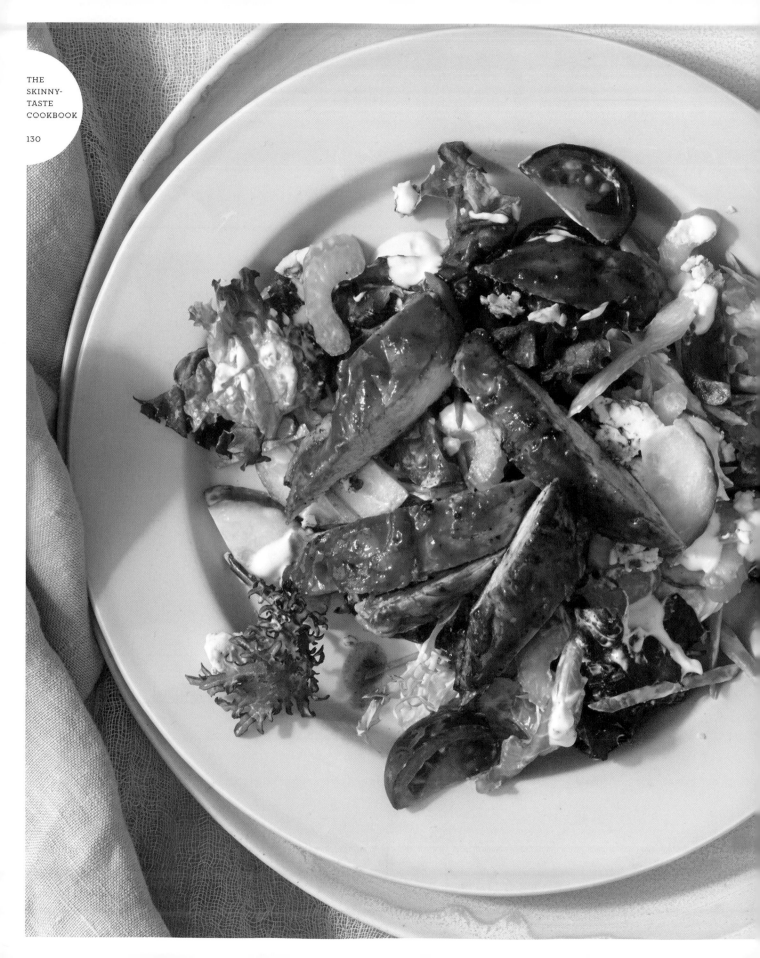

Heat a large nonstick skillet over high heat. Spray the pan with oil. Add the chicken and cook until browned on each side and no longer pink, 6 to 8 minutes. Remove the pan from the heat and pour the hot sauce over the chicken, turning to coat well. Slice on an angle and set aside.

For the salad: Tear the lettuce into bite-size pieces. Put it into a large bowl with ½ cup of the dressing and toss. Divide the lettuce among 4 serving plates. Top with the cucumbers, carrots, celery, and tomatoes, and drizzle the remaining dressing on top. Top the salad with the sliced chicken and sprinkle with the blue cheese crumbles.

FOOD FACTS heating things up

Adding a little spice to your foods may help you eat less. Capsaicin, the component that gives peppers their kick, has been shown to rev metabolism and increase body temperature, both of which can help burn more calories. Research also suggests that it helps quell appetite, cut cravings, and reduce the number of calories consumed at a meal. However, many of these benefits were seen in people who don't normally consume capsaicin—so if you normally like it hot, you may not reap all these pepper perks.

<u>skinny</u>**scoop**

Leftover buttermilk? Freeze it! Then thaw it overnight in the refrigerator or defrost it in the microwave. Freezing may cause the milk to separate. Before using in your recipe, be sure to mix it well to reincorporate.

Curried Chicken Salad

MAKES 5 CUPS · SERVES 5

GF **Q**

The first time I made this chicken salad, I dreamed about it for the next several days. It's spicy, savory, and sweet, and has lots of great texture. The best part is that it's made with fat-free Greek yogurt instead of mayonnaise, so there's no guilt! And it's even better the next day, so it's perfect to make ahead for lunch during the week.

2 teaspoons olive oil

¼ cup chopped onion

½ tablespoon curry powder*

1 pound boneless, skinless chicken breasts, cut into ½-inch cubes

¼ teaspoon kosher salt

Freshly ground black pepper

2 tablespoons 0% Greek yogurt

¼ teaspoon ground cinnamon

¾ cup dried cranberries*

1 large sweet apple, peeled and finely chopped (1½ cups)

¼ cup slivered almonds

2 tablespoon chopped fresh cilantro

¼ cup sliced scallions

PERFECT PAIRINGS

I like to serve this chicken salad cold on a large romaine lettuce leaf, which adds a nice amount of crunch and stands in for bread. You can also serve it over a bed of greens or in a whole wheat wrap.

Read the label to be sure this product is gluten-free.

In a large, heavy nonstick skillet, heat the olive oil over medium heat. Add the onion and curry powder and cook, stirring, until golden, 3 to 4 minutes. Increase the heat to medium-high, add the chicken, salt, and a pinch of black pepper, and cook, stirring frequently, until just cooked through, about 5 minutes. Transfer the chicken to a large bowl and let cool.

When cool, add the yogurt, cinnamon, cranberries, apple, almonds, cilantro, and scallions. Toss together to coat.

PER SERVING	(1 CUP)
CALORIES	233
FAT	7 g
SATURATED FAT	1 g
CHOLESTEROL	58 mg
CARBOHYDRATE	22 g
FIBER	2.5 g
PROTEIN	21 g
SUGARS	16 g
SODIUM	168 mg

Wild Salmon Salad
with Balsamic-Caper Vinaigrette

SERVES 4

GF **Q**

Wild salmon, green beans, capers, and baby greens topped with shaved Parmesan and balsamic vinegar—it's a heart-healthy salad loaded with mega omegas! I try to eat salmon at least once a week, and if there are any leftovers from the night before, this is usually what's for lunch the next day! When I worked full-time in the city, this was one of my favorite go-to lunches. I would pack the shaved Parmesan cheese and dressing on the side, and anxiously await lunchtime.

BALSAMIC-CAPER VINAIGRETTE

8 teaspoons balsamic vinegar

4 teaspoons extra-virgin olive oil

⅛ teaspoon kosher salt

Freshly cracked black pepper

4 teaspoons capers, drained

SALAD

¾ teaspoon kosher salt

½ pound green beans, trimmed and halved

1 pound skin-on wild salmon fillet, cut into 4 pieces

Freshly ground black pepper

Cooking spray or oil mister

6 cups mixed baby arugula and spinach

¼ cup shaved Parmesan cheese

For the balsamic-caper vinaigrette: In a small bowl, whisk together the vinegar and oil. Season with the salt and a pinch of black pepper. Toss in the capers and set aside.

For the salad: Bring a medium pot of water with ½ teaspoon of the salt to a boil. Add the green beans and cook until crisp-tender, 8 to 10 minutes. Drain and run under cold water to stop the cooking. Drain again and set aside.

Heat a grill pan or skillet over high heat. Season the salmon with the remaining ¼ teaspoon salt and a pinch of black pepper, lightly spray the pan with oil, and put the salmon in the pan. Sauté until cooked through, about 5 minutes on each side. Transfer to a plate and remove the skin.

Place 1½ cups of mixed greens on each of 4 plates. Divide the green beans among the plates, sprinkle with the Parmesan, and put a piece of salmon on top. Drizzle the dressing over the top of each salad.

skinny**scoop**

If you're pressed for time, you can use canned salmon or even albacore tuna in place of the wild salmon.

PER SERVING	(3 OUNCES SALMON + 1¾ CUPS SALAD)
CALORIES	262
FAT	13.5 g
SATURATED FAT	2.5 g
CHOLESTEROL	62 mg
CARBOHYDRATE	9 g
FIBER	3.5 g
PROTEIN	27 g
SUGARS	3 g
SODIUM	305 mg

FABULOUS MAIN-DISH SALADS

BLT Salad with Avocado

SERVES 4

I have a confession: I LOVE real bacon. (Really, who doesn't?) I find a way to work real pork bacon into my life whenever a craving strikes. This salad is the answer to my BLT-loving prayers, with all the best flavors of the sandwich and none of the added calories of the bread. When I bring home the bacon (pun intended!), I always look for center-cut—it's leaner than standard strips because it's cut close to the bone. Could you use turkey bacon? Sure, it is perfectly suitable in this quick and easy salad.

12 slices lean center-cut bacon, at room temperature

4 Roma tomatoes, chopped

¼ cup light mayonnaise (I prefer Hellmann's Light)

⅛ teaspoon kosher salt

Freshly ground black pepper

6 cups chopped romaine lettuce

1 medium (4 ounces) Hass avocado, chopped

PERFECT PAIRINGS
This salad is perfect as is for lunch, but if you want to make this a light dinner, toss in 6 ounces of chopped grilled chicken (250 calories).

Put the bacon in a large skillet and set the skillet over low heat. Cook the bacon, turning often, until crisp. Transfer to a paper towel to drain and cool. Crumble the bacon.

In a medium bowl, combine the tomatoes and mayonnaise and season with the salt and a pinch of black pepper. Set aside for about 10 minutes to let the tomatoes release their juices as this will be the "dressing" to your salad.

To serve, place 1½ cups lettuce on each of 4 plates, then top each with about ½ cup of the tomato mixture. Top with the avocado and bacon, and serve.

PER SERVING	(2 GENEROUS CUPS)
CALORIES	197
FAT	13 g
SATURATED FAT	3 g
CHOLESTEROL	19 mg
CARBOHYDRATE	13 g
FIBER	5 g
PROTEIN	10 g
SUGARS	5 g
SODIUM	397 mg

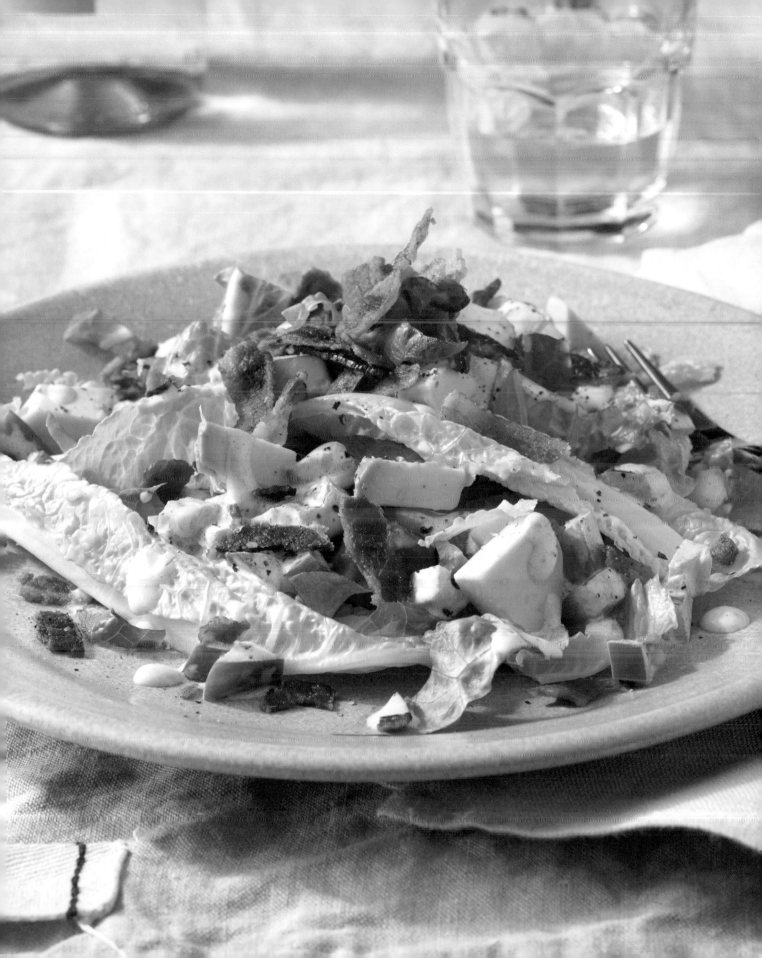

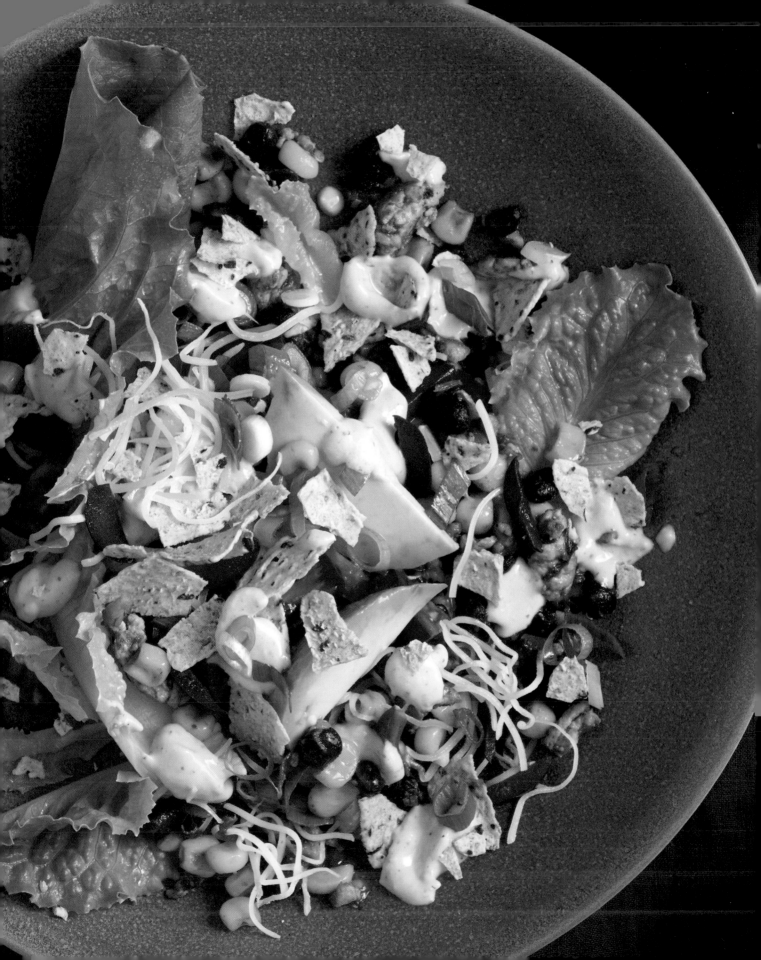

Turkey Santa Fe Taco Salad with Avocado Crema

SERVES 4

GF Q

Each bite of this salad is a fiesta in your mouth! Color, crunch, flavor, and spice—this is the whole package. But in my opinion, what really makes it off the hook is the zesty avocado crema. Not to mention, this satisfying dish is loaded with fiber and protein. The turkey-bean topping is so good that I usually double it and use the extras as a filling the next day for stuffed peppers, enchiladas, or even mixed in with some scrambled egg whites—delish!

TURKEY-BEAN TOPPING

½ pound 99% extra-lean ground turkey breast

½ teaspoon kosher salt

½ cup canned black beans,* rinsed and drained

2 tablespoons chopped pickled jalapeño pepper (or more to taste)

1 large tomato, chopped

1 garlic clove, minced

3 tablespoons chopped onion

2 tablespoons chopped fresh cilantro, plus more for garnish

1¼ teaspoons ground cumin

¼ cup frozen corn kernels

AVOCADO CREMA

1 medium (4 ounces) Hass avocado, chopped

¼ cup reduced-fat sour cream

1 tablespoon fresh lime juice

1 medium fresh jalapeño pepper, chopped

1½ tablespoons chopped fresh cilantro

¼ teaspoon plus ⅛ teaspoon kosher salt

Freshly ground black pepper

SALAD

5 cups shredded green leaf lettuce

½ cup shredded reduced-fat Mexican cheese blend (I recommend Sargento)

1 cup chopped tomatoes

2 tablespoons sliced black olives

2 tablespoons chopped scallions

1 ounce baked tortilla chips, crushed (heaping ½ cup)

Read the label to be sure this product is gluten-free.

For the turkey-bean topping: Heat a large skillet over medium-high heat. Add the ground turkey, season with ¼ teaspoon salt, and cook, using a wooden spoon to break the meat into small pieces, until no longer pink, 4 to 5 minutes. Add the beans, pickled jalapeño, tomato, garlic, onion, cilantro, and cumin. Stir

(recipe continues)

PER SERVING	(2 CUPS)
CALORIES	302
FAT	11.5 g
SATURATED FAT	4 g
CHOLESTEROL	45 mg
CARBOHYDRATE	25 g
FIBER	8 g
PROTEIN	25 g
SUGARS	7 g
SODIUM	526 mg

FABULOUS MAIN-DISH SALADS

well, reduce the heat to low, cover, and cook for 20 minutes to blend the flavors. Uncover and add the corn and ¼ teaspoon salt. Simmer until the liquid reduces and the corn is cooked through, 5 more minutes.

For the avocado crema: In a blender, combine half the avocado (reserve the other half for the salad), the sour cream, lime juice, ¼ cup water, the jalapeño, cilantro, salt, and black pepper to taste. Blend until smooth.

For the salad: Divide the lettuce among 4 serving plates. Add the turkey-bean topping, cheese, tomatoes, olives, scallions, and remaining avocado. Top with the avocado crema and crushed tortilla chips.

The Salad Solution

Want to add more vegetables and vitamins into your day? There's a simple solution: Eat more salads! Here are a few tips to keep in mind:

GO GREEN The darker the leaf, the more phytonutrients it contains. That means spinach greens are more antioxidant-packed than romaine lettuce, which is more nutritious than iceberg lettuce. Don't be afraid to try new greens or go for a mix of different leaves.

BE COLORFUL Phytochemicals, the beneficial nutrients in plants that offer a variety of health benefits, are what give plants their color, and each color represents a different health benefit. To make sure you're covering your bases, opt for a colorful spread in your salad bowl.

EAT SEASONALLY Eating what's in season offers a number of perks. In-season fruits and veggies are usually tastier because they're fresher. They can also be cheaper because they don't have to travel far distances to get to your plate.

PICK YOUR PROTEIN Make your salad more satisfying by topping it with some lean protein, which is shown to be more satiating than fat or carbs. Some healthy picks to consider: tofu, edamame, chicken, fish, egg whites, and beans.

ADD SOME CRUNCH Satisfy your senses by sprinkling on nuts or seeds; slicing up some sweet apples, pears, or jicama; or going with radishes, peppers, or water chestnuts.

GET YOUR HEALTHY FAT FIX Fat not only makes a salad more satisfying, it can also help boost your absorption of certain nutrients. Good sources of healthy fat include avocados, olive oil, nuts and seeds, and fatty fish like salmon.

GO FOR WHOLE GRAINS Get an extra hit of fiber and B vitamins by topping your greens with grains like quinoa, farro, barley, or couscous.

Baja Grilled Flank Steak Salad

SERVES 4

GF **Q**

Flank steak is a great choice for steak salads because it's lean and full-flavored. But because it's so lean, to get melt-in-your-mouth results, cook it medium-rare and thinly slice it across the grain. Although I really love veggies, I could probably never become a vegetarian because I love steak, too! But that's okay—I believe in everything in moderation, and by choosing lean cuts of beef, I know I'm getting a good dose of iron and nutrients without all the saturated fat I would get from fattier cuts.

SPICE RUB

1 teaspoon garlic powder

¾ teaspoon kosher salt

½ teaspoon ground cumin

½ teaspoon sweet paprika

¼ teaspoon dried oregano

¼ teaspoon chipotle chile powder or cayenne pepper

1 pound flank steak, trimmed of all external fat

LEMON-LIME DRESSING

2 tablespoons fresh lime juice

1 tablespoon fresh lemon juice

1 tablespoon extra-virgin olive oil

1 tablespoon minced scallions

1 tablespoon minced fresh cilantro

⅛ teaspoon kosher salt

Freshly cracked black pepper

SALAD

2 medium ears fresh corn or 1 cup thawed frozen corn kernels

1 large head romaine lettuce, cut lengthwise into 4 wedges

1 medium (4 ounces) Hass avocado, thinly sliced

1 cup heirloom cherry tomatoes, halved

¼ cup crumbled queso fresco or cotija cheese

For the spice rub: In a small bowl, combine the garlic powder, salt, cumin, paprika, oregano, and chipotle powder.

Generously season each side of the steak with the dry rub and, using your hands, rub it into the meat. Let sit for about 10 minutes.

For the lemon-lime dressing: In a medium bowl, whisk together the lime juice, lemon juice, olive oil, scallions, cilantro, salt, and a pinch of black pepper. Set aside.

Preheat a grill to medium-high (or preheat a grill pan over medium-high heat).

(recipe continues)

PER SERVING	(1 SALAD: 3 OUNCES STEAK, 1 WEDGE + ¾ CUP TOPPING)
CALORIES	356
FAT	21 g
SATURATED FAT	6.5 g
CHOLESTEROL	50 mg
CARBOHYDRATE	21 g
FIBER	7.5 g
PROTEIN	23 g
SUGARS	5 g
SODIUM	325 mg

FABULOUS MAIN-DISH SALADS

139

Summer corn is so sweet and delicious, you barely have to cook it—you can basically eat it raw, or just toss it on the grill for a minute or two. But if it's out of season, you can use thawed frozen corn in its place.

For the salad: If using fresh corn, grill the corn, turning often, until the corn is charred on all sides, 20 to 25 minutes. Set aside to cool.

Increase the heat of the grill or grill pan to high. Grill the steak for 5 to 7 minutes on each side for medium-rare, or longer to your taste. Remove the steak from the grill, cover, and let rest for 5 minutes. Cut the corn kernels off the cob and set aside.

Thinly slice the steak ¼ inch thick, across the grain and at an angle to the cutting board, then cut it crosswise into ½-inch pieces.

Put a romaine wedge on each of 4 serving plates, top each with one-fourth of the grilled steak. Dividing evenly, top with the avocado, corn, tomatoes, and cheese. Drizzle the dressing over the salads.

FOOD FACTS like it lean?

Flank is one of 24 cuts of beef that meets government standards for "lean" (five cuts of beef are considered "extra lean"). It's also nutrient-rich because it packs a powerhouse of essential nutrients (iron, niacin, and potassium) in a reasonable number of calories: A 3.5-ounce serving of cooked flank steak has 155 calories, 7 grams of total fat, and about 3 grams of saturated fat.

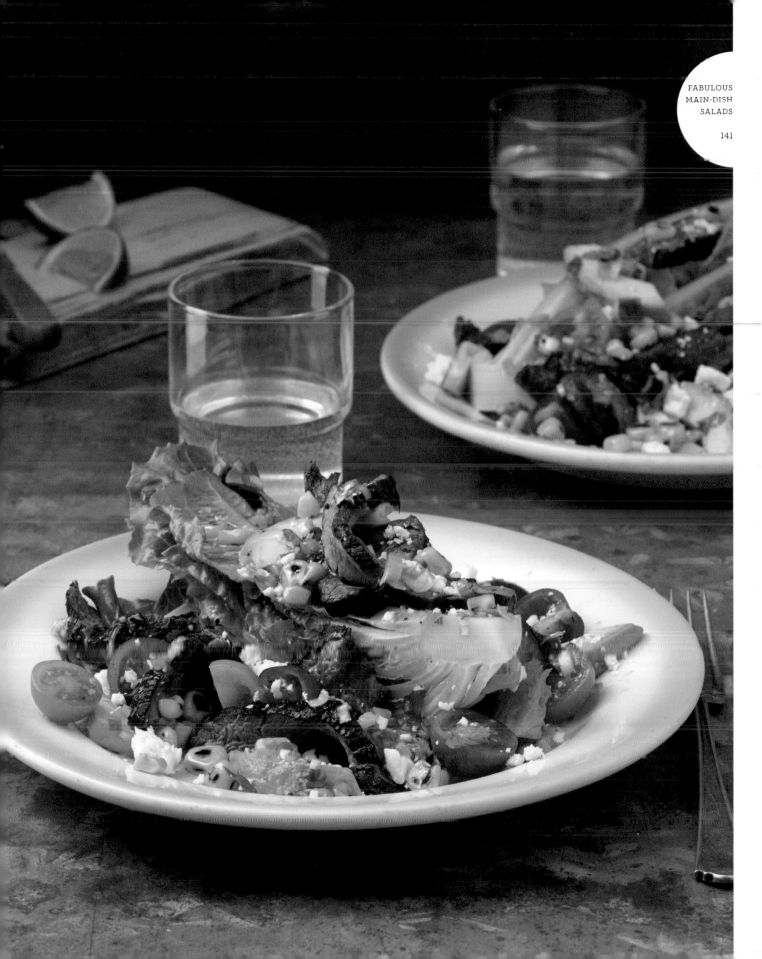

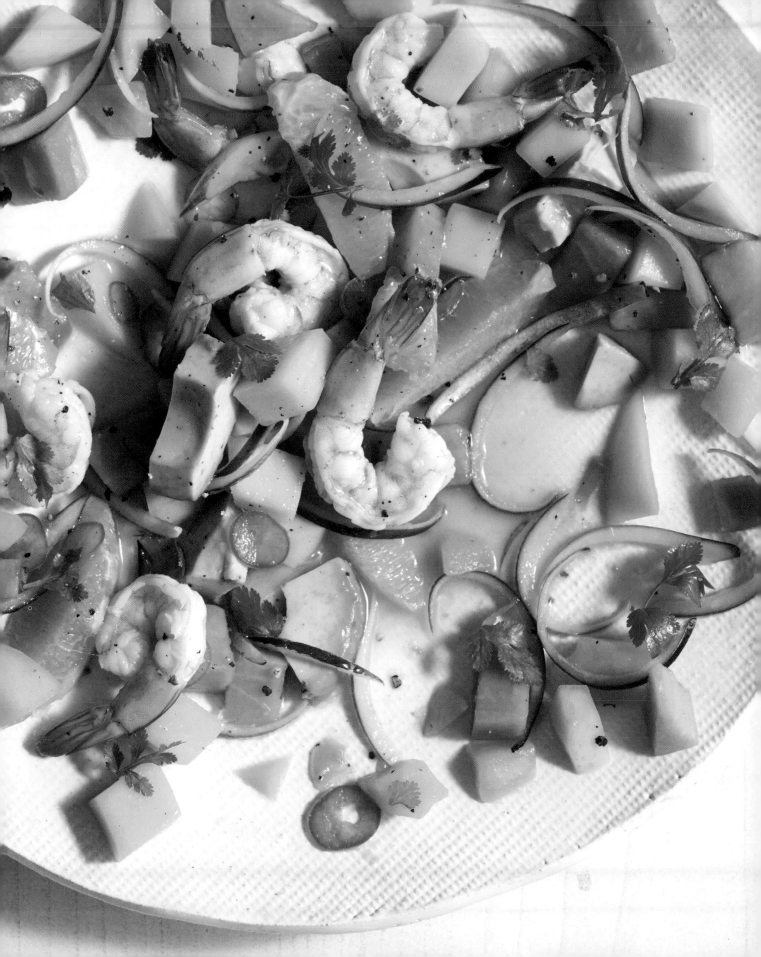

Chilled Caribbean Shrimp Salad

SERVES 5

GF Q

Easy, delicious, and no cooking involved—this is the perfect dish for those warm summer nights when you don't want to heat up the kitchen. I'm a big fan of tropical fruit, probably because I spent many of my summers as a teen in Puerto Rico, where I fell in love with the island, culture, and, especially, the tropical fruit. Mangoes used to litter my cousin's backyard, and I would eat them every chance I could.

¼ medium red onion, thinly sliced

Kosher salt

1 tablespoon extra-virgin olive oil

2½ tablespoons fresh lime juice

2 oranges, peeled and divided into segments

1 pound cooked and peeled large shrimp

1 mango, cut into 1-inch chunks

1½ cups chopped fresh papaya

1 medium fresh jalapeño pepper, thinly sliced

2 tablespoons chopped fresh cilantro

1 medium (4 ounces) Hass avocado, cut into 1-inch chunks

Freshly ground black pepper

Put the onions in a large bowl and season with ¼ teaspoon salt. Add the olive oil and lime juice. Set aside for 5 minutes.

Set aside 3 segments of the orange, then put the remaining orange pieces in the bowl with onions. Add the shrimp, mango, papaya, jalapeño, and cilantro, and season with another ¼ teaspoon of salt and black pepper to taste.

Squeeze the juice from the remaining orange segments over the salad and refrigerate until chilled, at least 30 minutes. When ready to serve, sprinkle a pinch of salt and pepper over the avocado, and gently toss into the salad.

FOOD FACTS a plus for papayas
Papayas, which can range in size from 1 to 20 pounds, are loaded with nutrients, including potassium, vitamins A and C, and fiber. In fact, 1 cup of papaya contains enough vitamin C to satisfy a woman's daily requirements and comes close to taking care of a man's daily goal, too.

skinny scoop

To make this ahead, simply leave out the avocado, then add it just before you're ready to serve. If you can't find papaya, try substituting cantaloupe or honeydew melon.

PER SERVING	(SCANT 1¾ CUPS)
CALORIES	236
FAT	7.5 g
SATURATED FAT	1 g
CHOLESTEROL	177 mg
CARBOHYDRATE	24 g
FIBER	5 g
PROTEIN	21 g
SUGARS	17 g
SODIUM	347 mg

FABULOUS MAIN-DISH SALADS

143

Roast Beef and Watercress Pasta Salad

SERVES 4

(GF) (Q)

Yesterday's roast is transformed into a fabulous (and mayo-less) pasta salad! Karina, my older daughter, loves when I make Sunday Night Roast Beef (page 211) for dinner, so I usually try to make it for her when she's home from college. But unless we're having company to join us for dinner, a whole roast is usually too large for our family of four to eat in one night, so I came up with this recipe as a quick way to turn leftovers into a new meal. If I don't have leftovers, I still make this recipe, using sliced roast beef from the deli instead.

4 ounces uncooked spiral pasta (use brown rice pasta for gluten-free*)

¼ teaspoon kosher salt, plus more for the pot

1 tablespoon extra-virgin olive oil

4 cups (2½ ounces) watercress or baby arugula

6 ounces thinly sliced roast beef, cut into strips

1 cup halved grape or cherry tomatoes

3 tablespoons capers, drained

2½ tablespoons balsamic vinegar

⅛ teaspoon freshly ground black pepper

¼ cup freshly shaved Parmigiano-Reggiano cheese

Read the label to be sure this product is gluten-free.

Cook the pasta to al dente in a pot of salted boiling water according to package directions. Drain and rinse under cold water.

Transfer the pasta to a large bowl and toss with the olive oil. Add the watercress, roast beef, tomatoes, capers, vinegar, salt, and black pepper. Just before serving, top with shaved Parmesan.

PER SERVING	(1¾ CUPS)
CALORIES	260
FAT	8.5 g
SATURATED FAT	3 g
CHOLESTEROL	33 mg
CARBOHYDRATE	25 g
FIBER	2 g
PROTEIN	20 g
SUGARS	4 g
SODIUM	344 mg

Grilled Portobello Spinach Salad

SERVES 4

V GF

There's a fabulous family-style Italian restaurant in my neighborhood called Nick's that makes the best salads and brick-oven pizzas. One of the salads I love is made with grilled portobello mushrooms topped with freshly shaved Parmigiano-Reggiano. That's where I got the inspiration for this salad. Portobello mushrooms are large and substantial, so they make a great meat substitution.

MUSHROOMS

¼ cup balsamic vinegar

1 tablespoon olive oil, plus more for the grill

1 teaspoon dried basil

1 teaspoon dried oregano

1 tablespoon minced garlic

⅛ teaspoon kosher salt

Freshly ground black pepper

4 portobello mushroom caps (12 ounces total)

BALSAMIC VINAIGRETTE

1 tablespoons balsamic vinegar

3 tablespoons olive oil

⅛ teaspoon kosher salt

Freshly ground black pepper

SALAD

6 cups baby spinach

⅛ teaspoon kosher salt

Freshly ground black pepper

¼ cup sun-dried tomatoes (not oil-packed), thinly sliced

½ cup shaved Parmigiano-Reggiano cheese

For the mushrooms: In a large bowl, whisk together the vinegar, olive oil, basil, oregano, garlic, salt, and black pepper to taste. Add the mushroom caps and toss well. Let sit at room temperature for about 30 minutes, turning a few times.

For the balsamic vinaigrette: In a medium bowl, whisk together the vinegar, olive oil, salt, and black pepper to taste.

Preheat a grill to medium (or preheat a grill pan over medium heat). Brush the grill grate or spray the pan with oil. Put the mushrooms on the grill, reserving the marinade for basting. Grill until tender, basting frequently, 5 to 7 minutes on each side. Transfer to a cutting board.

For the salad: In a large bowl, toss the spinach with the balsamic vinaigrette, and season with the salt and black pepper to taste. Divide the spinach among 4 plates and top with the sun-dried tomatoes. Slice the mushroom caps on an angle, put one on each salad, and then top with the Parmesan.

PERFECT PAIRINGS

I like to serve this over baby spinach, but it would also be great over arugula or mixed baby greens. If you like, you can grill some chicken breasts along with the mushrooms to add to the salad.

PER SERVING	(1½ CUPS SALAD + 1 MUSHROOM CAP)
CALORIES	217
FAT	17 g
SATURATED FAT	4 g
CHOLESTEROL	0 mg
CARBOHYDRATE	11 g
FIBER	2.5 g
PROTEIN	8 g
SUGARS	7 g
SODIUM	232 mg

FABULOUS MAIN-DISH SALADS

Greek Chickpea Salad

SERVES 4

Believe it or not, I started including chickpeas in my salads only a few years ago, but now it's a regular thing! They add great texture to this Mediterranean-inspired salad and make it a great meatless option. I chop all the vegetables the same size as the chickpeas and let them marinate for a few hours or overnight so they absorb all the flavors from the lemon, herbs, and olives. Just before serving, I add the cucumbers and top it with feta so the cucumbers stay crunchy and the feta doesn't get lost.

2 garlic cloves, minced

1 tablespoon olive oil

3 tablespoons fresh lemon juice

½ teaspoon kosher salt

2 cups canned chickpeas,* rinsed and drained

¼ cup chopped red onion

1 cup quartered grape or cherry tomatoes

½ cup chopped orange bell pepper

2 tablespoons chopped fresh parsley

½ teaspoon fresh oregano leaves or ¼ teaspoon dried

¼ cup Kalamata olives, pitted and chopped

1½ cups seeded, chopped cucumber

⅓ cup crumbled feta cheese

Read the label to be sure this product is gluten-free.

In a large bowl, combine the garlic, olive oil, lemon juice, and salt. Add the chickpeas, red onion, tomatoes, bell pepper, parsley, oregano, and olives and toss well. For best results, let marinate a few hours or overnight in the refrigerator to allow the flavors to meld. Just before serving, toss in the cucumbers and feta cheese.

FOOD FACTS chickpeas boost satiety
Chickpeas (aka garbanzo beans) are loaded with fiber and protein—the right combo to help tame your appetite. In a study done by Australian researchers, people who ate a diet rich in chickpeas—100 grams (about ½ cup) per day—for 3 months reported feeling more satiated and consumed fewer calories during that time. Once the study participants resumed their normal diet again, they consumed more processed snack food.

PER SERVING	(1¼ CUPS)
CALORIES	204
FAT	9 g
SATURATED FAT	2.5 g
CHOLESTEROL	11 mg
CARBOHYDRATE	25 g
FIBER	1.5 g
PROTEIN	8 g
SUGARS	3 g
SODIUM	518 mg

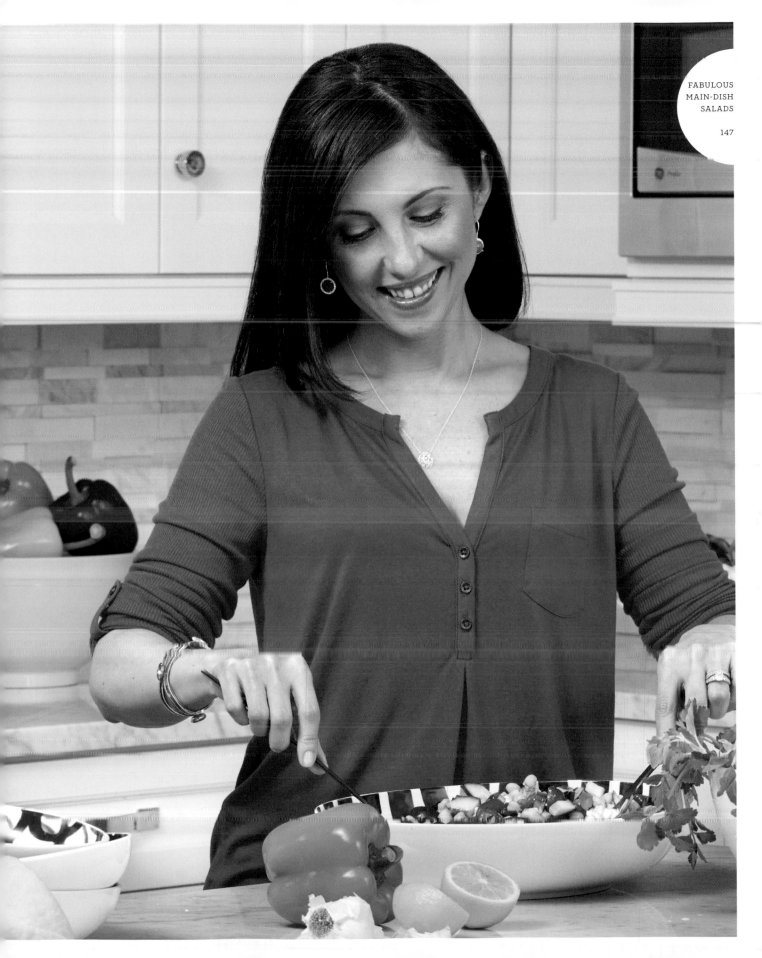

PERFECT POULTRY

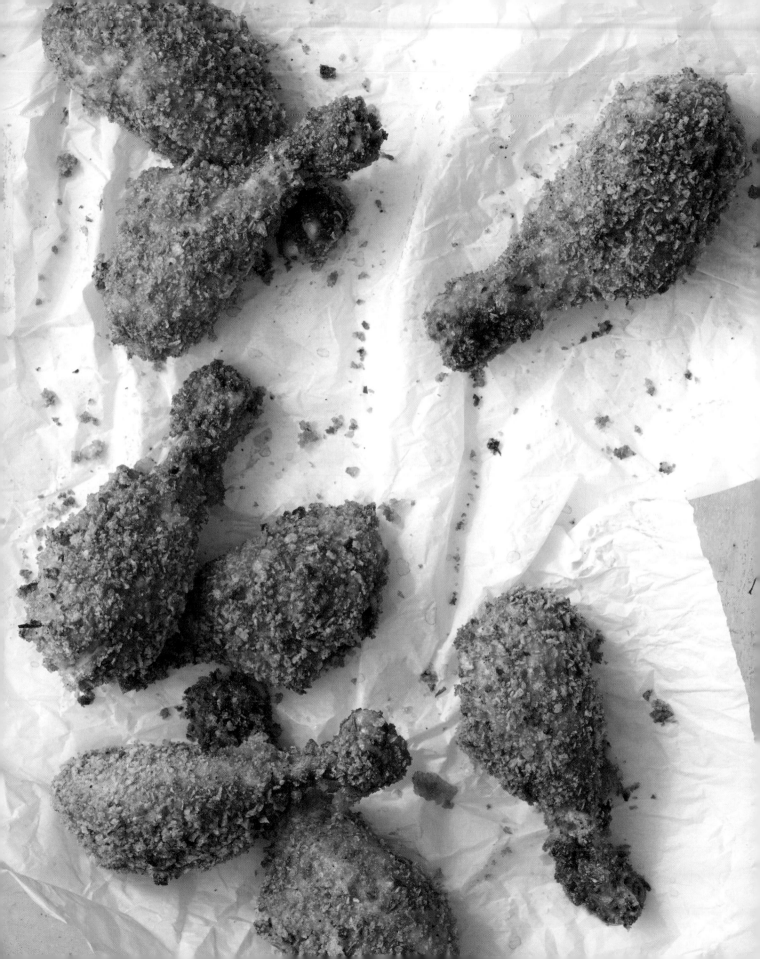

Buttermilk Oven "Fried" Chicken

SERVES 4

Fried chicken is one of my biggest weaknesses, so naturally I've been perfecting this lighter version for years. I've managed to achieve the same crispy golden texture you get from frying from my oven. Yep, it's skinnier, easier, quicker, and (bonus) there's no greasy mess to clean up. Soaking the chicken overnight (sometimes two nights) in a buttermilk bath is a must for meat that's moist and juicy. To easily remove the skin from the drumsticks, use one paper towel to grasp the joint end and a second one to pull off the skin.

CHICKEN

8 chicken drumsticks (about 3½ ounces each), skinned

½ teaspoon kosher salt

½ teaspoon sweet paprika

½ teaspoon poultry seasoning

¼ teaspoon garlic powder

⅛ teaspoon freshly ground black pepper

1 cup buttermilk

Juice of ½ lemon

Cooking spray or oil mister

COATING

⅔ cup panko bread crumbs

½ cup crushed cornflake crumbs

2 tablespoons grated Parmesan cheese

1½ teaspoons kosher salt

1 teaspoon dried parsley flakes

1½ teaspoons sweet paprika

½ teaspoon onion powder

½ teaspoon garlic powder

¼ teaspoon chili powder

For the chicken: In a medium bowl, season the chicken with the salt, paprika, poultry seasoning, garlic powder, and black pepper. Pour the buttermilk and lemon juice over the chicken and refrigerate for 6 to 8 hours, preferably overnight.

Preheat the oven to 400°F. Place a rack on a baking sheet and lightly spray with oil.

For the coating: In a shallow bowl, combine the panko, cornflake crumbs, Parmesan, salt, parsley, paprika, onion powder, garlic powder, and chili powder.

Remove the chicken from the buttermilk, dredge each piece in the crumb mixture, and put the pieces onto the prepared baking sheet. Spray the tops of the chicken with oil.

Bake until golden brown and cooked through, 40 to 45 minutes.

PERFECT PAIRINGS
Serve this with corn on the cob, **Cheesy Cauliflower "Mash" (page 269)**, or **Seasoned Sweet Potato Wedges (page 277)** and a side of **Confetti Slaw (page 303)**.

PER SERVING	(2 DRUMSTICKS)
CALORIES	294
FAT	8.5 g
SATURATED FAT	2.5 g
CHOLESTEROL	182 mg
CARBOHYDRATE	12 g
FIBER	1 g
PROTEIN	41 g
SUGARS	2 g
SODIUM	709 mg

PERFECT POULTRY

151

Chicken Rollatini Stuffed with Zucchini and Mozzarella

SERVES 4

I came up with this recipe a few summers back when my garden produced an overabundance of zucchini. I make stuffed chicken breasts so many different ways, and this is one of my favorites. It's easier than you think—there are no strings or toothpicks required.

Cooking spray or oil mister

1 tablespoon plus 1 teaspoon olive oil

4 garlic cloves, chopped

1½ cups packed shredded zucchini

¼ cup plus 2 tablespoons grated Romano or Parmesan cheese

½ teaspoon plus ⅛ teaspoon kosher salt

Freshly ground black pepper

¾ cup shredded part-skim mozzarella (3 ounces)

8 thin chicken breast cutlets (4 ounces each)

½ cup Italian seasoned whole wheat bread crumbs, homemade (see page 110) or store-bought

Juice of 1 lemon

Preheat the oven to 450°F. Lightly spray a baking dish with oil.

Heat a large skillet over medium-high heat. Add 1 teaspoon of the oil and the garlic. Cook, stirring, until golden, about 1 minute. Add the zucchini, ¼ cup of the Romano, ⅛ teaspoon of the salt, and black pepper to taste. Cook, stirring, until the zucchini is tender, 3 to 4 minutes. Remove the pan from the heat and let cool to room temperature. Add the mozzarella and mix well.

Wash and dry the chicken and arrange on a cutting board. Spread each cutlet with 3 tablespoons zucchini-cheese mixture. Loosely roll up and set aside, seam side down.

In a small bowl, combine the bread crumbs and remaining 2 tablespoons Romano. In a separate bowl, combine the remaining 1 tablespoon of olive oil, the lemon juice, the remaining ½ teaspoon salt, and a pinch of black pepper.

Dip the rolled chicken in the lemon mixture, then into the bread crumbs, rolling to coat evenly. Place the chicken seam side down in the prepared baking dish. Spray the tops of the chicken with oil. Bake until cooked through, 25 to 30 minutes. Serve hot.

PER SERVING	(2 ROLLS)
CALORIES	402
FAT	16 g
SATURATED FAT	6 g
CHOLESTEROL	127 mg
CARBOHYDRATE	15 g
FIBER	1 g
PROTEIN	47 g
SUGARS	2 g
SODIUM	867 mg

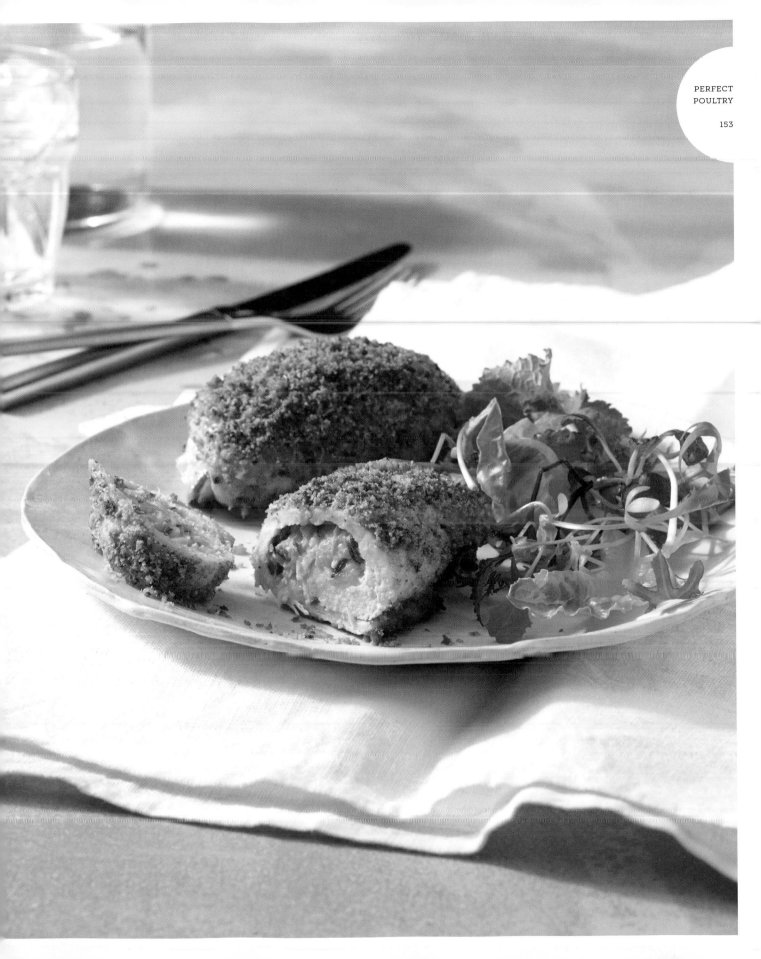

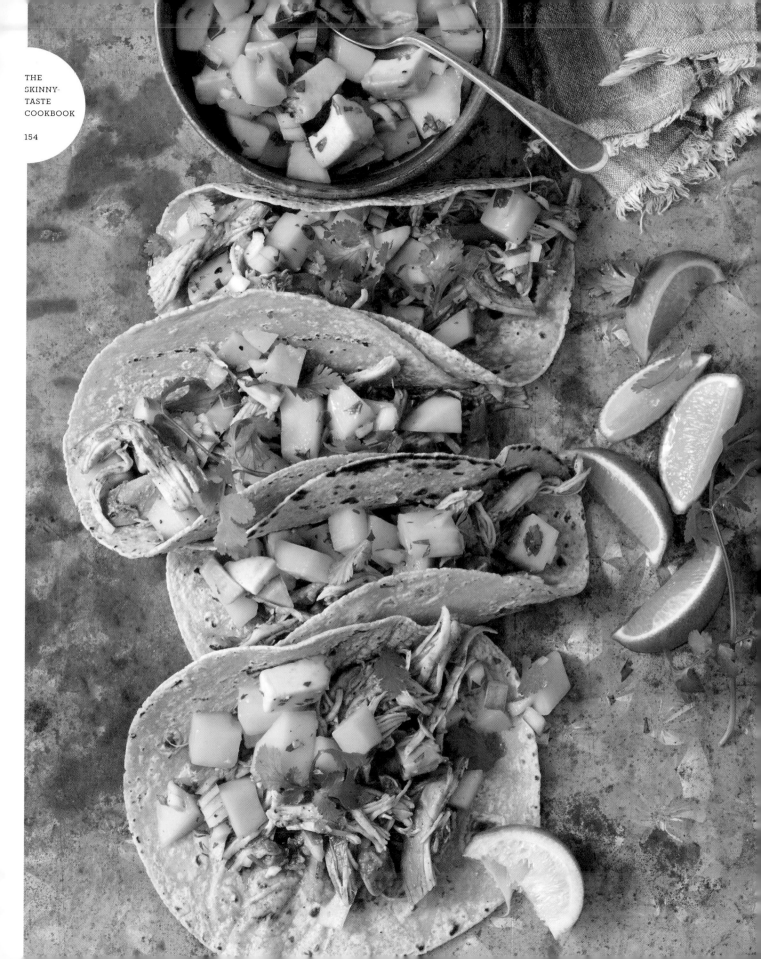

Slow-Cooker Jerk Chicken Tacos with Caribbean Salsa

SERVES 6

GF **SC**

Who says tacos have to be Mexican? These chicken tacos get their heat from the wonderful flavors of Jamaican jerk spices, and then they're topped with a fresh mango-avocado salsa.

CHICKEN

3 garlic cloves, crushed

2 tablespoons jerk seasoning*

Kosher salt

1½ pounds boneless chicken breasts

1 tablespoon lime juice (from ½ lime)

¼ cup fresh orange juice

1 tablespoon chopped fresh cilantro

CARIBBEAN SALSA

1 large mango, diced into ½-inch pieces

½ medium (2 ounces) Hass avocado, diced into ½-inch pieces

1 tablespoon chopped red onion

1 tablespoon chopped fresh cilantro

1½ tablespoons fresh lime juice

⅛ teaspoon kosher salt

Freshly ground black pepper

12 Mission extra-thin yellow corn tortillas

Read the label to be sure this product is gluten-free.

For the chicken: Combine the garlic, jerk seasoning, and ¼ teaspoon salt and spread it over the chicken. Put the chicken, the lime and orange juices, and cilantro in the slow cooker. Cover and cook on high for 2 hours.

For the Caribbean salsa: Meanwhile, in a medium bowl, combine the mango, avocado, red onion, cilantro, lime juice, salt, and black pepper to taste. Refrigerate until ready to serve.

Remove the chicken from the slow cooker and shred it with two forks. Pour any liquid in a slow cooker into a bowl, then return the chicken to the slow cooker. Add ½ cup of the reserved liquid, just enough to moisten the chicken, and season with ⅛ teaspoon salt and black pepper to taste.

Heat the tortillas in a skillet set over medium-high for about 30 seconds. Fill each with ⅓ cup of the chicken and 2 tablespoons of salsa.

skinny**scoop**

Although any brand of jerk seasoning will do, I really like Walkerswood Jerk Seasoning, which I purchase on Amazon. It's very spicy—a little goes a long way! If you don't enjoy too much spice, get the mild variety, which is what I use.

PER SERVING	(2 TACOS)
CALORIES	???
FAT	6 g
SATURATED FAT	1 g
CHOLESTEROL	73 mg
CARBOHYDRATE	28 g
FIBER	4.5 g
PROTEIN	27 g
SUGARS	11 g
SODIUM	490 mg

PERFECT POULTRY

155

Naked Persian Turkey Burgers

SERVES 5

(Q) (FF)

This bunless burger isn't just *any* burger. It's a moist, delicious spin on kofta, a Middle Eastern meatball that's full of fresh herbs, spices, and even some veggies. My secret to making turkey burgers perfectly moist every time is adding shredded zucchini—it works like a charm! To serve them, I place each burger on a bed of lettuce and top it with a chopped salad that's sort of like a Persian pico de gallo.

PERSIAN SALAD

2½ cups chopped English cucumbers

1½ cups quartered small heirloom cherry tomatoes

⅓ cup chopped red onion

2 teaspoons finely chopped fresh mint

2½ tablespoons fresh lemon juice

1 tablespoon extra-virgin olive oil

¼ teaspoon kosher salt

Freshly ground black pepper

BURGERS

¾ cup grated zucchini

1¼ pounds 93% lean ground turkey

⅓ cup finely chopped red onion

2 garlic cloves, minced

¼ cup unseasoned whole wheat bread crumbs

¼ cup chopped fresh parsley

1 tablespoon finely chopped fresh mint

1 teaspoon ground cumin

½ teaspoon ground coriander

¼ teaspoon ground allspice

¼ teaspoon chili powder

¼ teaspoon kosher salt

Freshly ground black pepper

Cooking spray or oil mister

5 cups chopped romaine lettuce

5 tablespoons grated feta cheese

For the Persian salad: In a large bowl, combine the cucumbers, tomatoes, red onion, mint, lemon juice, olive oil, salt, and black pepper to taste. Mix well, cover, and refrigerate for at least 1 hour.

For the burgers: Squeeze any liquid out of the zucchini with a paper towel. Put the zucchini in a large bowl and add the ground turkey, red onion, garlic, bread crumbs, parsley, mint, cumin, coriander, allspice, chili powder, salt, and black pepper to taste. Form into 5 equal, flattened patties about 1 inch thick. Refrigerate until ready to cook.

(recipe continues)

PER SERVING	(1 BURGER + FETA, ¾ CUP SALAD)
CALORIES	277
FAT	15 g
SATURATED FAT	4.5 g
CHOLESTEROL	92 mg
CARBOHYDRATE	13 g
FIBER	3 g
PROTEIN	25 g
SUGARS	5 g
SODIUM	313 mg

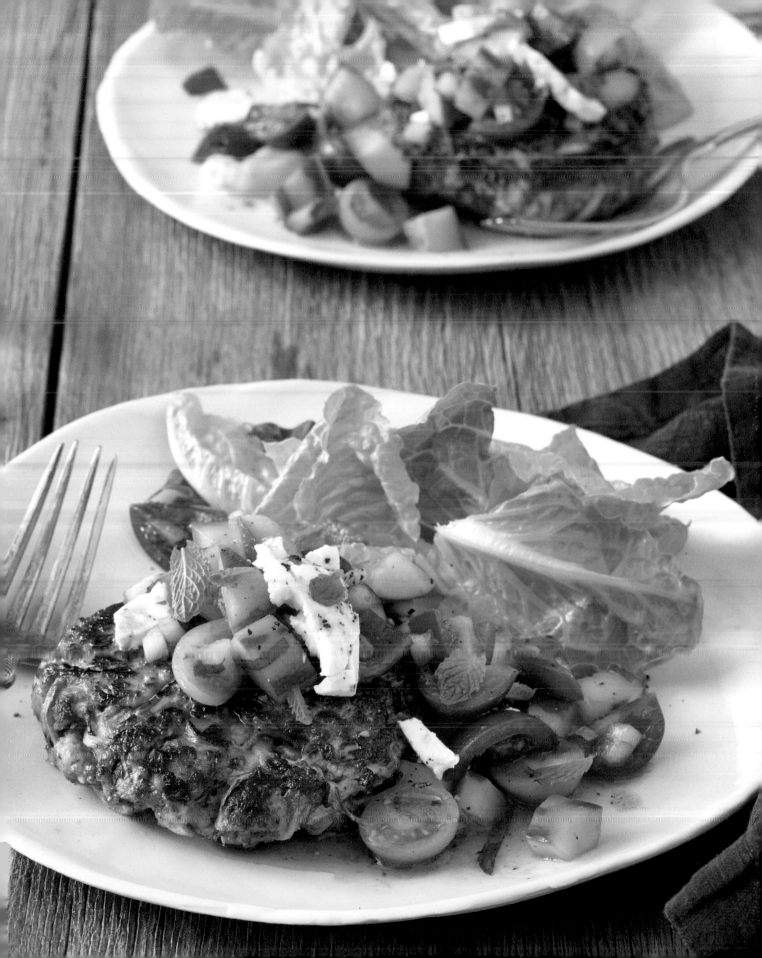

Heat a large nonstick skillet over medium-high heat. Lightly spray the pan with oil. Put the burgers in the pan and reduce the heat to medium-low. Cook until browned, about 4 minutes on each side.

To serve, put 1 cup of lettuce on each of 5 serving plates. Put a turkey burger on each plate along with about ¾ cup of the salad, then sprinkle 1 tablespoon feta on each.

Italian Sausage with Peppers and Onions

SERVES 4

GF **Q**

On those busy nights when I've been out all day and have no idea what to make for dinner, I usually wind up making this dish. Whether I make it outside on the grill in the summer or indoors in the winter, it's a year-round favorite in my home. I make this lean by swapping out fatty pork sausage for leaner chicken sausage, which tastes just as good (if not better).

1 teaspoon olive oil

1 large red bell pepper, cut into ¼-inch-wide strips

1 large yellow or orange bell pepper, cut into ¼-inch-wide strips

1 medium onion, thinly sliced

¼ teaspoon dried oregano

1 sprig of fresh rosemary

Kosher salt and freshly ground black pepper

14 ounces fresh sweet or hot Italian chicken sausages* (I recommend Premio or Al Fresco)

Read the label to be sure this product is gluten-free.

Preheat the grill or the broiler to medium heat.

Heat a large skillet over medium-low heat. Add the olive oil, peppers, and onion, tossing to coat well. Add the oregano, rosemary, and a pinch of salt and black pepper to taste. Cover the pan and cook, stirring occasionally, until the vegetables are soft, 18 to 20 minutes.

Grill or broil the sausages, turning, until golden and cooked through, 12 to 15 minutes. Transfer to a cutting board and slice into ½-inch pieces. Add to the cooked peppers and onions and cover until ready to serve.

skinny**scoop**

If you want to make the whole thing outside on the grill, use a cast-iron pan to cook the onions and peppers (covered and over medium heat), turning every 3 to 5 minutes until they are soft, then grill the sausage until cooked through.

PERFECT PAIRINGS
This can be served with a crusty piece of whole wheat Italian bread and **My House Salad, Made with Love (page 267)**, or turn it into a sandwich by tucking it all into a whole wheat baguette.

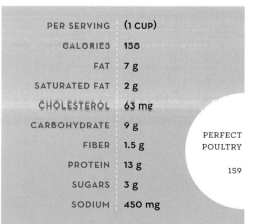

PER SERVING	(1 CUP)
CALORIES	150
FAT	7 g
SATURATED FAT	2 g
CHOLESTEROL	63 mg
CARBOHYDRATE	9 g
FIBER	1.5 g
PROTEIN	13 g
SUGARS	3 g
SODIUM	450 mg

PERFECT POULTRY

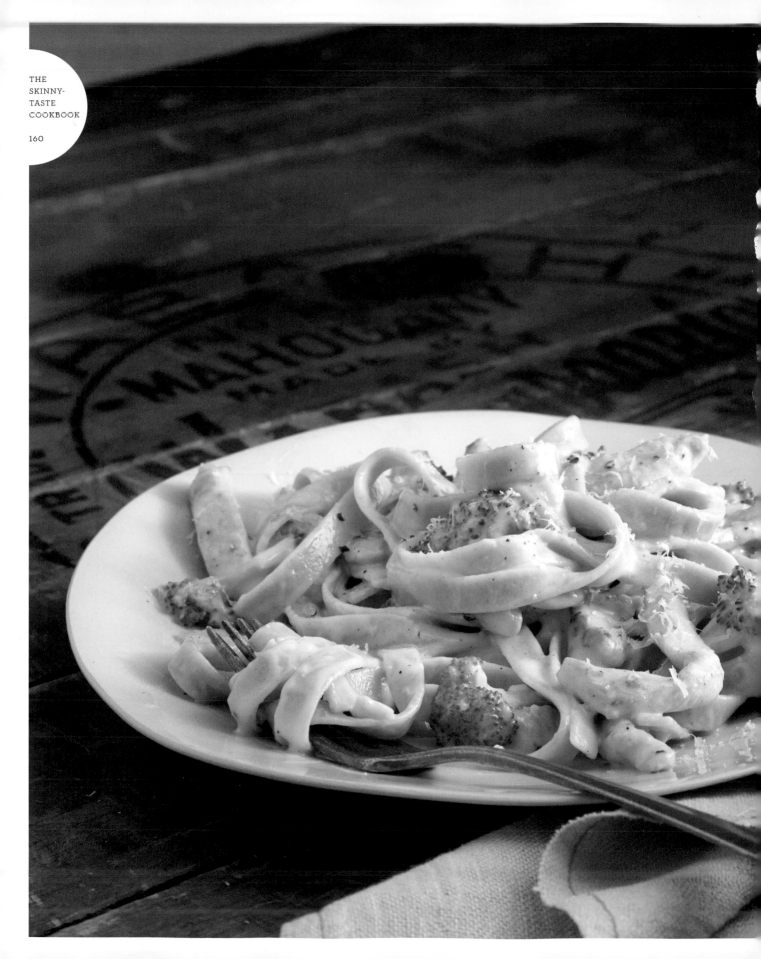

Fettuccine Alfredo with Chicken and Broccoli

SERVES 5

Q

You may not be all that surprised to learn that fettuccine Alfredo is the most requested recipe makeover on Skinnytaste. It's such a decadent, flavorful dish, although certainly not a simple one to skinny-fy, as it traditionally consists of nothing more than butter, cream, white pasta, and cheese. My skinny solution: Use whole-grain pasta, add lean protein and vegetables, and use the best-quality cheese to make up for the lack of butter. That way, you'll feel totally satisfied and you can enjoy a dish that's full of flavor without all the extra fat and calories. I'm *so* confident that you'll love it, because I've put a lot of time, effort, and heart into it!

Cooking spray or oil mister

1 pound thin chicken breast cutlets, cut into thin strips

1 teaspoon garlic salt

Freshly cracked black pepper

9 ounces whole wheat fettuccine (I recommend DeLallo)

2 teaspoons kosher salt

3 cups (8 ounces) small broccoli florets

1 cup 2% milk

2 tablespoons ⅓-less-fat cream cheese

1 tablespoon unsalted butter

1 tablespoon minced shallot

1 garlic clove, minced

1 tablespoon all-purpose flour

5 ounces (scant ⅔ cup) Swanson 33% less sodium chicken broth

⅓ cup freshly grated Parmigiano-Reggiano cheese

¼ cup freshly grated Pecorino Romano cheese (plus more for serving, optional)

1 tablespoon finely minced fresh parsley

Heat a large, deep nonstick skillet over high heat. Spray the skillet with oil. Season the chicken with the garlic salt and black pepper to taste, and add half of the chicken to the pan. Cook until the chicken is golden on the outside and cooked through, about 2 to 3 minutes on each side. Transfer to a large plate. Spray the pan and repeat with the remaining chicken and set aside. Remove the skillet from the heat and let cool.

Cook the pasta to al dente in a pot of salted boiling water according to package directions, adding the broccoli in the last 1½ to 2 minutes of cooking. Reserving ¼ cup of the cooking water, drain the pasta and broccoli in a large colander and return it to the cooking pot.

(recipe continues)

PER SERVING	(GENEROUS 1½ CUPS)
CALORIES	430
FAT	10.5 g
SATURATED FAT	5 g
CHOLESTEROL	82 mg
CARBOHYDRATE	44 g
FIBER	5.5 g
PROTEIN	36 g
SUGARS	4 g
SODIUM	610 mg

Meanwhile while the pasta cooks, in a blender, combine the milk and cream cheese and blend until smooth; set aside.

Set the skillet over medium-low heat and add the butter. Once melted, add the shallot and garlic and cook, stirring, until golden, about 1 minute. Sprinkle in the flour and cook, stirring, for 1 minute. Whisk in the chicken broth, then whisk in the milk-cream cheese mixture. Increase the heat to medium-high and bring to a boil, whisking occasionally. Reduce the heat to low and simmer the cream sauce until thickened, 2 to 3 minutes.

Once the pasta is cooked and drained, set the pot over medium-high heat and add 2 tablespoons of the reserved pasta water. Add the chicken, cream sauce, and Parmesan and toss well. Season with a pinch of black pepper to taste. If needed, add the remaining 2 tablespoons reserved pasta water to loosen the sauce.

To serve, divide the pasta among 5 serving plates. Sprinkle with the Romano and garnish with the parsley. Serve hot with extra black pepper and grated Romano on the side, if desired.

Chicken Cordon Bleu Meatballs

SERVES 6

FF

Who says meatballs have to be Italian? Not me! I thought it would be fun to use the flavors of Chicken Cordon Bleu in a meatball, and I was right! Each meatball is stuffed with ham and light Swiss cheese and baked in the oven, then finished in a creamy white wine sauce. I'm not sure what I like best—the oozing cheese that comes out from the center of each meatball or the decadent sauce they're simmered in.

MEATBALLS

Cooking spray or oil mister

1½ pounds 93% lean ground chicken

¼ cup seasoned whole wheat bread crumbs, homemade (see page 110) or store-bought

¼ cup grated Parmesan cheese

¼ cup finely chopped fresh parsley

1 large egg

1 large garlic clove, crushed

½ teaspoon kosher salt

2 (1-ounce) slices lean deli ham, cut into 6 pieces each

3 slices reduced-fat Swiss cheese, cut into 4 pieces each (2.2 ounces total)

SAUCE

1 tablespoon unsalted butter

1 tablespoon all-purpose flour

¼ cup white wine

1 cup Swanson 33% less sodium chicken broth

½ cup 1% milk

1 tablespoon Dijon mustard

1 teaspoon fresh lemon juice

⅛ teaspoon kosher salt

Freshly ground black pepper

1 teaspoon finely chopped fresh parsley

Preheat the oven to 425°F. Spray a large nonstick baking sheet with oil.

For the meatballs: In a large bowl, combine the ground chicken, bread crumbs, Parmesan, parsley, egg, garlic, and salt. Form 12 meatballs using slightly wet hands to prevent them from sticking. Stuff each meatball by making a hole in the middle and placing one piece each of ham and Swiss cheese in the center. Seal the meatballs well by pinching them closed. Place on the prepared baking sheet and bake 20 minutes, or until almost cooked through.

(recipe continues)

PER SERVING	(2 MEATBALLS + ¼ CUP SAUCE)
CALORIES	312
FAT	12 g
SATURATED FAT	5 g
CHOLESTEROL	133 mg
CARBOHYDRATE	7 g
FIBER	0.5 g
PROTEIN	38 g
SUGARS	2 g
SODIUM	663 mg

PERFECT PAIRINGS
To balance out the richness
of this dish, serve it with
**Lemon-Roasted Asparagus
(page 278)**.

For the sauce: Meanwhile, in a large, deep nonstick skillet with a fitted lid, melt the butter over medium heat. Sprinkle in the flour and cook, whisking constantly, for about 1 minute. Whisk in the wine and cook for 1 minute, then whisk in chicken broth and milk. Bring to a boil, then simmer until it thickens slightly, about 5 minutes. Whisk in the mustard and lemon juice, and season with the salt and a pinch of black pepper; remove from the heat and keep covered.

When the meatballs come out of the oven, add them to the skillet with the sauce. Cover and simmer the meatballs over medium-low heat until the meatballs are cooked through and the chicken is no longer pink, about 5 minutes.

To serve, place 2 meatballs on each of 6 serving plates and top with the sauce and parsley.

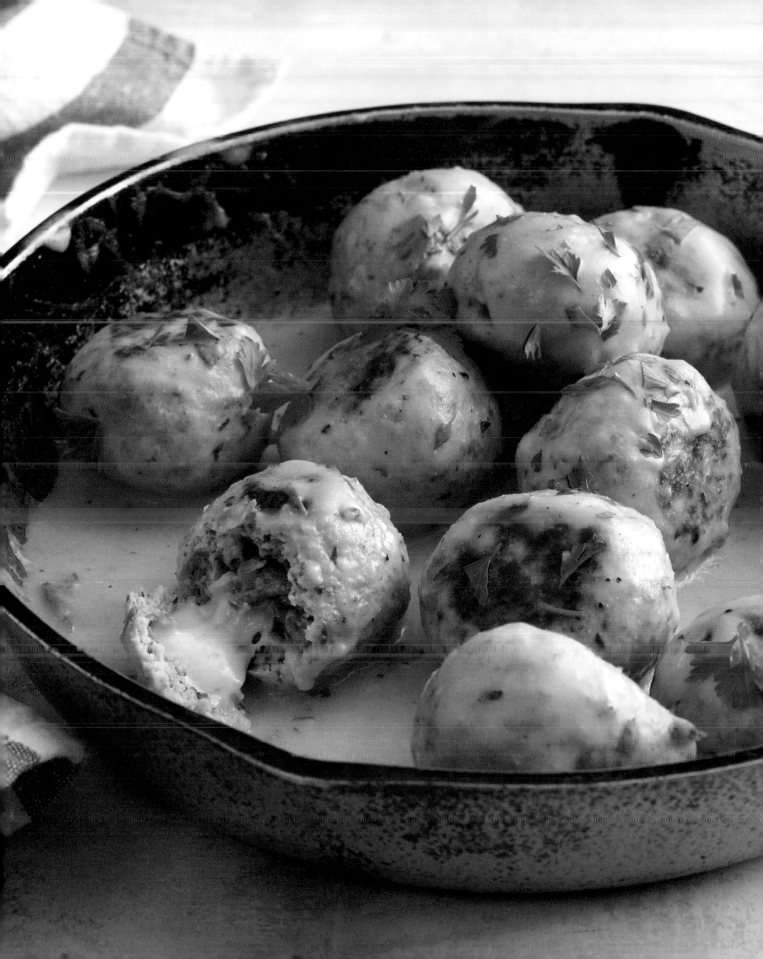

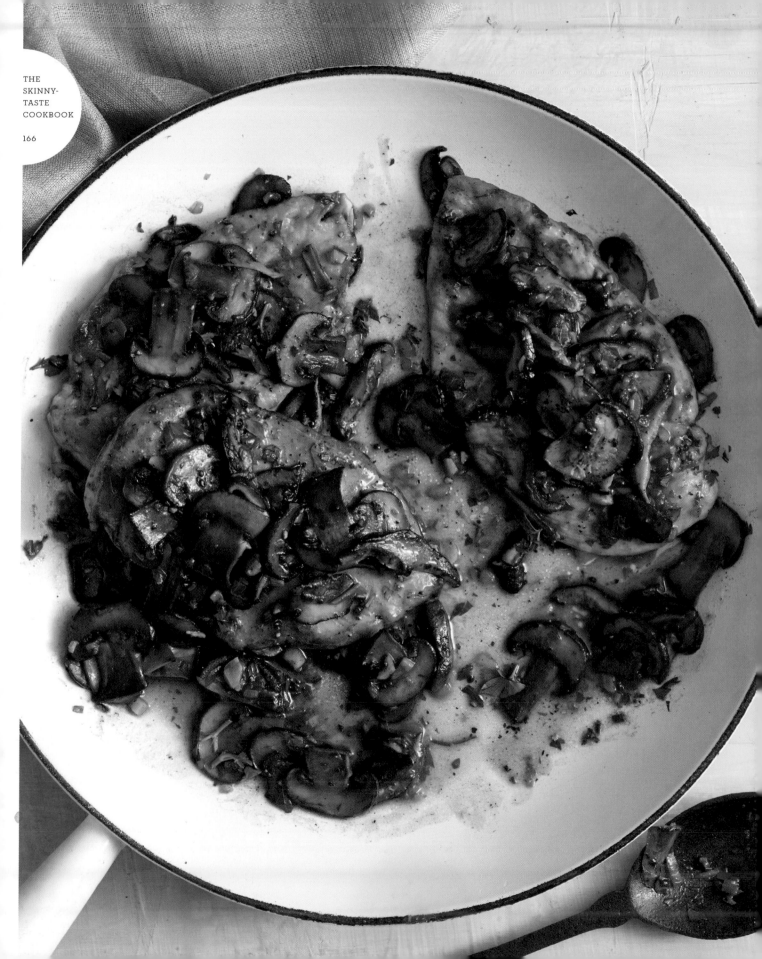

Chicken Marsala on the Lighter Side

SERVES 4

Q

Chicken Marsala is one of those dishes that's found on just about every Italian restaurant menu, but the dish is usually swimming in butter. So I've lightened it up, resulting in a tender chicken dish with a rich pan sauce made with a touch of Marsala wine and fresh parsley. Trust me, you'll be happy you decided not to order out!

2 large boneless, skinless chicken breasts (8 ounces each)

Kosher salt

Freshly ground black pepper

¼ cup plus 1 teaspoon all-purpose flour

1 tablespoon unsalted butter

2 teaspoons olive oil

3 garlic cloves, minced

¼ cup finely chopped shallots

8 ounces sliced cremini mushrooms

3 ounces sliced shiitake mushrooms

⅓ cup Marsala wine

½ cup Swanson 88% fat-free chicken broth

2 tablespoons chopped fresh parsley

Preheat the oven to 200°F.

Slice the chicken breasts in half horizontally to make 4 cutlets. Put each cutlet between two sheets of plastic wrap and lightly pound them until they are about ¼ inch thick. Season with ½ teaspoon salt and a pinch of black pepper.

Place an 18-inch-long length of wax paper on the counter. Put the flour in a shallow bowl and lightly dredge the chicken pieces in the flour, shaking off any excess. Put the chicken on the wax paper; reserve the 1 teaspoon remaining flour to use later.

Heat a large nonstick skillet over medium-high heat. Add ½ tablespoon of the butter and 1 teaspoon of the olive oil to the pan and swirl the pan until the butter has melted. Add the chicken and cook until slightly golden on both sides, about 3 minutes per side. Transfer to a baking dish and place in the oven to keep warm.

(recipe continues)

PERFECT PAIRINGS
You can serve this with noodles, roasted potatoes, or a simple vegetable, such as **Sautéed Broccoli Rabe with Garlic and Oil (page 284).**

PER SERVING	(1 BREAST + MUSHROOMS AND SAUCE)
CALORIES	241
FAT	8 g
SATURATED FAT	2.5 g
CHOLESTEROL	80 mg
CARBOHYDRATE	10 g
FIBER	1 g
PROTEIN	26 g
SUGARS	2 g
SODIUM	428 mg

Add the remaining ½ tablespoon butter and 1 teaspoon olive oil to the skillet. Add the garlic and shallots and cook until soft and golden, about 2 minutes. Add the mushrooms, season with ⅛ teaspoon salt and a pinch of black pepper, and cook, stirring occasionally, until golden, about 5 minutes. Sprinkle in the reserved 1 teaspoon of flour and cook, stirring, for about 30 seconds. Add the Marsala wine, chicken broth, and parsley. Cook, stirring and scraping up any browned bits from the bottom of the pan with a wooden spoon, until thickened, about 2 minutes.

Return the chicken to the skillet with the mushrooms, reduce heat to low, cover, and simmer in the sauce to let the flavors blend, about 4 to 5 minutes.

To serve, put a piece of chicken on each of 4 serving plates. Spoon the mushrooms and sauce evenly over the top, and serve hot.

Spaghetti "Squashta" with Turkey Bolognese

SERVES 6

GF **Q**

This quick slimmed down Bolognese sauce is the perfect topping for spaghetti squash—my favorite low-calorie solution to pasta. A great big bowl of "squashta," as my husband calls it, is under 250 calories! My kids prefer to have real pasta, so I just boil some pasta for them instead.

2 ounces pancetta, chopped

½ tablespoon unsalted butter

½ cup chopped (1 small) onion

1 celery stalk, minced

1 medium carrot, minced

1.3 pounds 93% lean ground turkey

Kosher salt

Fresh cracked pepper

¼ cup white wine

½ tablespoon tomato paste

¾ cup 1% milk

1 (28-ounce) can crushed tomatoes (I recommend Tuttorosso)

1 bay leaf

2 medium spaghetti squash

¼ cup chopped fresh basil

In a large Dutch oven, sauté the pancetta over medium heat until the fat melts, about 3 minutes. Reduce heat to medium-low, add the butter, onion, celery, and carrot and cook until soft, 5 to 6 minutes. Increase the heat to medium-high, add the turkey, and season with ¾ teaspoon salt and pepper to taste. Cook until no longer pink, 7 to 8 minutes, breaking the meat up with a wooden spoon. Add the wine and cook until reduced; 2 to 3 minutes. Add the tomato paste, milk, tomatoes, and bay leaf. Bring to a boil, reduce heat to low, and simmer, covered, 20 to 25 minutes, stirring occasionally.

Meanwhile, using a sharp knife, pierce the squash 8 or 9 times. Microwave on high for 6 minutes. Turn the squash and cook until the shell is tender, 5 to 8 minutes depending on the size. Let cool for 5 minutes. Halve the squash lengthwise. (There should be no resistance, but if there is, microwave it a few more minutes.) Remove the seeds and use a fork to scrape out the spaghetti-like strands of squash.

Remove and discard bay leaf; stir in the basil. To serve, put 1 cup spaghetti squash in each of 6 serving bowls and top each with a generous ¾ cup of sauce.

skinny scoop

You can also bake the squash in the oven. See page 268 for instructions.

PER SERVING	(1 CUP SQUASH + GENEROUS ¾ CUP SAUCE)
CALORIES	301
FAT	12 g
SATURATED FAT	4 g
CHOLESTEROL	84 mg
CARBOHYDRATE	23 g
FIBER	5 g
PROTEIN	25 g
SUGARS	9 g
SODIUM	916 mg

PERFECT POULTRY

169

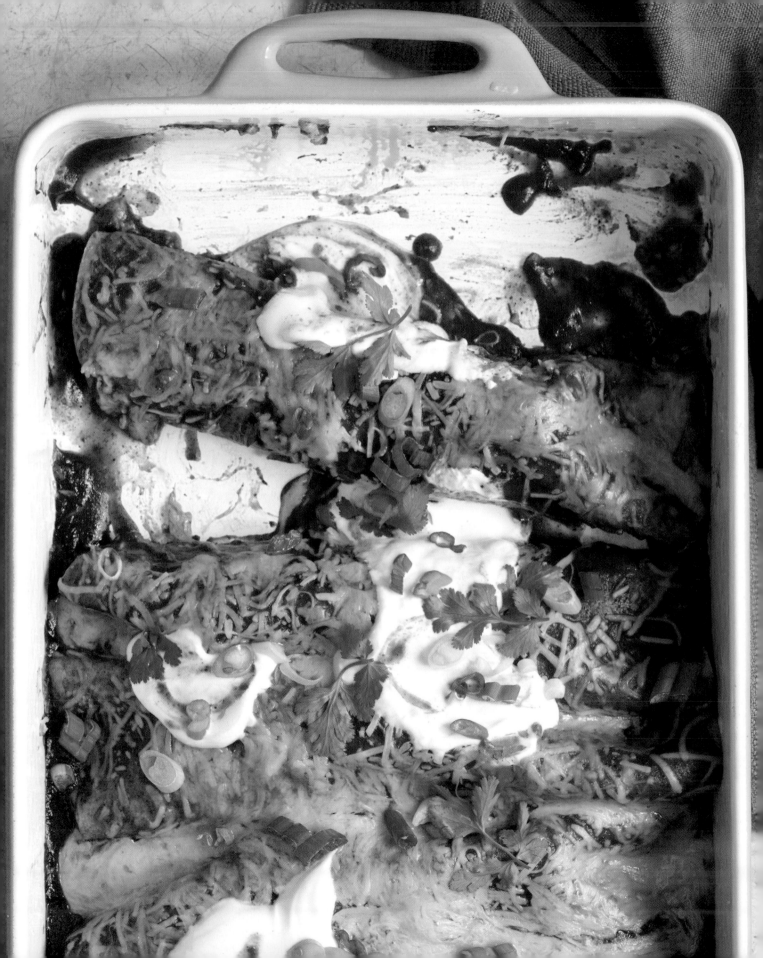

So-Addicted Chicken Enchiladas

SERVES 8

Enchiladas are on my top-three list of Mexican favorites, right along with chiles rellenos and carnitas tacos. Stuffed tortillas smothered in a spicy sauce topped with melted cheese—that's a recipe for delicious! I'm not exactly sure just how authentic my enchiladas are, but I really don't care because they are so darn good. But are they skinny? Of course!

1 teaspoon canola or olive oil

1 cup chopped onion

2 large garlic cloves, minced

½ cup canned tomato sauce

⅓ cup reduced-sodium chicken broth

9 ounces cooked, shredded chicken breast (see page 80)

¼ cup plus 1 tablespoon chopped fresh cilantro

1 teaspoon McCormick Mexican-style chili powder

1 teaspoon ground cumin

½ teaspoon dried oregano

¾ teaspoon kosher salt

Cooking spray or oil mister

8 (7- or 8-inch) low-carb, whole wheat flour tortillas (such as La Tortilla Factory)

1½ cups Best Enchilada Sauce from Scratch (recipe follows) or store-bought sauce

1 cup shredded reduced-fat Mexican cheese blend (such as Sargento)

2 tablespoons chopped scallions, for garnish

4 tablespoons light sour cream, for serving (optional)

Preheat the oven to 400°F.

In a medium nonstick skillet, heat the oil over low heat. Add the onion and garlic and cook, stirring, until soft, about 2 minutes. Add the tomato sauce, chicken broth, cooked chicken, ¼ cup of the cilantro, the chili powder, cumin, oregano, and salt. Simmer until the flavors blend and the sauce reduces, 4 to 5 minutes. Remove the pan from the heat.

Spray a 13 × 9-inch glass baking dish with oil. Put ⅓ cup chicken mixture into each tortilla, roll them up, and place seam side down in the baking dish. Top with the enchilada sauce, then sprinkle the top with the cheese. Cover the dish with foil, being careful it does not touch the cheese. Bake until hot and the cheese is melted, 20 to 25 minutes.

To serve, put an enchilada on each of 8 serving plates, sprinkle with the scallions and the remaining 1 tablespoon cilantro, and serve with light sour cream on the side, if desired.

PERFECT PAIRINGS

I serve these with cilantro lime rice—combine ¾ cup cooked brown rice with a squeeze of lime juice and a tablespoon chopped fresh cilantro—and a simple side salad.

PER SERVING	(1 ENCHILADA)
CALORIES	194
FAT	8 g
SATURATED FAT	2 g
CHOLESTEROL	77 mg
CARBOHYDRATE	21 g
FIBER	9.5 g
PROTEIN	18 g
SUGARS	5 g
SODIUM	640 mg

Best Enchilada Sauce from Scratch

MAKES ABOUT 4 CUPS

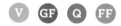

I have a serious weakness for enchiladas. As long as I have some tortillas, cheese, and my homemade enchilada sauce, I can turn any leftover into a delicious enchilada. Store-bought sauce is just not an option for me, and you'll see why after you try this simple homemade recipe. It makes enough for 16 to 18 enchiladas, so use what you need and freeze whatever you don't.

skinnyscoop

I like to freeze this in 1-quart freezer bags so I can quickly thaw what I need to whip up a Mexican fiesta any time I want!

½ teaspoon olive oil

4 garlic cloves, minced

1½ cups Swanson 33% less sodium chicken broth*

3 cups canned tomato sauce

2 tablespoons chopped chipotle chile in adobo sauce (or more to taste)

1 teaspoon McCormick Mexican-style chili powder (or to taste)

1 teaspoon ground cumin

½ teaspoon kosher salt

⅛ teaspoon freshly ground black pepper

Read the label to be sure this product is gluten-free.

Heat a medium nonstick saucepan over medium heat. Add the oil and garlic and cook, stirring, until golden, about 1 to 1½ minutes. Add the chicken broth, tomato sauce, chipotle chile, chili powder, cumin, salt, and black pepper. Bring to a boil, reduce the heat to low, and simmer until the flavors blend, 7 to 10 minutes. Serve immediately, or let cool and refrigerate in an airtight container for up to 3 days, or keep frozen for up to 3 months.

PER SERVING	(ABOUT ¼ CUP)
CALORIES	20
FAT	0 g
SATURATED FAT	0 g
CHOLESTEROL	0 mg
CARBOHYDRATE	4 g
FIBER	1 g
PROTEIN	1 g
SUGARS	2 g
SODIUM	121 mg

Roasted Poblanos Rellenos with Chicken

SERVES 5

GF FF

Meet my new favorite chile relleno! Okay, so this isn't exactly like a traditional chile relleno: stuffed with cheese, battered in egg, and deep-fried. I gave these babies a much-needed healthy makeover, and they turned out awesome! This recipe is a little more labor-intensive than others, so I recommend making this on the weekend or when you have more time. You can even prepare it a day ahead and bake when ready to eat—and it freezes well once baked, so it's perfect for make-ahead meals for the week.

5 poblano peppers

1 medium jalapeño pepper

SAUCE

4 medium vine tomatoes, quartered

½ onion, chopped

3 garlic cloves

2 tablespoons chopped fresh cilantro

1 teaspoon olive oil

1 teaspoon ground cumin

¾ teaspoon kosher salt

FILLING

1 teaspoon olive oil

½ cup diced onion

4 garlic cloves, minced

¼ cup finely chopped fresh cilantro

8 ounces cooked, shredded chicken breast (see page 80)

1 cup canned small white beans,* drained and lightly mashed

¾ cup Swanson 33% less sodium chicken broth*

½ teaspoon ground cumin

½ teaspoon garlic powder

¼ teaspoon kosher salt

Freshly ground black pepper

1¼ cups shredded reduced-fat Colby-Jack cheese blend

2 tablespoons fresh cilantro leaves, for garnish

Read the label to be sure this product is gluten-free.

Using a small, sharp knife, cut a slit lengthwise along one side of each poblano pepper, then make a small crosswise slit along the top to create a T-shape, being careful not to cut off the stem. Carefully cut out and remove the core and scoop out the seeds. Holding the peppers with tongs, roast them and the jalapeño over an open flame, such as the grill, broiler, or gas stovetop, turning often, until the skin is completely blistered and blackened. Transfer to a paper bag (or place in a bowl and cover with plastic wrap) and let steam for 10 to 15 minutes. Use

(recipe continues)

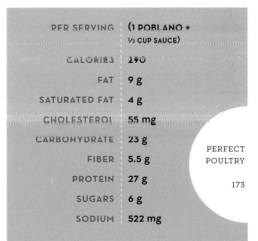

PER SERVING	(1 POBLANO + ⅕ CUP SAUCE)
CALORIES	290
FAT	9 g
SATURATED FAT	4 g
CHOLESTEROL	55 mg
CARBOHYDRATE	23 g
FIBER	5.5 g
PROTEIN	27 g
SUGARS	6 g
SODIUM	522 mg

a table knife to scrape off the charred skins, being careful not to tear the peppers.

For the sauce: In a blender, combine the stemmed, roasted jalapeño pepper including the seeds, the tomatoes, onion, garlic, cilantro, and ¼ cup water. Blend until smooth.

In a large, deep nonstick skillet, heat the oil over medium heat. Add the pureed tomato mixture, cumin, and salt. Simmer, uncovered, stirring occasionally, until slightly thickened and the color turns deep red, 20 to 25 minutes.

Preheat the oven to 350°F.

Pour 1¼ cups of the sauce into the bottom of a 9 × 13-inch baking dish (or pour ¼ cup of sauce into each of 5 individual 8-ounce oval baking dishes).

For the filling: In a large nonstick skillet, heat the oil over medium heat. Add the onion, garlic, and cilantro. Cook, stirring, until soft, about 2 minutes. Add the chicken, beans, broth, cumin, garlic powder, salt, and black pepper to taste, and cook until the liquid has reduced, about 5 minutes.

Carefully stuff about ⅔ cup of the filling into each poblano pepper. Place the peppers seam side up on top of the sauce in the baking dish(es) and top each with ¼ cup Colby-Jack cheese. Cover the dish tightly with foil. (You can stop here and refrigerate if you want to prepare this ahead.)

Bake until hot and bubbling, 20 to 30 minutes (or 30 to 40 minutes if the stuffed peppers were refrigerated). Serve hot with the remaining warm sauce on the side and garnished with cilantro.

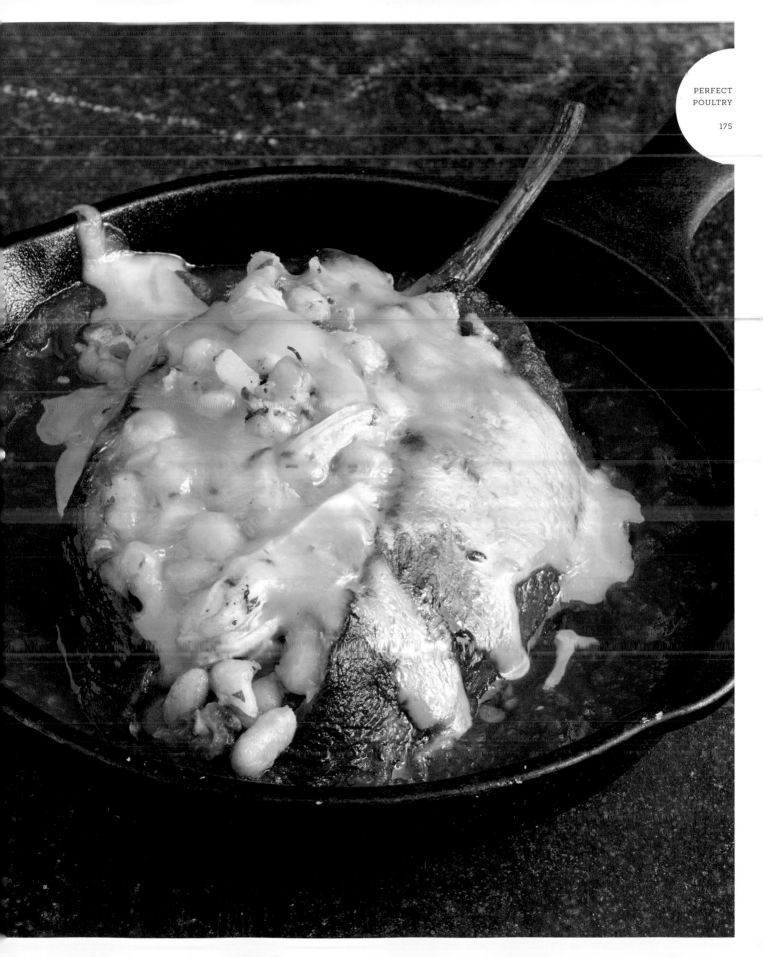

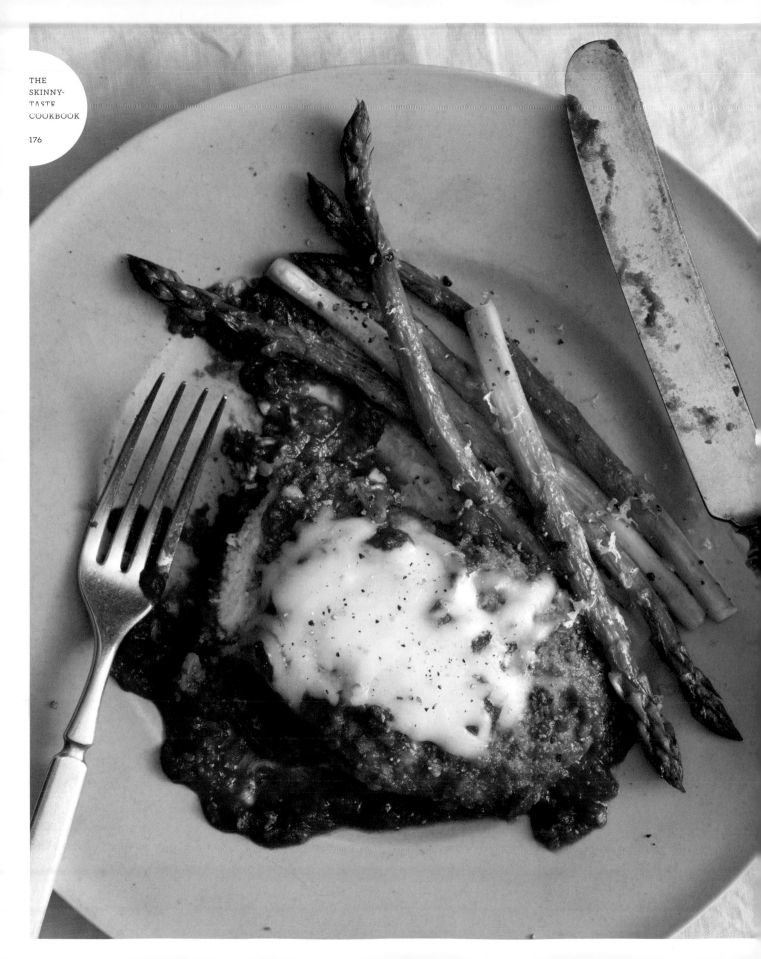

Skinny Chicken Parmesan

SERVES 6

FF

Chicken Parmesan is one of the first dishes I learned to lighten up and one of my most popular recipes on Skinnytaste. If you're familiar with my blog, you'll notice some subtle differences. This iteration starts in the oven, and then finishes on the stove in a skillet full of marinara, so it's saucier than my previous version.

Cooking spray or oil mister

3 boneless, skinless chicken breasts (8 ounces each), fat trimmed

¾ teaspoon kosher salt

½ cup seasoned whole wheat bread crumbs, homemade (see page 110) or store-bought

3 tablespoons grated Parmesan cheese

2 teaspoons melted unsalted butter

1 tablespoon olive oil

2 cups Quickest Marinara Sauce (page 94) or store-bought marinara sauce

9 tablespoons part-skim mozzarella cheese

Preheat the oven to 450°F. Lightly spray a large baking sheet with oil.

Slice the chicken breasts in half horizontally to make 6 cutlets. Season both sides with salt.

In a shallow bowl, combine the bread crumbs and Parmesan. In a small bowl, combine the butter and olive oil. Brush the butter and oil on both sides of the chicken, dredge the chicken in the bread crumb mixture, and put the chicken on the prepared baking sheet. Lightly spray oil on top of the chicken.

Bake until golden on the bottom, about 20 minutes. Turn the chicken over and bake until the center is cooked through and the bottom is golden, 5 to 6 minutes.

Meanwhile, in a large, deep covered skillet, cook the marinara sauce over medium heat until heated through, 2 to 3 minutes.

Place the baked chicken in the skillet and top each piece with 1½ tablespoons of the mozzarella. Cover the pan and cook until the cheese melts, 3 to 4 minutes. Serve hot.

PERFECT PAIRINGS
Serve this over whole wheat pasta or along with **Lemon-Roasted Asparagus (page 278)**, pictured opposite. You can also serve it on a whole wheat baguette or Italian bread to make it a skinny hero.

PER SERVING	(1 CUTLET WITH SAUCE AND CHEESE)
CALORIES	174
FAT	7 g
SATURATED FAT	2.5 g
CHOLESTEROL	62 mg
CARBOHYDRATE	5 g
FIBER	1 g
PROTEIN	22 g
SUGARS	1 g
SODIUM	407 mg

PERFECT POULTRY

Asian Peanut Noodles with Chicken

SERVES 6

GF **Q**

What's my skinny secret to satisfy those noodle cravings while maintaining my waistline? For starters, I loaded up this dish with plenty of noodle-size vegetables. For the peanut sauce, I was able to cut the fat substantially by swapping the peanut butter for Better'n Peanut Butter. While nothing beats the taste of all-natural peanut butter spread over a slice of bread, I find Better'n Peanut Butter a suitable alternative when I'm cooking a dish that requires the same peanut taste without the fat. It's all-natural, with 85 percent less fat and 40 percent fewer calories. You can find it online, at Trader Joe's, and at natural foods stores.

PEANUT SAUCE

1 cup Swanson 33% less sodium chicken broth*

5 tablespoons Better'n Peanut Butter

2 tablespoons honey

2 tablespoons soy sauce (or tamari* for gluten-free)

1 tablespoon Sriracha sauce

1 tablespoon grated fresh ginger

2 garlic cloves, crushed

CHICKEN AND VEGETABLES

1 pound boneless, skinless chicken breast, cut into thin strips

Kosher salt

Freshly cracked black pepper

1 tablespoon Sriracha sauce (or to taste)

1 tablespoon soy sauce (or tamari* for gluten-free)

Juice of ½ lime

4 garlic cloves, crushed

1 tablespoon grated fresh ginger

½ tablespoon sesame oil

¾ cup chopped scallions

1¼ cups shredded carrots

1¼ cups broccoli slaw

8 ounces rice noodles

2 tablespoons chopped unsalted roasted peanuts

6 lime wedges

6 sprigs of fresh cilantro, for garnish

Read the label to be sure this product is gluten-free.

For the peanut sauce: In a small saucepan, combine the chicken broth, Better'n Peanut Butter, honey, soy sauce, Sriracha, ginger, and garlic. Bring to a simmer over medium-low heat and cook, stirring occasionally, until the flavors blend and the sauce is slightly thickened, 8 to 10 minutes.

For the chicken: Season the chicken strips with ⅛ teaspoon of the salt and a pinch of black pepper, then transfer it to a large

(recipe continues)

PER SERVING	(ABOUT 1⅓ CUPS)
CALORIES	359
FAT	6 g
SATURATED FAT	1 g
CHOLESTEROL	48 mg
CARBOHYDRATE	53 g
FIBER	4 g
PROTEIN	22 g
SUGARS	9 g
SODIUM	670 mg

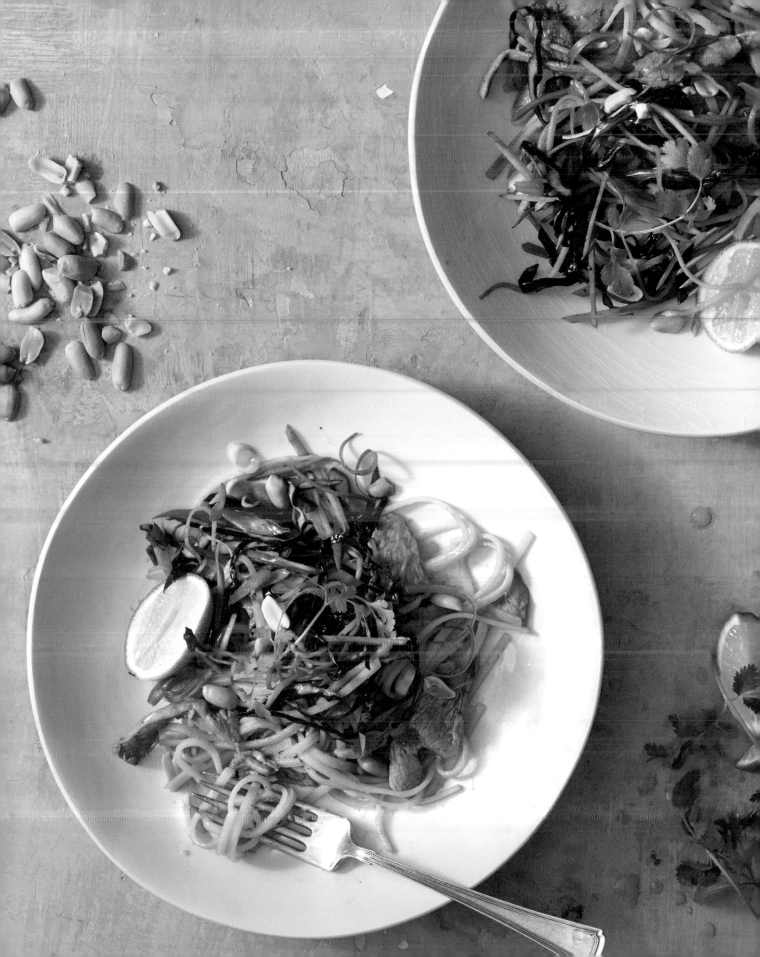

bowl and add the Sriracha, soy sauce, lime juice, 2 of the garlic cloves, and the ginger.

Heat a large nonstick skillet or wok over high heat. Add the sesame oil, then add the chicken. Cook, stirring, until cooked through, 2 to 3 minutes. Transfer to a plate. Add the remaining 2 garlic cloves, the scallions, carrots, and broccoli slaw, and season with a pinch of salt. Cook, stirring, until the vegetables are crisp-tender, 1 to 2 minutes. Transfer to a plate.

Cook the noodles in a large pot of water according to package instructions. Drain and put them in the hot wok. Add the chicken and peanut sauce and cook, tossing everything together, for 1 minute.

Divide the noodles and chicken evenly among 6 bowls (about 1 cup each). Top each with ⅓ cup vegetables and 1 teaspoon peanuts. Serve with a lime wedge and a sprig of cilantro, for garnish.

Orecchiette with Sausage, Baby Kale, and Bell Pepper

SERVES 5

GF **Q**

Weeknights are usually pretty hectic in my home. Madison keeps me super busy and wants my full, undivided attention, so I like to make meals as quick and simple as possible. Speed is what I love about this yummy pasta dish. In the same amount of time it takes to boil the water, the sausage and vegetables are cooked. Plus, this dish is a great way to incorporate healthy greens in your diet without having to do much prep work.

2¾ teaspoons kosher salt

1 teaspoon olive oil

1 medium onion, chopped

1 medium red bell pepper, chopped

5 garlic cloves, chopped

Freshly cracked black pepper

14 ounces fresh sweet or hot Italian chicken sausage,* casings removed

6 cups baby kale

10 ounces whole wheat pasta such as orecchiette (use brown rice pasta for gluten-free)

¼ cup grated Pecorino Romano cheese, plus more for serving (optional)

¼ teaspoon crushed red pepper flakes (optional)

Read the label to be sure this product is gluten-free.

Bring a large pot of water and 2 teaspoons of the salt to a boil.

Meanwhile, heat a large, deep nonstick skillet over medium heat. Add the olive oil, onion, bell pepper, garlic, the remaining ¾ teaspoon salt, and black pepper to taste. Cook, stirring, until soft, 4 to 5 minutes. Add the sausage and cook, using a wooden spoon to break the meat into small pieces as it browns, 6 to 8 minutes. Add the kale, cover, and cook 2 to 3 minutes. Uncover, stir, and cook until the kale is wilted, about 3 more minutes.

Add the pasta to the boiling water and cook to al dente according to the package directions. Drain, reserving 1 cup of the pasta water, and add the cooked pasta to the skillet. Add ⅓ cup of the reserved pasta water. Increase the heat to

(recipe continues)

skinny scoop

I never cared for whole wheat pasta until I discovered DeLallo pasta. It has a great texture, plus they come in tons of fancy pasta shapes.

PER SERVING	(ABOUT 1½ CUPS)
CALORIES	412
FAT	11 g
SATURATED FAT	3.5 g
CHOLESTEROL	67 mg
CARBOHYDRATE	57 g
FIBER	2.5 g
PROTEIN	23 g
SUGARS	3 g
SODIUM	658 mg

PERFECT POULTRY

181

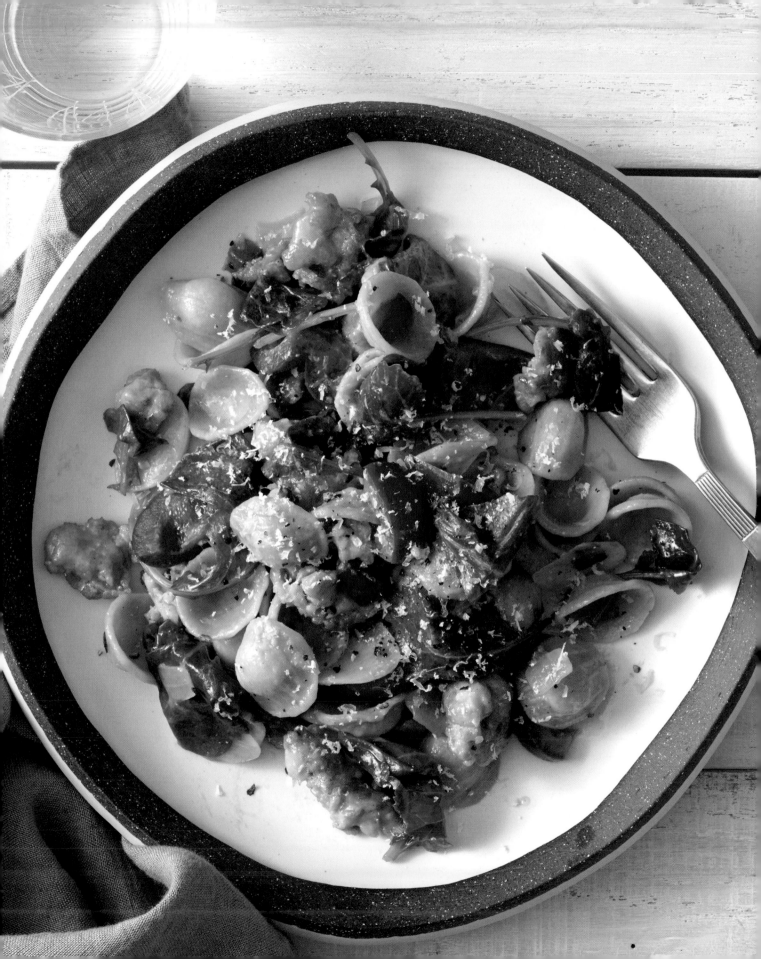

medium-high heat, add the ¼ cup Romano and pepper flakes (if using), and toss well. Cook for another 1 to 2 minutes, adding more of the reserved water, if needed. Transfer the pasta to a large bowl. Serve immediately with grated cheese, if desired.

FOOD FACTS kale, a super green
Why should you love kale? Let us count the reasons. First, it's loaded with immune-boosting vitamin C, and it also chips in some vitamin A, vitamin K, and calcium. Then there are all the phytochemicals: quercetin, kaempferol, and sulforaphane, which protect against a variety of diseases. And don't forget it's a source of alpha-linolenic acid, the plant form of omega-3 fatty acids.

Poultry Labels 101

Historically, *everyone* got their chicken straight from the farm. Back then, you could tell a lot about your future dinner by seeing where it was raised. Now, most of us depend on food labels in the supermarket to tell us the kind of life our chicken lived, but let's face it, label lingo can be a bit confusing. Fortunately, we've created a poultry primer to help you make a beeline to the right bird:

CAGE-FREE: The birds weren't kept in cages, and could roam freely around their shelter, which may have been entirely indoors.

FREE RANGE OR FREE ROAMING: The birds lived in a shelter that had continuous access to the outdoors, although there's no guarantee that they spent much time out there or that the outside area was all that large or even fully open. Animals are not required to be outside for any period of time—they just need to have access available to them.

HORMONE-FREE: This is actually a little misleading, as the USDA prohibits the use of hormones in poultry. That means you don't have to bother paying extra for a package that claims "hormone-free" chicken.

NATURAL: Natural chicken has no artificial colors or ingredients and has been minimally processed. Although this labeling is voluntary,

most companies that produce natural products will say so on their packaging.

NO ANTIBIOTICS: This label means the chicken was raised without the use of antibiotics, which are used to treat sick animals or prevent disease when animals are susceptible to infection. Low doses of antibiotics are also added to chicken feed for long periods of time to promote rapid growth. Most of the antibiotics used to treat animals are the same ones used to treat humans.

USDA ORGANIC: Organic chickens have had access to the outdoors and direct sunlight, have been fed 100 percent organic feed, and have never been given antibiotics or growth hormones. The government does on-site inspections of organic chicken farms in order to verify that they're complying with all of these rules. The USDA makes no claims that organically produced food is safer or more nutritious than conventionally produced food.

Chicken Pasta Caprese

SERVES 5

GF **Q**

Imagine a big bowl of pasta tossed with sweet garden tomatoes, lots of fresh basil, sautéed chicken breast, and small chunks of mozzarella that start to melt when tossed with the hot pasta—good stuff! This is a summertime favorite in my home and a great way to use up all those glorious end-of-summer tomatoes. I personally love using unusal pasta shapes such as Casarecce shown in the photo or Gemelli, but ziti or penne would also work just fine.

1 pound skinless, boneless chicken breasts, cut into ½-inch cubes

½ teaspoon dried basil

Kosher salt

Freshly ground black pepper

Cooking spray or oil mister

9 ounces pasta (use brown rice pasta for gluten-free)

4 teaspoons extra-virgin olive oil

6 garlic cloves, coarsely chopped

2½ cups halved grape tomatoes

¼ cup thinly sliced fresh basil

4 ounces part-skim mozzarella cheese, cut into cubes

Heat a large nonstick skillet over high heat. Season the chicken with the dried basil, ¼ teaspoon of salt, and black pepper to taste. Spray the skillet with oil and add the chicken. Cook until the chicken is cooked through, about 3 minutes on each side. Transfer the chicken to a plate.

Cook the pasta to al dente in a pot of salted boiling water according to package directions. Drain, reserving about ½ cup of the pasta water.

Meanwhile, increase the heat under the skillet to high, add the olive oil and garlic, and cook, stirring, until golden, being careful not to burn it, about 1 minute. Add the tomatoes, ⅛ teaspoon salt, and black pepper to taste, and reduce the heat to medium-low. Cook, stirring, until the tomatoes become tender, 5 to 6 minutes.

Add the pasta to the tomatoes. If the pasta seems too dry, add some of the reserved pasta water. Add the chicken and toss well. Remove the pan from the heat, stir in the fresh basil and cheese, and serve hot.

PER SERVING	(1¾ CUPS)
CALORIES	402
FAT	10.5 g
SATURATED FAT	3.5 g
CHOLESTEROL	73 mg
CARBOHYDRATE	43 g
FIBER	2.5 g
PROTEIN	33 g
SUGARS	4 g
SODIUM	337 mg

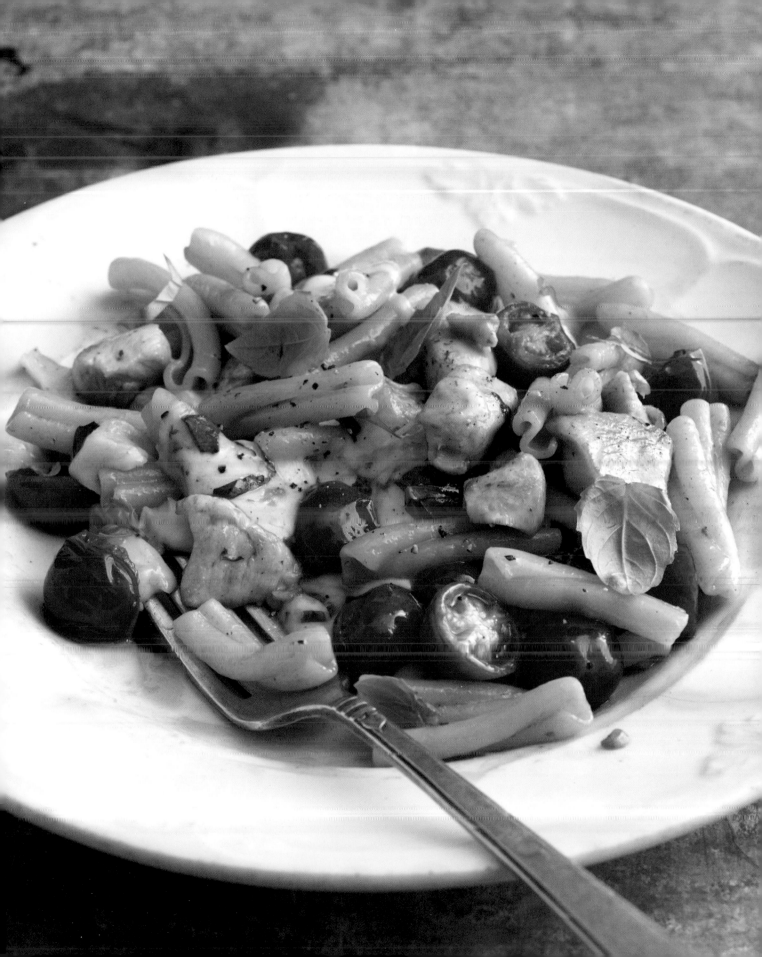

Cajun Chicken Pasta on the Lighter Side

SERVES 5

GF **Q**

When I'm ragin' for Cajun, I love to make this colorful pasta dish loaded with yummy vegetables and sautéed chicken in a light creamy sauce that has a bit of a kick! A few years back I was asked to remake this dish, which is popular at a chain restaurant. I love a challenge, so I was happy to tackle it, and it has since become one of the most popular dishes on Skinnytaste—it's that good!

⅓ cup fat-free milk

1 tablespoon all-purpose flour (or sweet rice flour for gluten-free)

3 tablespoons light cream cheese

8 ounces linguine (use brown rice pasta for gluten-free*)

Kosher salt

1 pound boneless, skinless chicken breasts, sliced into strips

1¼ teaspoons Cajun seasoning (or more to taste)

1 teaspoon garlic powder

⅛ teaspoon freshly cracked black pepper

Cooking spray or oil mister

1 tablespoon olive oil

1 medium red bell pepper, thinly sliced

1 medium yellow bell pepper, thinly sliced

½ medium red onion, sliced

3 garlic cloves, minced

8 ounces mushrooms, sliced

2 medium tomatoes, chopped

1 cup Swanson 33% less sodium chicken broth*

2 medium scallions, chopped

*Read the label to be sure this product is gluten-free.

In a blender, make a slurry by combining the milk, flour, and cream cheese. Set aside.

Cook the pasta to al dente in a pot of salted water according to package directions. Drain and set aside.

Meanwhile, heat a large heavy nonstick skillet over medium-high heat. Season the chicken with 1 teaspoon Cajun seasoning, ½ teaspoon of the garlic powder, and ¼ teaspoon salt. Spray the pan with oil and add half of the chicken. Cook until cooked through, about 3 minutes on each side. Transfer to a plate and repeat with the remaining chicken.

PER SERVING	(1½ CUPS)
CALORIES	375
FAT	7.5 g
SATURATED FAT	2 g
CHOLESTEROL	63 mg
CARBOHYDRATE	47 g
FIBER	4 g
PROTEIN	30 g
SUGARS	6 g
SODIUM	475 mg

Add the olive oil to the skillet and reduce the heat to medium. Add the bell peppers, onion, and garlic, cook, stirring, until almost tender, 3 to 4 minutes. Add the mushrooms and tomatoes and cook, stirring, until the vegetables are tender, 3 to 4 more minutes. Add the remaining ½ teaspoon garlic powder and season with ½ teaspoon salt and the black pepper. Reduce the heat to medium-low, add the chicken broth and the slurry, and cook, stirring, until it begins to thicken, about 2 minutes.

Return the chicken strips to the skillet. Adjust with ⅛ teaspoon salt and the remaining ¼ teaspoon Cajun seasoning, or more to taste, and cook until heated through, about 1 minute. Add the linguine and toss well to coat.

To serve, divide the pasta and chicken among 5 serving plates and sprinkle with the scallions.

skinny**scoop**

Have all your vegetables prepped and ingredients ready before you start cooking. That way, it will all come together in about the same amount of time it takes to cook the pasta.

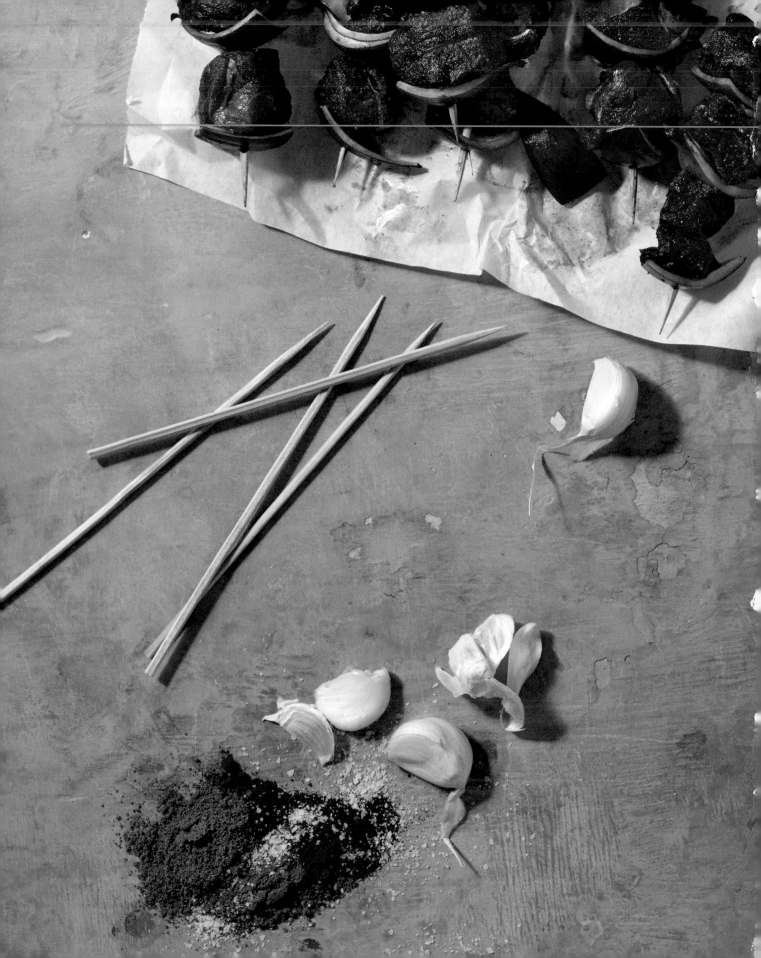

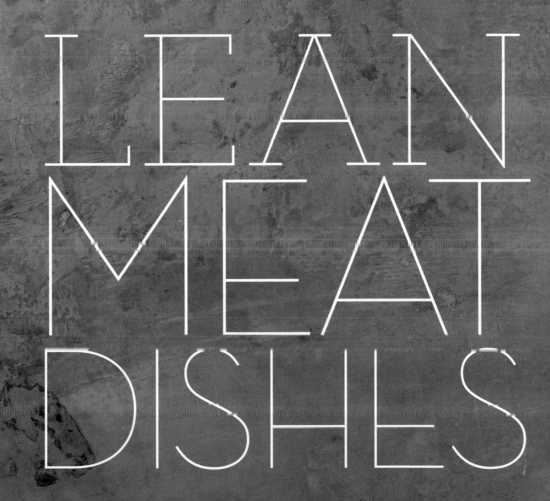

LEAN MEAT DISHES

Mongolian Beef and Broccoli

SERVES 4

GF **Q**

Two dishes—Mongolian beef and beef and broccoli—combine in this easy and lighter alternative to Chinese takeout. It's made with lean strips of sirloin beef, broccoli florets, and scallions in a sweet and savory light stir-fry sauce. Fortunately, nothing is quicker than stir-fry, perfect for weeknights.

2 teaspoons cornstarch

3 tablespoons plus 2 teaspoons reduced-sodium soy sauce (use tamari* for gluten-free)

2 teaspoons rice wine

4 teaspoons sesame oil

1 pound sirloin steak, trimmed of fat, thinly sliced against the grain

¼ teaspoon kosher salt

4 cups broccoli florets

4 medium scallions, cut into 1-inch pieces; white and greens separated

1 tablespoon minced garlic

½ teaspoon minced fresh ginger

2 tablespoons packed dark brown sugar

1 tablespoon oyster sauce*

PERFECT PAIRINGS
Serve this with ¾ cup cooked brown jasmine rice, or if you have leftover brown rice, whip up **Vegetable Fried Brown Rice (page 273)**.

Read the label to be sure this product is gluten-free.

In a shallow glass container, whisk together the cornstarch, 2 teaspoons of the soy sauce, the rice wine, and 1 teaspoon of the sesame oil. Season the steak with salt, add to the marinade, and turn to coat. Let sit at room temperature for 30 minutes.

Bring a large pot of water to a rolling boil. Add the broccoli and cook until bright green and crisp-tender, about 1 minute. Drain and run under cold water to stop the cooking.

Heat a large nonstick wok or skillet over high heat. Add 1 teaspoon of the oil, then half of the beef. Cook for 30 seconds without disturbing, flip, and cook another 30 seconds, moving the meat around until browned on all sides. Transfer to a plate and repeat with 1 teaspoon oil and the remaining beef.

Heat the remaining 1 teaspoon sesame oil in the wok and add the scallion whites, garlic, and ginger. Cook until fragrant, about 30 seconds. Add the broccoli, brown sugar, remaining 3 tablespoons soy sauce, and the oyster sauce and cook, stirring, for 30 seconds. Add the beef and cook, stirring, 30 more seconds. Remove from the heat and stir in the scallion greens.

PER SERVING	(ABOUT 1⅓ CUPS)
CALORIES	256
FAT	10 g
SATURATED FAT	2.5 g
CHOLESTEROL	76 mg
CARBOHYDRATE	15 g
FIBER	0.5 g
PROTEIN	28 g
SUGARS	7 g
SODIUM	768 mg

skinny **scoop**

Since brown rice takes
a while to cook, I always
start that first, and then
proceed with prepping my
vegetables. To save even
more time, you can prepare
your rice a day ahead and
keep it refrigerated.

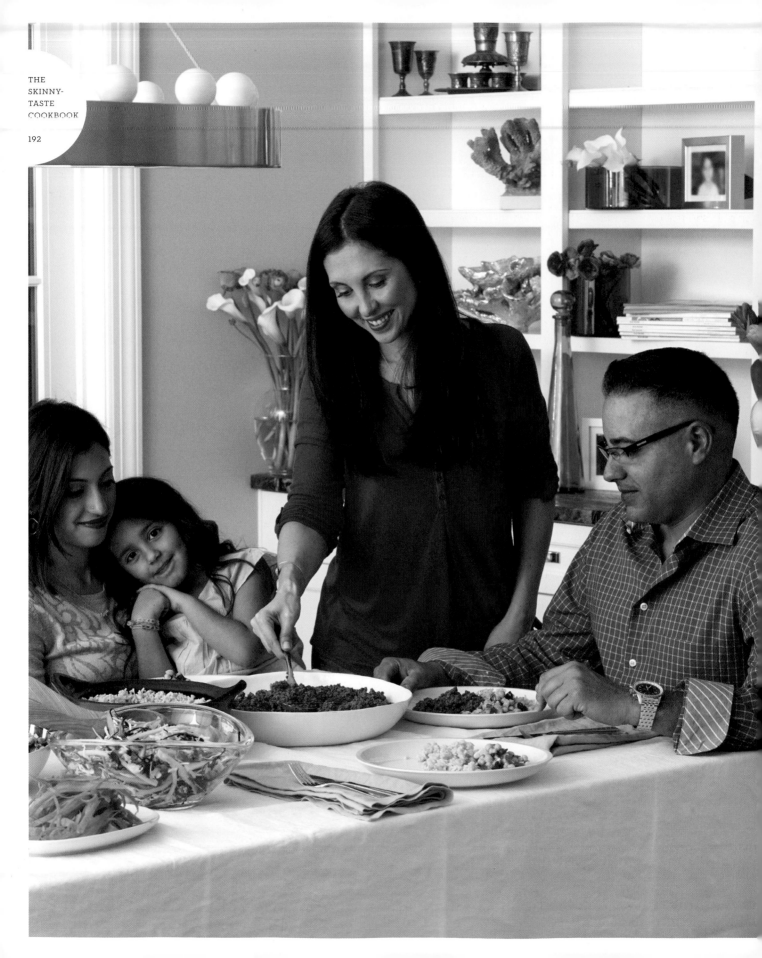

Slow-Cooker Picadillo

SERVES 10

GF FF SC

At least once a month—if not more—it's Picadillo Night at my house. My whole family loves when I whip up this flavorful Cuban dish, and I love it because it's so easy and inexpensive. I grew up on this dish, which was one of Mom's specialties. Throughout the years, I've adapted her version by using leaner beef; and rather than making it on the stove, I find it convenient to make this in the slow cooker, which helps make the meat very tender. Some people also add raisins, but my family prefers it without them.

2½ pounds 93% lean ground beef

2 teaspoons kosher salt

Freshly ground black pepper

1 cup finely chopped onion

1 cup chopped red bell pepper

3 garlic cloves, minced

¼ cup finely chopped fresh cilantro

1 small tomato, chopped

¼ cup drained alcaparrado (olives, pimientos, and capers) or pitted green olives

1 (8-ounce) can tomato sauce

1 tablespoon of the brine from the alcaparrado or olives

1½ teaspoons ground cumin, plus more as needed

¼ teaspoon garlic powder

2 bay leaves

Set a large, deep skillet over medium-high heat, add the beef, and season it with the salt and a pinch of black pepper. Cook, using a wooden spoon to break the meat into small pieces as it browns, 4 to 5 minutes. Drain the liquid from the pan. Add the onion, bell pepper, and garlic to the meat and cook until fragrant, 3 to 4 minutes.

Transfer the mixture to a slow cooker and add the cilantro, tomato, alcaparrado, tomato sauce, brine, cumin, garlic powder, bay leaves, and 1¼ cups water. Cover and cook on high for 3 to 4 hours or on low for 6 to 8 hours.

To serve, taste for cumin and add more as needed. Discard the bay leaves. Serve a generous ½ cup per person.

skinny**scoop**

Alcaparrado is a mixture of olives, pimiento strips, and capers, and it is used in many Latin dishes. Pimiento-stuffed Spanish Manzanilla olives can also be used in their place.

PERFECT PAIRINGS

Serve this over brown rice with a simple cabbage salad, like my **Confetti Slaw (page 285)**, pictured on page 192, or served with tortillas to make tacos. This also makes a great filling for stuffed peppers or empanadas.

PER SERVING	(GENEROUS ½ CUP)
CALORIES	207
FAT	8.5 g
SATURATED FAT	3.5 g
CHOLESTEROL	74 mg
CARBOHYDRATE	5 g
FIBER	1 g
PROTEIN	28 g
SUGARS	3 g
SODIUM	477 mg

LEAN MEAT DISHES

Colombian Carne Asada with Ají Picante

SERVES 6

GF **Q**

Carne asada is a marinated grilled steak dish that is a beloved staple in Colombia, where my mom was born. Whenever we get together for family barbecues, this is usually on the menu. The steaks are served with *ají picante*, a popular condiment that you can make as mild or as spicy as you like. It's a fantastic complement that adds a touch of heat, freshness, and acidity, and it can be used in everything from soups and stews to steaks and empanadas.

STEAK

1½ pounds flank steak

1 teaspoon ground cumin

½ teaspoon dried oregano

½ teaspoon kosher salt

Freshly cracked black pepper

1 tablespoon olive oil

3 garlic cloves, crushed

3 scallions, cut into 1-inch lengths

¾ cup Corona Light beer

AJÍ PICANTE

2 tablespoons fresh lime juice

½ tablespoon distilled white vinegar

¼ cup finely chopped scallions

¼ cup finely chopped fresh cilantro (stems and leaves)

¼ cup seeded and finely chopped tomato

1 tablespoon finely minced fresh jalapeño or serrano pepper

¼ teaspoon plus ⅛ teaspoon kosher salt

Cooking spray or oil mister

skinny**scoop**

I never throw away the stems of the cilantro! They add so much flavor and texture to the *ají* sauce.

For the steak: Using sharp knife, lightly score the steak about ⅛ inch deep on both sides in a crisscross pattern at ½-inch intervals. Put the steak in a shallow glass baking dish.

In a small bowl, combine the cumin, oregano, salt, and a few turns of black pepper. Rub the olive oil and garlic over both sides of the steak, and then rub in the spice mix. Add the scallions and beer, turn the steak over a few times to coat both sides, cover the dish, and refrigerate for at least 3 hours, turning occasionally, or as long as overnight.

For the ají picante: In a medium jar or container with a fitted lid, combine ¼ cup water, the lime juice, vinegar, scallions, cilantro, tomato, jalapeño, and salt. Refrigerate until ready to use and up to 2 days.

(recipe continues)

PER SERVING	(3 OUNCES STEAK + 2 TABLESPOONS SAUCE)
CALORIES	208
FAT	9.5 g
SATURATED FAT	3 g
CHOLESTEROL	78 mg
CARBOHYDRATE	3 g
FIBER	0.5 g
PROTEIN	25 g
SUGARS	1 g
SODIUM	233 mg

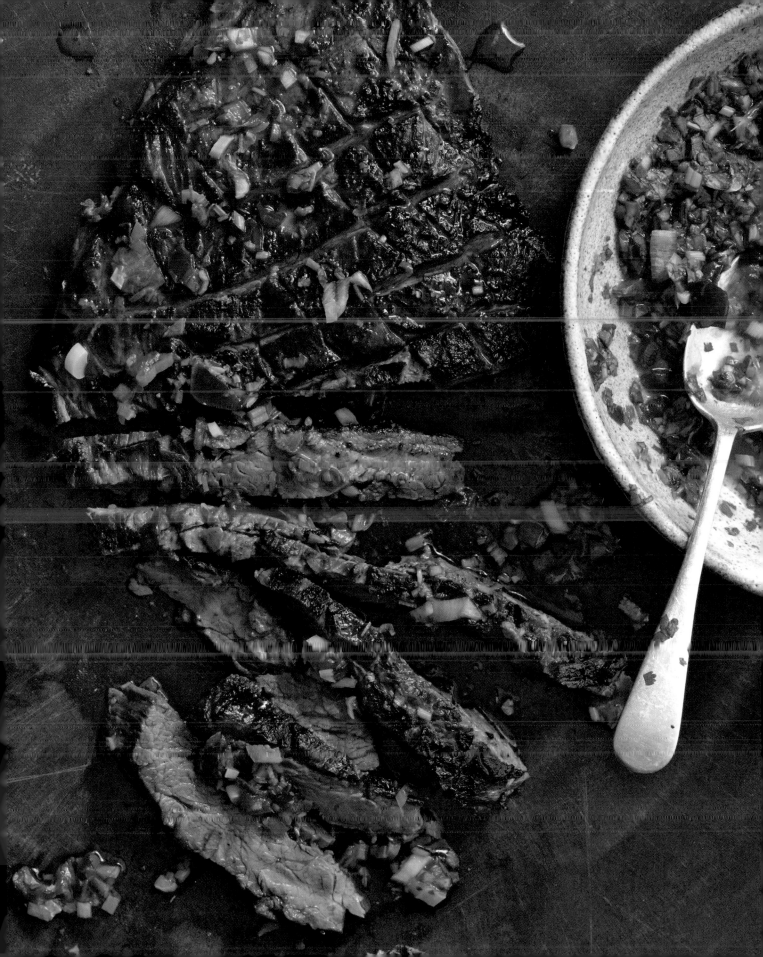

Typically, my family serves
this with small potatoes or
grilled arepas, which are
Colombian corn cakes; but
you can serve it with grilled
corn on the cob, rice, or on
top of a bed of greens to
make a steak salad. Or try it
with **Grilled Mexican Corn
Salad (page 289)**.

Preheat a grill to high.

Lightly oil the grate. Remove the steaks from the marinade,
discarding the marinade, and grill to desired doneness, 3 to
4 minutes per side for medium-rare, turning the steaks a
quarter-turn after 1½ minutes to form crisscross grill marks,
if desired. Transfer the steaks to a cutting board and let rest
5 minutes. Thinly slice the steaks across the grain. Transfer to a
platter and serve with *ají picante* on the side.

Steak Out!

You can have your meat and it eat, too—you just have to pick the leanest and healthiest types.
Here's how.

CHECK THE CUT: There are plenty of lean cuts
of meat (those containing less than 10 grams
of total fat and 4.5 grams or less saturated fat
per 3.5-ounce serving), but in general, round
and sirloin steaks are your best bet. Tenderloin
(aka filet mignon) and flank steak are also good
choices. And, of course, you can always consult
with the butcher.

MAKE THE GRADE: The three different "grades"
of beef indicate the amount of marbling or fat
the cut contains. Prime has the most fat, choice
has less, and select has the least. Choose select
and choice cuts more often than not; they're
not only lower in calories and fat, they're also
less expensive.

Slow-Cooker Mexican Pork Carnitas

SERVES 10

GF **FF** **SC**

Taco night is a weekly event in my home, and this spicy pork makes the perfect filling. Pork shoulder is often sold with the bone in. To save time, I have my butcher remove the bone for me, but you can leave it in and increase the cooking time to 10 hours. This makes enough for several dinners, so it's super economical and can be used so many different ways, from tacos to salads, or even served over rice.

2 pounds boneless pork shoulder roast, trimmed

½ teaspoon kosher salt

DRY ADOBO RUB

1¼ teaspoons ground cumin

½ teaspoon garlic powder

½ teaspoon dried oregano

½ teaspoon plus ¼ teaspoon kosher salt

¼ teaspoon ground black pepper

6 garlic cloves, crushed with a garlic press

½ cup low-sodium chicken broth*

2 bay leaves

2 chipotle peppers in adobo sauce, minced (or more if you like it spicy)

¼ teaspoon ground cumin

Read the label to be sure this product is gluten-free.

Season the pork all over with the salt. Set a large nonstick pan over medium-high heat, add the pork, and brown on all sides for about 10 minutes. Remove from the heat.

For the dry arobo rub: In a small bowl, combine 1 teaspoon of the cumin, the garlic powder, oregano, ½ teaspoon of the salt, and the black pepper.

Using a sharp paring knife, insert the knife into the pork about 1 inch deep and insert the crushed garlic, rubbing any excess over the pork. Rub the pork all over with the dry adobo rub.

Pour the chicken broth into the slow cooker and add the bay leaves, chipotle peppers, and pork. Cover and cook on low for 8 hours. After 8 hours, transfer the pork to a large dish. Discard the bay leaves. Shred the pork using two forks and return it to the slow cooker with the juices. Add the remaining ¼ teaspoon cumin and the ¼ teaspoon salt. Serve.

PERFECT PAIRINGS
Serve this pork on warmed tortillas and top with some **Confetti Slaw (page 285)**. We also like to serve it over cilantro lime rice (combine ¾ cup cooked brown rice with a squeeze of lime juice and 1 tablespoon chopped fresh cilantro).

PER SERVING	(ABOUT 3 OUNCES PORK)
CALORIES	112
FAT	3 g
SATURATED FAT	1 g
CHOLESTEROL	50 mg
CARBOHYDRATE	1 g
FIBER	0 g
PROTEIN	19 g
SUGARS	0 g
SODIUM	213 mg

LEAN
MEAT
DISHES

197

Teriyaki-Glazed Grilled Pork Chops with Pineapple Salsa

SERVES 5

GF

The homemade pineapple-teriyaki glaze is really the star of this dish. It's so good you may even want to double the recipe and keep it in your refrigerator—it's great on everything from burgers to salmon and steak! I love pork chops, but lean chops can sometimes be tricky to cook because they dry out if not cooked properly. Marinating them in pineapple juice, which is acidic, and cooking them on the grill for about 6 minutes on each side yields perfectly juicy chops. If pork isn't your thing, you can replace it with skinless chicken breasts or lean sirloin steaks instead.

PORK CHOPS

¼ cup pineapple juice

4 teaspoons reduced-sodium soy sauce (or tamari* for gluten-free)

1 large garlic clove, crushed

½ teaspoon grated fresh ginger

5 boneless pork loin chops (4 ounces each), trimmed of fat

TERIYAKI SAUCE

1 teaspoon cornstarch

3 tablespoons reduced-sodium soy sauce (or tamari* for gluten-free)

¼ cup pineapple juice

2 tablespoons dark brown sugar

½ teaspoon grated fresh ginger

1 small garlic clove, minced

PINEAPPLE SALSA

1⅓ cups fresh pineapple, cut into ½-inch cubes

1 fresh jalapeño pepper, finely chopped

2 tablespoons finely chopped red onion

1 tablespoon finely chopped fresh cilantro

Cooking spray or oil mister

Read the label to be sure this product is gluten-free.

For the pork chops: In a small bowl, combine the pineapple juice, soy sauce, garlic, and ginger. Put the pork chops in a container and pour the marinade over them. Let sit for about 30 minutes.

For the teriyaki sauce: In a small bowl, whisk together the cornstarch and 3 tablespoons cold water until dissolved. In a small saucepan, combine the soy sauce, pineapple juice, brown sugar, ginger, and garlic. Bring to a boil over medium-low heat and cook until reduced and thickened, about 4 minutes. Add

(recipe continues)

PER SERVING	(1 CHOP + ⅓ CUP SALSA)
CALORIES	214
FAT	6 g
SATURATED FAT	2 g
CHOLESTEROL	63 mg
CARBOHYDRATE	15 g
FIBER	1 g
PROTEIN	24 g
SUGARS	11 g
SODIUM	520 mg

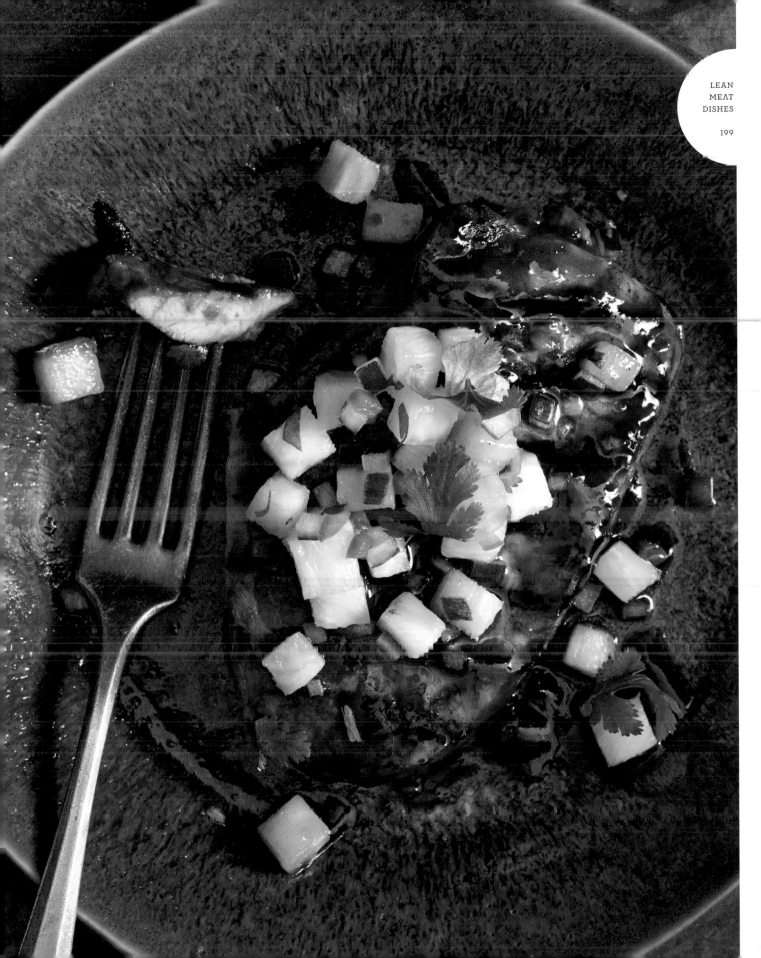

PERFECT PAIRINGS
Try this with stir-fried vegetables, **Roasted Sesame Green Beans (page 272)**, or a side of **Vegetable Fried Brown Rice (page 273)**.

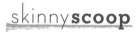

When it comes to fruit, I always prefer fresh, but if you're pressed for time, you can use precut to make the salsa. Look for pineapple that is packed in pineapple juice; you can use the juice from the can to make the marinade.

the cornstarch mixture and cook until thickened, about 2 more minutes. Remove the pan from the heat and set aside to cool.

For the pineapple salsa: In a small bowl, combine the pineapple, jalapeño, red onion, and cilantro. Set aside.

Preheat a grill to medium-high (or preheat a grill pan over medium-high heat).

Remove the chops from the marinade, discarding the marinade. Oil the grill grates or spray a grill pan with oil. Grill the chops until no longer pink, 6 to 7 minutes per side. Spoon 1 tablespoon of the teriyaki sauce over each chop in the final 30 seconds of cooking time.

To serve, put a chop on each of 5 serving dishes and top each with ⅓ cup pineapple salsa.

Skinny Salisbury Steak with Mushroom Gravy

SERVES 8

FF

The name "Salisbury steak" reminds me of frozen TV dinners from way back when, but these are nothing like those tasteless meat patties you may have grown up eating. This dish is moist and flavorful, with a delicious mushroom gravy that is wonderful over Cheesy Cauliflower "Mash."

1½ teaspoons olive oil

¾ cup finely chopped onion

1 pound 93% lean ground beef

1 pound 93% lean ground turkey

½ cup fine dried bread crumbs

1 large egg

1 large egg white

2 cups Swanson beef stock

¼ teaspoon plus ⅛ teaspoon kosher salt

⅛ teaspoon freshly ground black pepper, plus more for seasoning

2 tablespoons all-purpose flour

2 tablespoons tomato paste

1 teaspoon red wine vinegar

2 teaspoons Worcestershire sauce

½ teaspoon mustard powder

8 ounces sliced white mushrooms

2 tablespoons chopped fresh parsley, for garnish

Heat a large, deep nonstick skillet over medium heat. Add the oil and onion and cook, stirring, until golden, about 5 minutes.

In a large bowl, combine half of the cooked onion, the ground beef, ground turkey, bread crumbs, whole egg, egg white, ¼ cup of the beef stock, ¼ teaspoon of the salt, and the black pepper. Form into 8 oval patties that are about ¾ inch thick.

In a bowl, whisk together the flour and remaining 1¾ cups beef stock. Stir in ¼ cup water, the remaining cooked onion, tomato paste, vinegar, Worcestershire sauce, and mustard powder.

Wipe down the skillet and heat over medium-high heat. Working in batches so you don't overcrowd the pan, cook the patties until browned, 2 to 3 minutes per side. Transfer to a plate.

Add the mushrooms to the skillet, season with the remaining ⅛ teaspoon salt and black pepper to taste, and cook, stirring, until slightly browned, 2 to 3 minutes. Return the patties to the skillet and pour in the sauce. Reduce the heat to low, cover, and simmer, stirring occasionally, until the meat is tender, 25 minutes. Serve hot with parsley sprinkled on top.

PERFECT PAIRINGS
Try this with **Cheesy Cauliflower "Mash" (page 269)** and some steamed corn or peas on the side.

PER SERVING	(1 STEAK + ⅓ CUP GRAVY)
CALORIES	245
FAT	11 g
SATURATED FAT	3.5 g
CHOLESTEROL	100 mg
CARBOHYDRATE	10 g
FIBER	8.5 g
PROTEIN	26 g
SUGARS	3 g
SODIUM	339 mg

LEAN MEAT DISHES

201

Grilled Lamb Chops with Mint Yogurt Sauce

SERVES 4

GF **Q**

Lamb loin chops are perfect for weeknight meals because they take less than 15 minutes to cook. They're also a lot less expensive than lamb rib chops and they're much leaner if trimmed—it's a win-win! Mint and lamb are a perfect combination, so this yogurt sauce makes a great complement to the meat. I like to marinate the chops for a few hours prior to cooking and prepare the yogurt sauce ahead of time to let the flavors settle. Don't worry if you don't have the time—it will still taste great.

MINT YOGURT SAUCE

¾ cup 1% Greek yogurt

1 teaspoon extra-virgin olive oil

1 teaspoon fresh lemon juice

2 tablespoons finely chopped fresh mint

1½ tablespoons finely chopped fresh chives

½ teaspoon kosher salt

Freshly cracked black pepper

LAMB CHOPS

8 lamb loin chops (3½ ounces each), fat trimmed

1 teaspoon kosher salt

½ teaspoon freshly ground black pepper

2 tablespoons fresh lemon juice

4 garlic cloves, crushed

1 tablespoon fresh rosemary

½ teaspoon dried oregano

Cooking spray or oil mister

PERFECT PAIRINGS
This pairs perfectly with the **Roasted Winter Beets and Red Potatoes (page 279)**.

For the mint yogurt sauce: In a medium bowl, combine the yogurt, olive oil, lemon juice, mint, chives, salt, and black pepper to taste. Cover and refrigerate a few hours to let the flavors develop.

For the lamb chops: Season both sides of the lamb chops with the salt and black pepper to taste. Place the chops in a large bowl and pour the lemon juice over them. Add the garlic, rosemary, and oregano. Cover with plastic wrap and marinate at room temperature for 1 hour, or as long as overnight in the refrigerator.

Preheat a grill to medium-high (or preheat a grill pan over medium-high heat). Oil the grill grates or spray the grill pan with oil. Grill the chops until a thermometer inserted in the side of each chop registers 145°F for medium-rare or higher to your taste, 4 to 6 minutes on each side.

Serve the lamb chops with the mint yogurt sauce on the side.

PER SERVING	(2 CHOPS + 3½ TABLESPOONS SAUCE)
CALORIES	248
FAT	10 g
SATURATED FAT	4 g
CHOLESTEROL	91 mg
CARBOHYDRATE	3 g
FIBER	0 g
PROTEIN	34 g
SUGARS	1 g
SODIUM	541 mg

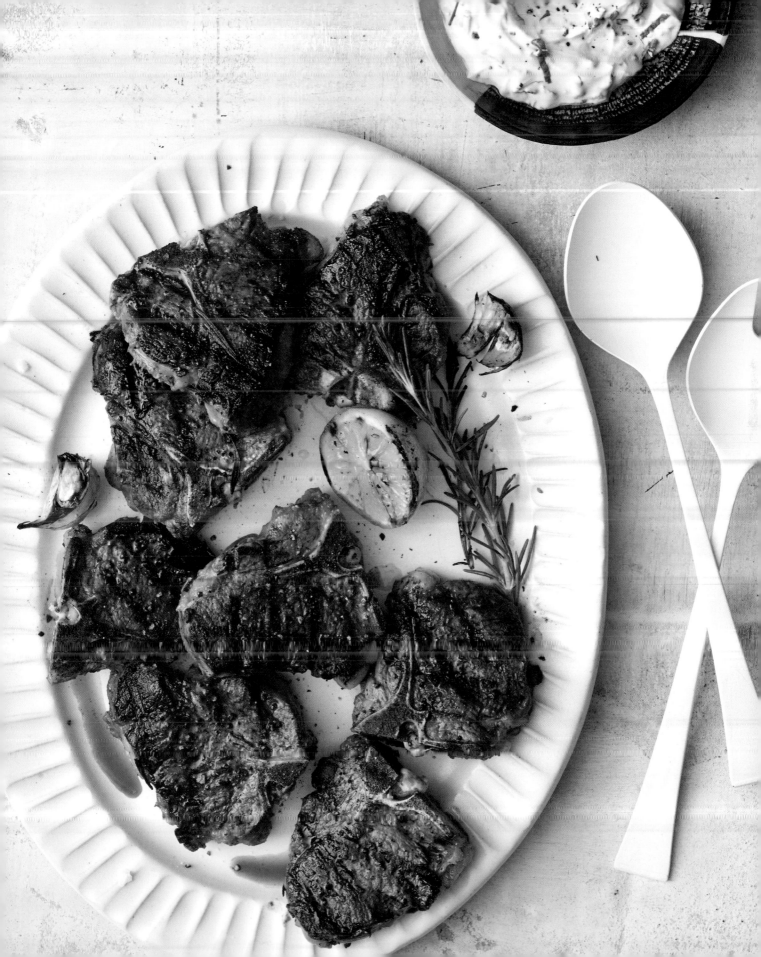

FOOD FACTS
score a point for pork
Pork tenderloin is just as
lean as a skinless chicken
breast, and it's also the most
tender cut. Just be sure not to
overcook it or you'll dry it out.

Cubano-Style Stuffed Pork Tenderloin

SERVES 4

GF

When I was in my early twenties I discovered a Cuban luncheonette in Queens called El Sitio that made the *best* Cubano sandwiches! Although it's been years since my last visit, a craving for that sandwich still arises. Inspired by that sandwich, this pork dish is my Cubano skinny solution.

PORK

1 pound pork tenderloin

1 tablespoon yellow mustard

2 ounces thinly sliced deli ham*

2 ounces reduced-fat Swiss cheese, sliced

2 thin slices dill pickle, about 4 inches long, patted dry

1 teaspoon olive oil

DRY RUB

1 teaspoon dark brown sugar

¾ teaspoon kosher salt

1 teaspoon garlic powder

½ teaspoon chili powder*

½ teaspoon ground cumin

¼ teaspoon dried oregano

⅛ teaspoon freshly ground black pepper

Read the label to be sure this product is gluten-free.

Preheat the oven to 425°F.

For the pork: Cut a lengthwise slit down the center of the tenderloin to within ½ inch of the bottom and open the tenderloin so it lies flat. On each half, make another lengthwise slit down the center to within ½ inch of the bottom and open it up. Wrap with plastic wrap. Pound with a mallet until ¼-inch thick. Remove the plastic wrap and spread the mustard on one side. Layer the ham on the mustard, and lay the Swiss cheese and pickles along the center of the pork. Starting with a long side, roll the pork up jelly-roll style. Tie the roast at 1½- to 2-inch intervals with kitchen string. Rub with the olive oil.

For the dry rub: In a medium bowl, combine the brown sugar, salt, garlic powder, chili powder, cumin, oregano, and black pepper. Rub the mixture over the pork, discarding any excess. Put the pork in a shallow baking dish.

Roast until a thermometer inserted in the pork registers 160°F, about 35 minutes. Transfer to a cutting board. Let rest 10 minutes before removing the string and slicing into 8 pieces.

PERFECT PAIRINGS
The Latina in me likes to serve this with rice, but a great big salad on the side is also perfect. Try **My House Salad, Made with Love (page 267)**.

PER SERVING	(2 SLICES)
CALORIES	185
FAT	5 g
SATURATED FAT	1.5 g
CHOLESTEROL	85 mg
CARBOHYDRATE	3 g
FIBER	0.5 g
PROTEIN	31 g
SUGARS	1 g
SODIUM	537 mg

LEAN MEAT DISHES

Grilled Lamb Skewers with Harissa Dipping Sauce

MAKES 12 SKEWERS • SERVES 6

GF **Q**

If I'm throwing a backyard party, I like to grill all kinds of different skewers and let everyone dig in. There's something fun and casual about forgoing forks and eating food right off a stick. These lamb skewers are a favorite for their exotic flavors and spicy harissa dipping sauce. Harissa is a traditional accompaniment to Moroccan and North African food. In a pinch, you can purchase jarred harissa, but making it yourself gives you complete control over how spicy you want it. Leftovers can be refrigerated and used on everything from eggs and burgers to couscous and soups.

LAMB

1½ pounds trimmed boneless leg of lamb, cut into 1-inch cubes

½ tablespoon olive oil

3 garlic cloves, crushed

1 tablespoon finely chopped fresh cilantro

2¼ teaspoons ground cumin

½ teaspoon sweet paprika

¾ teaspoon kosher salt

12 wooden skewers, soaked in water for 30 minutes

1 medium red onion, quartered and layers separated

HARISSA

1 tablespoon olive oil

2 large garlic cloves, peeled

1 (12-ounce) jar roasted peppers in water, drained

1 teaspoon fresh lemon juice

1½ teaspoons kosher salt

1 teaspoon crushed red pepper flakes (or to taste)

½ teaspoon ground coriander

½ teaspoon ground cumin

½ teaspoon sweet paprika

PERFECT PAIRINGS
Serve this with a Persian salad (see recipe in **Naked Persian Turkey Burgers [page 156]**) or try this with my **Quinoa Tabbouleh (page 287)**.

PER SERVING	(2 SKEWERS + 2½ TABLESPOONS HARISSA)
CALORIES	205
FAT	10 g
SATURATED FAT	3 g
CHOLESTEROL	71 mg
CARBOHYDRATE	4 g
FIBER	0 g
PROTEIN	24 g
SUGARS	2 g
SODIUM	721 mg

For the lamb: Place the lamb in a bowl and rub it with the olive oil, garlic, and cilantro. In a small bowl, combine the cumin, paprika, and salt and rub the mixture on the lamb. Marinate for 3 to 4 hours. Thread the lamb onto the skewers, 3 to 4 per skewer, with onion slices in between.

For the harissa: In a small skillet, heat the oil over medium heat. Add the garlic and cook, stirring, until golden and fragrant, 1 to 2 minutes. Transfer the garlic to a blender and add the roasted red peppers, lemon juice, salt, pepper flakes, coriander, cumin, and paprika. Blend until smooth.

Preheat a grill to high (or preheat a grill pan over high heat).

Grill the skewers 3 to 4 minutes per side. Transfer to a serving platter and serve with the harissa on the side.

skinny*scoop*

If you're not a fan of lamb, replace it with chicken breast or beef. To make a speedy harissa, I use jarred roasted peppers packed in water. If you want to roast the peppers yourself, use 2 red bell peppers, seeded and peeled after roasting (see page 233).

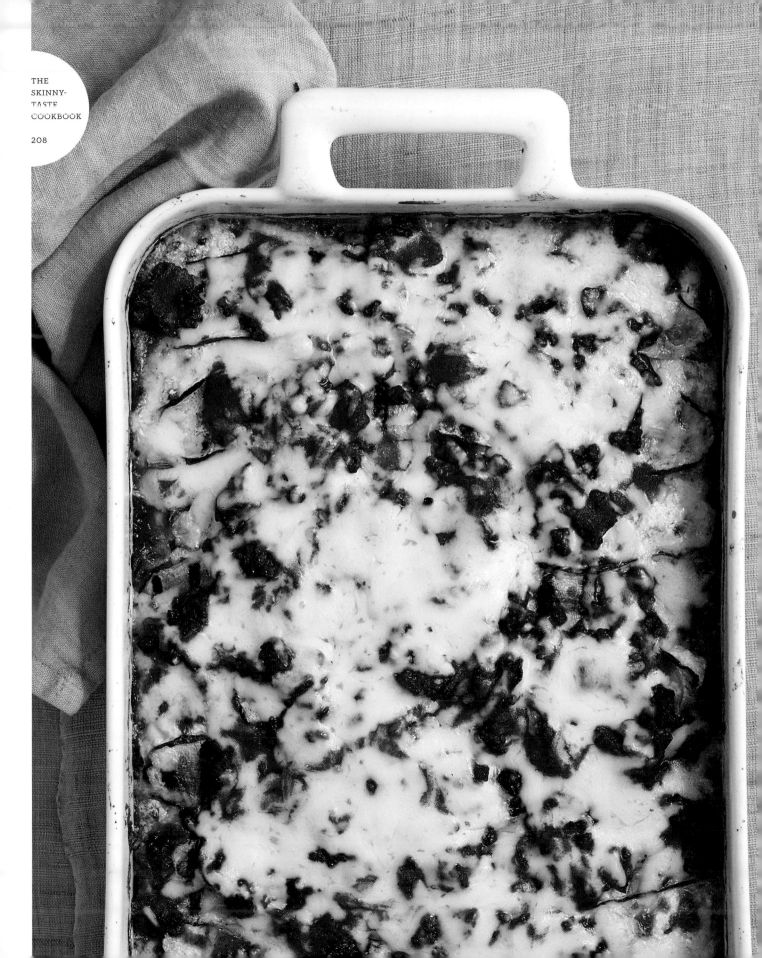

Noodle-less Zucchini Lasagna

SERVES 8

(GF) (FF)

Thinly sliced zucchini ribbons replace pasta in this delicious, low-carb, noodle-less dish. This lasagna totally satisfies my cravings for cheesy and indulgent Italian comfort food. It's perfect in the summer when I have tons of garden-fresh zucchini and herbs, but I also love making it during the colder months when I want something hot and comforting. Although it takes a little longer than most of my recipes, it's totally worth it!

1 pound 93% lean ground beef

1¼ teaspoons kosher salt

1 teaspoon olive oil

½ large onion, chopped

3 garlic cloves, minced

1 (28-ounce) can crushed tomatoes

2 tablespoons chopped fresh basil

Freshly ground black pepper

3 medium zucchini

Cooking spray or oil mister

1½ cups part-skim ricotta cheese

¼ cup grated Parmigiano-Reggiano cheese

1 large egg

4 cups shredded part-skim mozzarella cheese (16 ounces)

Heat a large, deep nonstick skillet over high heat. Add the meat, season with ½ teaspoon of the salt, and cook, using a wooden spoon to break the meat into small pieces as it browns, 4 to 5 minutes. Drain the meat in a colander and wipe the skillet with a paper towel.

Put the skillet over medium heat. Add the olive oil and onion and cook, stirring, until soft, 3 to 4 minutes. Add the garlic and cook 1 minute. Return the meat to the pan, add the tomatoes, basil, ¼ teaspoon of the salt, and the black pepper to taste. Reduce the heat to low, cover, and simmer, stirring occasionally, 25 minutes. Remove the lid and simmer uncovered 10 minutes, until thickened.

Meanwhile, slice the zucchini lengthwise with a mandoline into ⅛-inch-thick slices (you should have at least 30 to 35 long zucchini ribbons). Lightly salt the zucchini with the remaining ½ teaspoon salt and set aside for 15 minutes. Blot the zucchini with paper towels.

(recipe continues)

PER SERVING	(1 PIECE)
CALORIES	275
FAT	13 g
SATURATED FAT	7 g
CHOLESTEROL	84 mg
CARBOHYDRATE	13 g
FIBER	2.5 g
PROTEIN	26 g
SUGARS	5 g
SODIUM	648 mg

LEAN MEAT DISHES

Preheat a grill to medium heat (or preheat a grill pan over medium heat).

Oil the grill grates or spray the grill pan with cooking spray to avoid sticking. Grill the zucchini until cooked and slightly browned, 2 to 3 minutes on each side. Transfer to a plate lined with paper towels and press to absorb excess moisture.

Preheat the oven to 375°F.

In a medium bowl, combine the ricotta, Parmesan, and egg.

Spread ½ cup of the meat sauce in the bottom of a 9 × 13 × 2½-inch baking dish. Make a layer of the zucchini over the sauce to cover the bottom of the dish. Spread ½ cup of the ricotta mixture over the zucchini and sprinkle with 1 cup of the mozzarella. Make another layer of zucchini, top with 1½ cups meat sauce, ½ cup ricotta mixture, 1 cup mozzarella. Repeat the layers with the remaining ingredients for a total of 3 layers. Finish the lasagna by topping with the remaining zucchini and meat sauce. Cover the dish with foil.

Bake for 30 minutes, remove the foil, and bake 20 minutes uncovered. Add the remaining 1 cup mozzarella and bake uncovered until bubbling and the cheese is melted, 10 more minutes. Let stand for 5 to 10 minutes before cutting into 8 pieces.

Sunday Night Roast Beef and Gravy

SERVES 10

When it comes to roast beef, I have pretty big shoes to fill—my mom's was the best. The key to making perfect roast beef is to use a meat thermometer, so there's no guessing if it's cooked to your liking. I like mine a little on the rare side, so I take it out when the thermometer reads 135°F.

2½ pounds beef eye of round roast or top round roast, all fat trimmed off

Cooking spray or oil mister

3 garlic cloves, sliced into very thin slivers

¼ teaspoon kosher salt, plus more as needed

1 tablespoon Dijon mustard

½ teaspoon dried rosemary

¼ teaspoon freshly cracked pepper, plus more as needed

2 tablespoons all-purpose flour

2 cups Swanson beef stock

Remove the roast from the refrigerator about 1 hour before cooking to reach room temperature.

Preheat the oven to 500°F. Lightly spray a roasting pan with oil.

Using a sharp knife, pierce holes in the roast about ½ inch deep and insert slivers of garlic in each. Season with ¼ teaspoon of the salt, rub the mustard all over the roast, and sprinkle with the rosemary and pepper. Put the roast in the roasting pan.

Roast for 20 minutes. Reduce the oven temperature to 250°F and roast until a thermometer registers 135°F for rare, 140°F for medium-rare, 150°F for medium, and 155° to 160°F for well-done, about 1 hour 15 minutes or longer. Remove the roast from the oven and let rest 10 to 15 minutes. (The temperature will rise an additional 5° to 10°F as it sits.)

In a small saucepan, whisk together the flour and beef stock. Bring to a boil over medium heat and cook, whisking occasionally, until thickened, about 1 minute. Pour the pan drippings into the gravy and continue to cook, whisking, for 1 minute. Add a pinch of salt and black pepper to taste, if needed.

Using a good sharp carving knife, thinly slice the roast and serve with gravy.

PERFECT PAIRING
This dish works well with **Cheesy Cauliflower "Mash" (page 269)** and sautéed vegetables on the side. Try any leftovers in **Roast Beef Sandwiches with Creamy Horseradish Spread (page 81)** or in a **Roast Beef and Watercress Pasta Salad (page 144)**.

PER SERVING	(3 OUNCES BEEF + 3 TABLESPOONS GRAVY)
CALORIES	197
FAT	6 g
SATURATED FAT	2 g
CHOLESTEROL	87 mg
CARBOHYDRATE	2 g
FIBER	0 g
PROTEIN	33 g
SUGARS	0 g
SODIUM	291 mg

LEAN MEAT DISHES

211

FABULOUS FISH

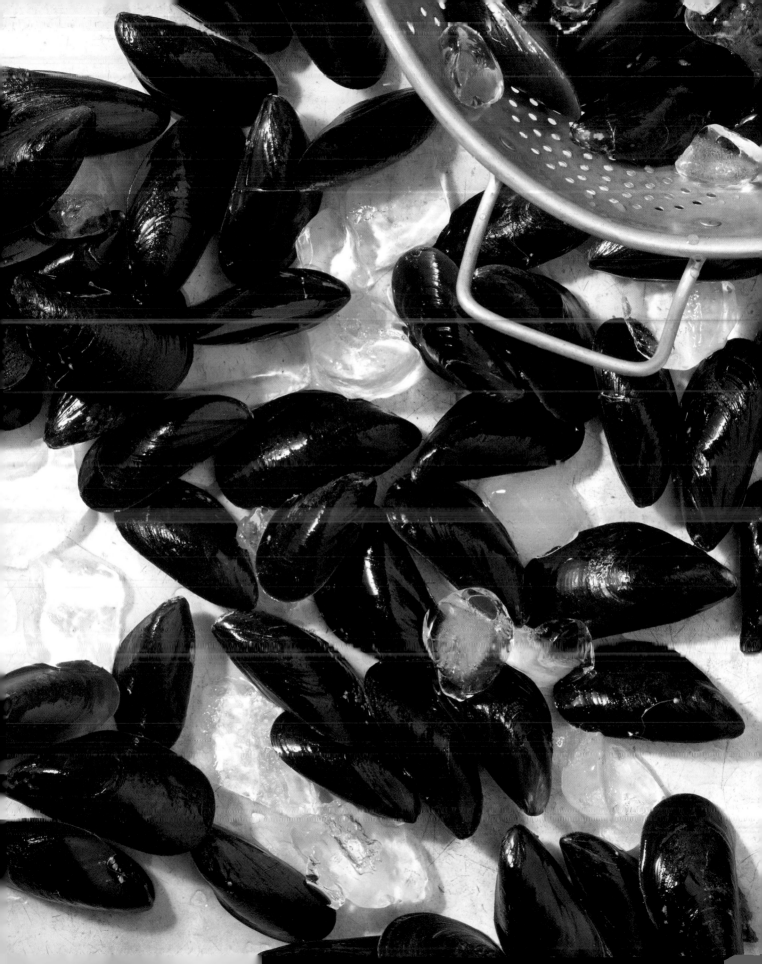

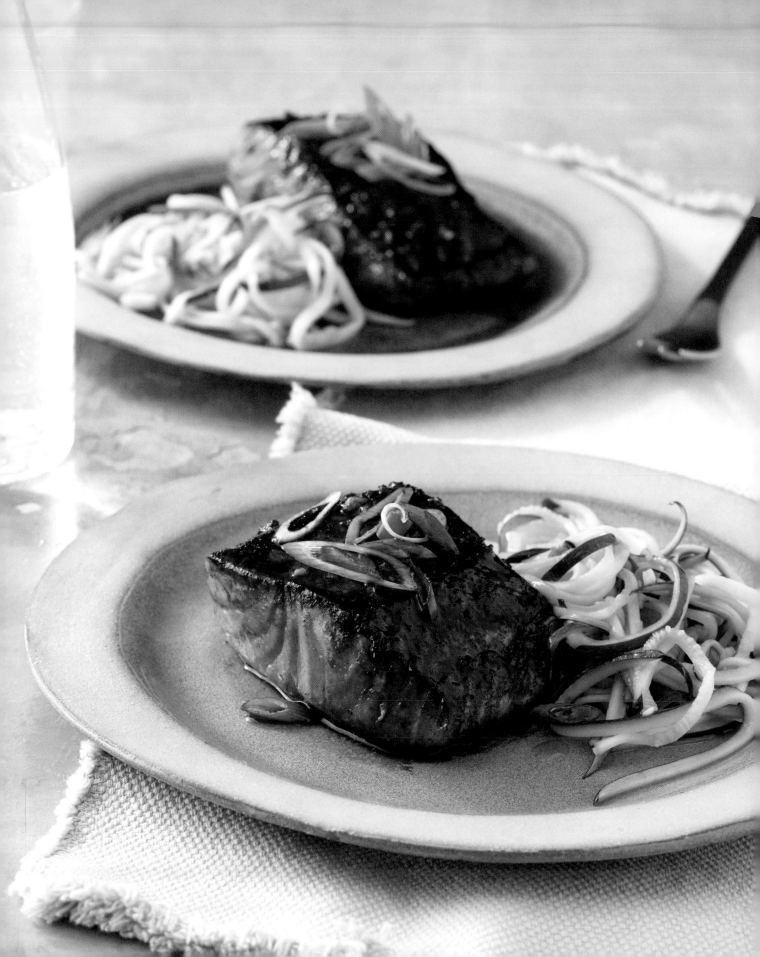

Sweet 'n' Spicy Sriracha-Glazed Salmon

SERVES 4

GF Q

This is one of my favorite ways to prepare salmon. The marinade in this recipe is the perfect combination of spicy, sweet, and savory—in fact, I also love to use it with steaks or chicken. The Sriracha sauce (aka rooster sauce) is a must, and you can find it in the Asian section of most supermarkets.

¼ cup reduced-sodium soy sauce (or tamari* for gluten-free)

2 tablespoons honey

1 tablespoon rice vinegar

1 tablespoon Sriracha sauce (or to taste)

1 tablespoon grated fresh ginger

1 tablespoon minced garlic

1 pound wild salmon fillet, cut into 4 (4-ounce) pieces

1½ teaspoons sesame oil

2 tablespoons finely chopped scallions, for garnish

*Read the label to be sure this product is gluten-free.

In a 1-gallon zip-top plastic bag, combine the soy sauce, honey, vinegar, Sriracha, ginger, and garlic. Add the salmon, toss to coat evenly, and refrigerate for at least 1 hour, or up to 8 hours, turning the fish once.

Remove the salmon from the bag, reserving the marinade. Heat a large sauté pan over medium high heat and add the sesame oil. Rotate the pan to coat the bottom evenly and add the salmon. Cook until one side of the fish is browned, about 2 minutes. Flip the salmon and cook until the other side browns, 2 more minutes. Reduce the heat to low and pour in the reserved marinade. Cover and cook until the fish is cooked through, 4 to 5 minutes.

Place a piece of salmon on each of 4 serving plates and sprinkle with the scallions.

PERFECT PAIRINGS

This is perfect served over brown rice with **Roasted Sesame Green Beans (page 272)**. For a fantastic, quick, low-carb option, I make zucchini noodles. Use a spiralizer or mandoline fitted with a julienne blade to cut the zucchini into spaghetti-like strands, then sauté them with a little sesame oil and garlic for 2 minutes.

PER SERVING	(1 PIECE)
CALORIES	229
FAT	8.5 g
SATURATED FAT	1.5 g
CHOLESTEROL	51 mg
CARBOHYDRATE	12 g
FIBER	0.5 g
PROTEIN	26 g
SUGARS	9 g
SODIUM	587 mg

Easy Broccolini Flounder Bake

SERVES 4

GF **Q**

A meal that takes 20 minutes to make—start to finish—sounds pretty appetizing, right? This simple cooking method is a favorite of mine for fish: I basically sauté some vegetables, season my fish, layer it all in a baking dish, bake, and voilà, dinner is ready! Flounder is a great choice for picky palates because it has a very mild taste, but you can use any fresh whitefish that's available in your area.

Cooking spray or oil mister

1 bunch broccolini (6 ounces)

3 teaspoons extra-virgin olive oil

Kosher salt

¾ cup halved cherry tomatoes

2 garlic cloves, minced

Pinch of crushed red pepper flakes

4 flounder fillets (about 4 ounces each)

Freshly ground black pepper

2 tablespoons fresh lemon juice

1 teaspoon chopped fresh oregano

2 tablespoons freshly grated Parmigiano-Reggiano cheese

skinny scoop

When you buy fish, ask your fishmonger what's freshest. I always use my nose to test its freshness. It shouldn't smell fishy; it should smell like the ocean. If you press the flesh of the meat with your finger (or ask the fishmonger to do so), the meat should spring back. If your finger leaves an indent, leave it at the store.

Preheat the oven to 450°F. Lightly spray a 9 × 13-inch baking dish with oil.

Trim 1 inch off the stems of the broccolini and halve the stalks lengthwise. Heat a large nonstick skillet over medium heat. Add 2 teaspoons of the olive oil, then add the broccolini. Season with ⅛ teaspoon salt and cook, stirring occasionally, until crisp-tender, about 4 minutes. Add the tomatoes and a pinch of salt and cook 1 minute. Add the garlic and pepper flakes and cook 1 more minute.

Season the flounder with ¼ teaspoon salt and black pepper, to taste. Put the fish in the prepared baking dish and drizzle with the remaining 1 teaspoon oil and the lemon juice, and sprinkle with the oregano.

Bake until the fish is partly cooked, about 5 minutes. Remove the baking dish from the oven, top the fish with the broccolini and Parmesan, and return the dish to the oven. Bake until the fish is cooked through and opaque, about 10 more minutes. Serve hot.

PER SERVING	(1 FILLET WITH ½ CUP VEGETABLES)
CALORIES	166
FAT	6 g
SATURATED FAT	1.5 g
CHOLESTEROL	58 mg
CARBOHYDRATE	4 g
FIBER	1.5 g
PROTEIN	23 g
SUGARS	1 g
SODIUM	228 mg

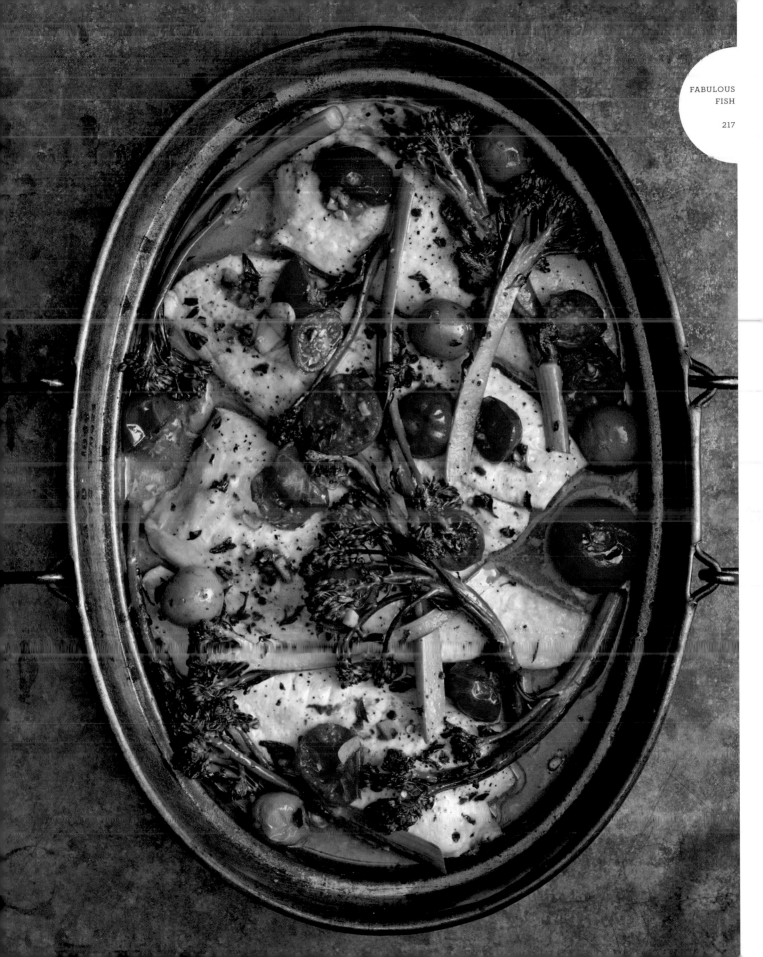

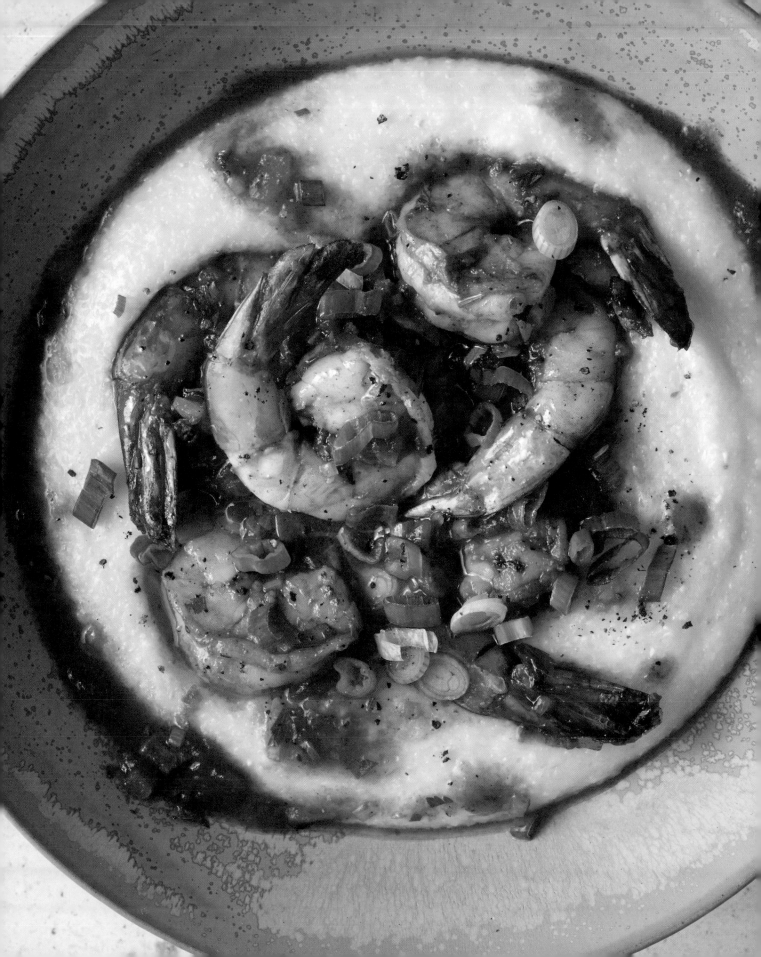

Kiss My (Shrimp and) Grits

SERVES 4

GF **Q**

The first time I had shrimp and grits was at the Sou'Wester restaurant at the stunning Mandarin Oriental hotel in DC, and it was love at first bite. It reminded me of creamy Italian polenta, only with a Southern twist. To give grits a lighter touch while keeping them creamy—with that wonderful cheese flavor (because, after all, that's what makes them so darn delicious)—I slowly simmer the grits in both fat-free milk and chicken broth. At the very end, I stir in some Havarti and pecorino cheese (a naturally low-fat cheese that packs a lot of flavor).

GRITS

2 cups reduced-sodium chicken broth*

1¼ cups fat-free milk

1 teaspoon kosher salt

1 cup quick-cooking grits (not instant)

½ tablespoon unsalted butter

1 ounce Havarti cheese, shredded (⅓ cup)

1 tablespoon grated Pecorino Romano cheese

SHRIMP

24 (about 1 pound) peeled and deveined jumbo shrimp

1 teaspoon Old Bay seasoning

1½ teaspoons olive oil

2 ounces lean smoked ham steak, finely chopped

¼ cup minced shallots

½ cup canned fire-roasted diced tomatoes with green chiles, drained (I recommend Muir Glen)

⅔ cup reduced-sodium chicken broth*

1 bay leaf

Freshly ground black pepper

1 tablespoon chopped fresh parsley

1 lemon wedge

3 tablespoons sliced scallions, for garnish

Read the label to be sure this product is gluten-free.

For the grits: In a medium pot, combine ¼ cup water, the chicken broth, milk, and salt and bring to a boil over medium heat. Slowly stir in the grits. Return to a boil, reduce the heat to the lowest setting, cover with a fitted lid, and simmer, stirring every 5 minutes or so to prevent the grits from sticking to the bottom, adding more water if necessary, until smooth like cream of wheat, 28 to 30 minutes. Stir in the butter and cheeses, remove the pan from the heat, and keep warm.

(recipe continues)

PER SERVING	(1 CUP GRITS + 6 SHRIMP AND SAUCE)
CALORIES	311
FAT	8 g
SATURATED FAT	3.5 g
CHOLESTEROL	85 mg
CARBOHYDRATE	39 g
FIBER	2.5 g
PROTEIN	22 g
SUGARS	6 g
SODIUM	756 mg

For the shrimp: Sprinkle the shrimp with the Old Bay. Heat a large sauté pan over high heat. Add 1 teaspoon of the olive oil and the shrimp and cook until browned, about 1 minute. Flip the shrimp and cook 1 more minute or until opaque. Transfer the shrimp to a plate.

Reduce the heat to medium-low and add the remaining ½ teaspoon oil and the ham. Cook until slightly browned, 3 to 4 minutes. Add the shallots and cook, stirring, until golden, 2 to 3 minutes. Add the drained tomatoes, chicken broth, bay leaf, and black pepper to taste. Increase the heat to medium and simmer until the sauce thickens and reduces slightly, 8 to 10 minutes. Remove the pan from the heat, add the shrimp and parsley, and finish with a squeeze of lemon juice. Stir well and discard the bay leaf.

Divide the grits among 4 serving plates and spoon the shrimp and sauce over the top of each. Sprinkle with the scallions and serve.

Skillet Lemon Sole with Tomatoes and Capers

SERVES 4

GF **Q**

When my mom prepared fish when I was a kid, she would bread and fry it nine times out of ten, probably because my father liked it that way. For those of you who think that's the only way fish tastes good, I'm here to tell you there are better ways! Poaching fish in a flavorful tomato broth with white wine and lemon and capers is my favorite method. It becomes juicy and flavorful, and is ready in less than 15 minutes. Even my youngest loves to eat fish this way—I just tell her it's chicken (wink, wink!).

2 teaspoons extra-virgin olive oil

2 garlic cloves, crushed

2½ cups chopped fresh tomatoes or no-salt-added canned petite diced tomatoes

¼ cup dry white wine

1 teaspoon herbes de Provence (or dried thyme)

1⅛ teaspoons kosher salt

Freshly ground black pepper

1 teaspoon fresh lemon juice

3 tablespoons capers, drained

4 fillets lemon sole (5 ounces each)

Heat a large, deep nonstick skillet over medium heat. Add the oil and garlic and cook, stirring, until golden, about 1 minute. Add the tomatoes, wine, herbes de Provence, ¾ teaspoon of the salt, and black pepper to taste. Cook until the wine reduces, 2 to 3 minutes. Add the lemon juice and capers. Lay the fish on top, season with the remaining ⅛ teaspoon salt and a pinch of black pepper, and cover; reduce the heat to medium-low and cook until the fish is opaque and flakes easily, about 10 minutes.

To serve, put a piece of fish on each of 4 serving plates and spoon the sauce on top.

PERFECT PAIRING
Summer Pearl Couscous (page 288) or **Lemon Roasted Asparagus (page 278)** would make the perfect side dish.

skinny**scoop**

Lemon sole is a flaky, whitefish found in the Atlantic. Despite its name, it does not taste like lemons at all, but it has a mild flavor with delicate, white flesh. If you can't find it, use any whitefish, including Pacific sole or Atlantic flounder. Garden tomatoes or canned tomatoes both work fine. If you want to add a little heat, you can add a pinch of crushed red pepper flakes.

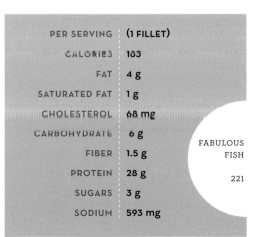

PER SERVING	(1 FILLET)
CALORIES	183
FAT	4 g
SATURATED FAT	1 g
CHOLESTEROL	68 mg
CARBOHYDRATE	6 g
FIBER	1.5 g
PROTEIN	28 g
SUGARS	3 g
SODIUM	593 mg

FABULOUS FISH

221

Mahi Mahi Fish Tacos with Spicy Avocado Cream

SERVES 5

GF **Q**

Fish tacos are the perfect summer dish, whether you're whipping them up for a quick weeknight dinner with the family or having some friends over for a casual meal after a long day at the beach. But rather than the battered, deep-fried versions you find at most taco stands, these delicious ones are gently poached in a flavorful combination of tomatoes, green chiles, cumin, garlic, and lime juice. I serve it with warmed corn tortillas, cabbage infused with cilantro and lime, and a spicy avocado cream sauce.

SLAW

2 cups shredded red cabbage

1 tablespoon roughly chopped fresh cilantro

2 tablespoons fresh lime juice

⅛ teaspoon kosher salt

AVOCADO CREAM

2 tablespoons reduced-fat sour cream

½ tablespoon fresh lime juice

½ medium (2 ounces) Hass avocado, chopped

½ small fresh jalapeño pepper, seeded

1 tablespoon chopped fresh cilantro

⅛ teaspoon kosher salt

Freshly ground black pepper

FISH

1 teaspoon olive oil

1 small onion, chopped

4 garlic cloves, minced

1 (10-ounce) can Ro*tel mild tomatoes, drained

1 (4.25-ounce) can diced green chiles

1 tablespoon chopped fresh cilantro

½ teaspoon ground cumin

½ teaspoon kosher salt

Freshly ground black pepper

1 pound mahi mahi fillet

½ lime

10 Mission white extra thin corn tortillas

For the slaw: In a large bowl, combine the cabbage, cilantro, lime juice, and salt. Toss well and set aside.

For the avocado cream: In a blender, combine 2 tablespoons water, the sour cream, lime juice, avocado, jalapeño, cilantro, salt, and black pepper to taste. Blend until smooth.

(recipe continues)

PER SERVING	(2 TACOS)
CALORIES	298
FAT	13 g
SATURATED FAT	4 g
CHOLESTEROL	47 mg
CARBOHYDRATE	23 g
FIBER	5 g
PROTEIN	20 g
SUGARS	5 g
SODIUM	577 mg

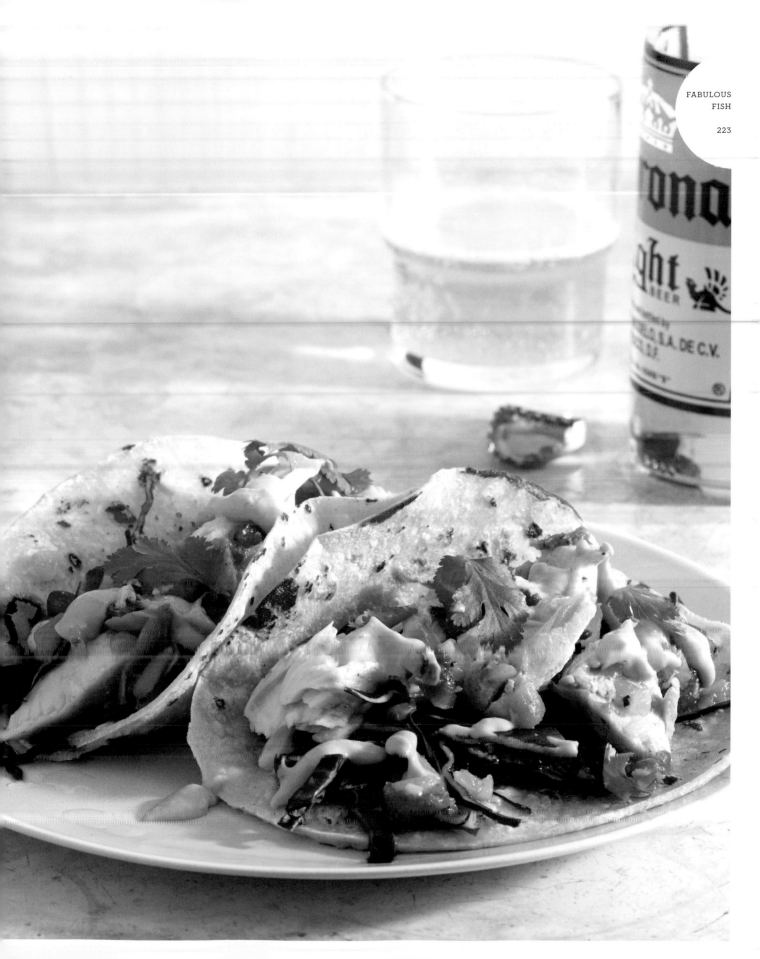

For the fish: In a large nonstick skillet, heat the olive oil over medium-high heat. Add the onion and cook, stirring, until translucent, 2 to 3 minutes. Add the garlic and cook until fragrant, about 1 minute. Add the tomatoes, chiles, cilantro, cumin, salt, and black pepper to taste. Cook for 1 minute. If it seems too dry, add about 3 tablespoons water. Reduce the heat to medium and put the mahi mahi in the skillet. Cover and cook until the fish is opaque in the center and flakes easily, 6 to 7 minutes. Using a wooden spoon, break up the fish and mix it into the tomatoes. Squeeze the lime over the fish.

To serve, heat the tortillas in a hot skillet set over high heat, 30 to 40 seconds on each side. Fill each tortilla with about ⅓ cup fish, top with about 3 tablespoons slaw, and drizzle with 1 tablespoon avocado cream.

Cilantro-Lime Shrimp

SERVES 6

GF **Q**

I find it hard to believe that there are people who don't like cilantro (Julia Child hated it!). The herb is a staple in my kitchen, and I love the flavor it adds to just about anything. If you're one of those people who detest cilantro, you can simply leave it out or replace it with another fresh herb, such as chives or parsley. Shrimp is another one of my kitchen staples—I always keep some stashed in my freezer for those nights when I don't plan ahead. It's the perfect go-to "skinny" protein when I need a quick, light meal.

1½ pounds peeled and deveined jumbo shrimp

¼ teaspoon plus ⅛ teaspoon ground cumin

¼ teaspoon kosher salt

Freshly ground black pepper

2 teaspoons extra-virgin olive oil

5 garlic cloves, crushed

2 tablespoons lime juice (from 1 medium lime)

3 to 4 tablespoons chopped fresh cilantro

Season the shrimp with the cumin, salt, and black pepper to taste.

Heat a large nonstick skillet over medium-high heat. Add 1 teaspoon of the oil to the pan, then add half of the shrimp. Cook them undisturbed for about 2 minutes. Turn the shrimp over and cook until opaque throughout, about 1 minute. Transfer to a plate. Add the remaining 1 teaspoon oil and the remaining shrimp to the pan and cook, undisturbed, for about 2 minutes. Turn the shrimp over, add the garlic, and cook until the shrimp is opaque throughout, about 1 minute. Return the first batch of shrimp to the skillet, mix well so that the garlic is evenly incorporated, and remove the pan from the heat.

Squeeze the lime juice over all the shrimp. Add the cilantro, toss well, and serve.

FOOD FACTS cilantro: why you should learn to love it
People all over the world have been using cilantro for more than 3,000 years to boost health and ward off diseases, from diabetes to depression to high blood pressure. According to studies, the plant's powers likely come from its antioxidants (including flavonoids and polyphenols) and its essential oils.

PERFECT PAIRING
I usually serve this over rice or turn it into a big salad with sliced avocado. It's also delicious as weeknight shrimp tacos: Simply serve it with warmed corn tortillas and shredded cabbage.

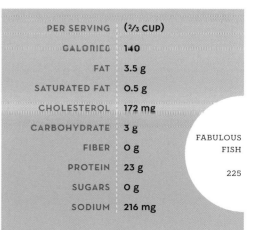

PER SERVING	(⅔ CUP)
CALORIES	140
FAT	3.5 g
SATURATED FAT	0.5 g
CHOLESTEROL	172 mg
CARBOHYDRATE	3 g
FIBER	0 g
PROTEIN	23 g
SUGARS	0 g
SODIUM	216 mg

FABULOUS FISH

225

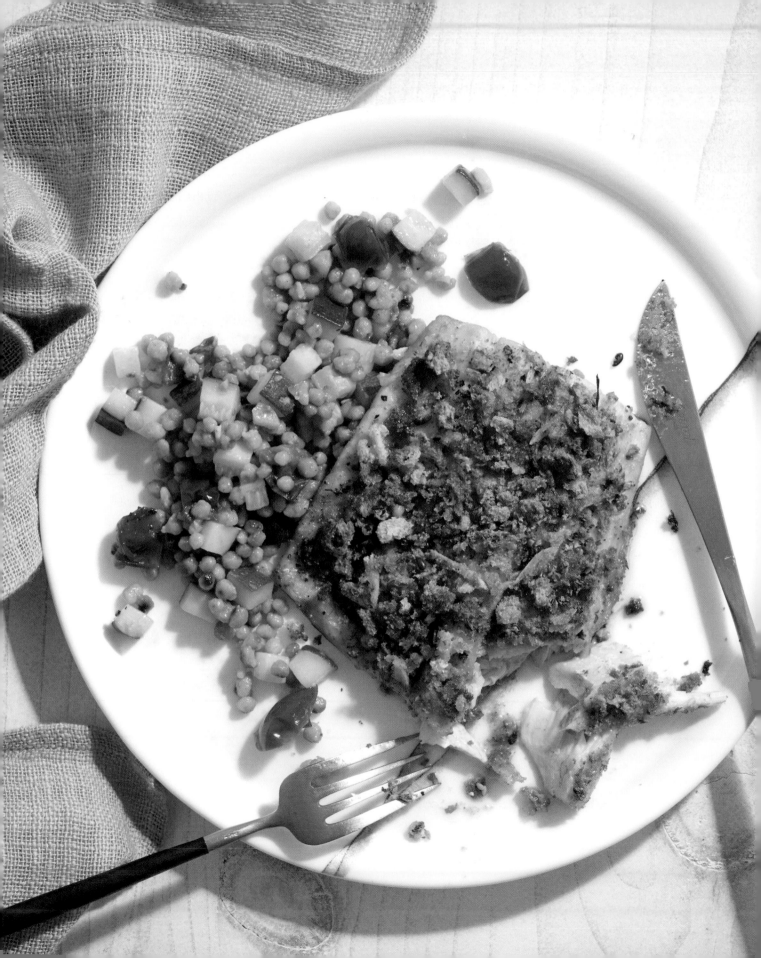

Striped Bass with Garlic Crumb Topping

SERVES 4

Q

This is my favorite foolproof method for preparing fish that is sure to please even the pickiest of fish eaters. But the real trick to making the best-tasting fish dishes is, of course, buying the fish fresh, preferably caught the same day. Striped bass is a great option for people who are picky because it's a mild-tasting fish, with a thick, meaty flesh and a large firm flake.

4 skin-on striped bass fillets (5 ounces each)

¼ teaspoon kosher salt

Freshly cracked black pepper

¼ cup white wine

1 tablespoon olive oil

1 tablespoon unsalted butter, melted

2 garlic cloves, crushed

2 tablespoons Italian seasoned whole wheat bread crumbs, homemade (page 110) or store-bought

Preheat the oven to 375°F.

Put the fish in a 9 x 13-inch baking dish and season with the salt and black pepper. Drizzle the white wine, olive oil, and melted butter over the fish, then top with the crushed garlic and bread crumbs.

Bake until the fish is opaque in the center and flakes easily, 12 to 15 minutes. Remove from the oven and set the oven on broil. Broil until the crumb topping is golden in color, watching close so it doesn't burn, 1 to 2 minutes.

PERFECT PAIRINGS
This is wonderful with **Summer Pearl Couscous (page 288)**, but if you're feeding a larger crowd, you can make this with **Tricolor Summer Penne (page 239)**.

skinny**scoop**

If striped bass is not in season or available, you can substitute it with halibut, sea bass, or cod.

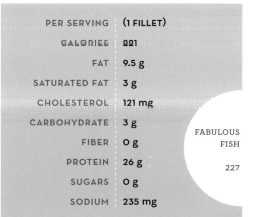

PER SERVING	(1 FILLET)
CALORIES	221
FAT	9.5 g
SATURATED FAT	3 g
CHOLESTEROL	121 mg
CARBOHYDRATE	3 g
FIBER	0 g
PROTEIN	26 g
SUGARS	0 g
SODIUM	235 mg

FABULOUS
FISH

227

Garlicky Lemon Shrimp and Broccolini Stir-Fry

SERVES 4

GF **Q**

Stir-frying is my favorite way to get a quick, healthy meal on the table in minutes! This one is made with lots of garlic—but don't worry, it doesn't overpower the dish. Instead, it creates a fragrant, tangy sauce that's delicious with the shrimp. Broccolini is sweet and tender and takes just a few minutes to cook, which makes it perfect for quick stir-fries. You can swap out the broccolini for other fast-cooking vegetables, such as asparagus, broccoli florets, or snap peas.

1 (6-ounce) bunch broccolini

½ cup reduced-sodium chicken broth*

2 tablespoons reduced-sodium soy sauce (or tamari* for gluten-free)

2 teaspoons cornstarch

1 tablespoon canola oil

1 pound peeled and deveined large shrimp

8 garlic cloves, chopped

3 tablespoons fresh lemon juice

Freshly ground black pepper

PERFECT PAIRING
Forget take-out. Try this stir-fry with **Vegetable Fried Brown Rice (page 273)** to make your own Asian-inspired dinner.

skinny**scoop**

If you buy shrimp with the shells on for this recipe, buy an extra ¼ pound so that you end up with 1 pound of peeled shrimp.

Read the label to be sure this product is gluten-free.

Trim 1 inch off the stems of the broccolini and thinly slice it lengthwise.

In a small bowl, combine the chicken broth and soy sauce. In a separate small bowl, whisk together the cornstarch and 2 tablespoons water.

Heat a large wok over high heat. Add ½ tablespoon of the oil, then add the shrimp. Cook, stirring, until opaque throughout, 1½ to 2 minutes. Transfer to a plate.

Add the remaining ½ tablespoon oil to the wok, reduce the heat to medium, and add the garlic and broccolini. Cook, stirring, until the garlic is golden and the broccolini is tender crisp, about 3 to 4 minutes. Increase the heat to high and add the soy sauce mixture. Bring to a boil and cook about 1½ minutes. Add the lemon juice, cornstarch mixture, and black pepper to taste. Bring to a simmer, add the shrimp, and stir well to coat. Serve hot.

PER SERVING	(ABOUT 1 CUP)
CALORIES	188
FAT	5.5 g
SATURATED FAT	0.5 g
CHOLESTEROL	172 mg
CARBOHYDRATE	9 g
FIBER	1.5 g
PROTEIN	28 g
SUGARS	1 g
SODIUM	525 mg

FOOD FACTS **shrimp, quite a catch!**
Shrimp delivers big nutrition benefits. A serving (3 ounces) offers
more than 11 grams of protein for just 60 calories and less than
1 gram of fat. They are also rich in the mineral selenium and
contain heart healthy omega 3 fats. And a study in *The American
Journal of Clinical Nutrition* found that even though shrimp are
high in dietary cholesterol, the shellfish can be included in a
heart-healthy diet because the dietary cholesterol doesn't affect
blood cholesterol levels.

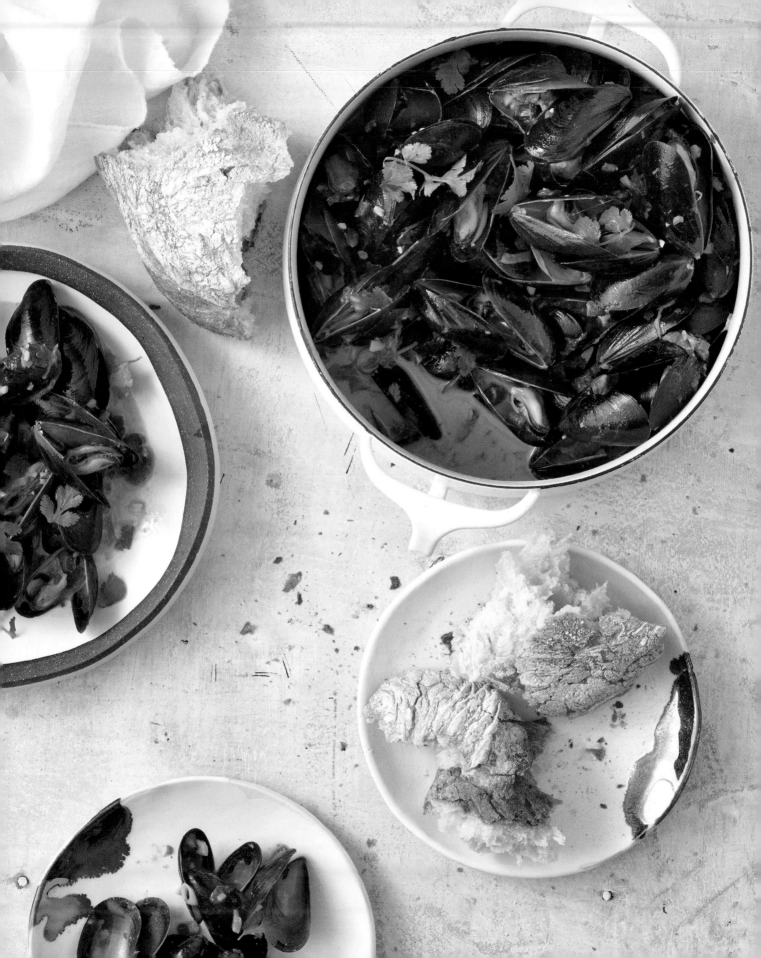

Thai Coconut Mussels

SERVES 5

GF **Q**

On the weekends I reenergize. I get more rest, play with my kids, visit the farmers' market, and recharge my body with delicious dishes like these aromatic mussels simmered in coconut milk with tomatoes, scallions, and ginger. My husband and I love the flavors of Thai cuisine and these mussels, which are inexpensive and take just minutes to prepare, are an ideal source of lean protein.

1 teaspoon coconut oil

½ cup finely chopped red bell pepper

3 medium scallions, thinly sliced

4 garlic cloves, minced

1 tablespoon chopped fresh ginger

1 (14.5-ounce) can petite diced tomatoes

1 (14-ounce) can light coconut milk (I recommend Thai Kitchen)

1 to 2 fresh red chiles, finely chopped (or ½ to ¾ teaspoon crushed red pepper flakes)

½ cup roughly chopped fresh cilantro

½ teaspoon kosher salt

3 pounds mussels, scrubbed and debearded (about 60 medium)

½ lime

In a large pot, heat the coconut oil over medium-low heat. Add the bell pepper and scallions and cook, stirring, until soft, 1 to 2 minutes. Add the garlic and ginger and cook until fragrant, about 1 minute. Add the tomatoes, coconut milk, chiles, ¼ cup of the cilantro, and salt. Cover and simmer for 10 minutes to blend the flavors.

Add the mussels, cover, and cook until the mussels open, 5 to 7 minutes. Squeeze the lime over the mussels and top with the remaining ¼ cup cilantro. Divide the mussels and broth equally among 5 bowls and serve.

PERFECT PAIRINGS
To help soak up every last drop of this delicious broth, I serve the mussels over brown rice or with a crusty piece of bread.

skinny scoop

When purchasing mussels, look for uncracked, tightly closed shells or shells that close when lightly tapped. Scrub them with a stiff brush under cold running water to remove any sand. The shells will remain closed until you cook them; discard any shells that don't open. To debeard, use your fingers to firmly pull out the hairy filaments.

PER SERVING	(12 MUSSELS)
CALORIES	309
FAT	12.5 g
SATURATED FAT	5.5 g
CHOLESTEROL	54 mg
CARBOHYDRATE	21 g
FIBER	1.5 g
PROTEIN	33 g
SUGARS	5 g
SODIUM	918 mg

FABULOUS FISH

231

Spanish Seafood Stew

SERVES 4

Q

This dish was inspired by paella, one of my favorite Spanish dishes, but it's made without the rice, and in a fraction of the time, making it a perfect weeknight dinner option. There's no need to make your own fish stock, as the anchovies add great depth of flavor, not to mention omega-3 fats. And don't worry; the dish won't taste like anchovies. Any combination of fish and shellfish can be used. If you want to get a little fancy, try it with scallops and lobster tails. A crusty piece of bread is a must to soak up all that wonderful saffron-infused broth!

1 pound firm whitefish fillet (such as halibut, Pacific cod, or sea bass), cut into 4 pieces

20 medium shrimp, peeled and deveined

¼ teaspoon kosher salt

Freshly ground black pepper

1 teaspoon extra-virgin olive oil

1 small link (1.75 ounces) dried chorizo, cut into ¼-inch-thick slices

1 small onion, finely chopped

3 garlic cloves, minced

2 anchovy fillets, rinsed

1 medium tomato, finely chopped

1 teaspoon smoked paprika

2 cups Swanson 33% less sodium chicken broth

2 tablespoons tomato paste

3 bay leaves

About ¼ teaspoon saffron

1 cup frozen peas

1 large roasted red bell pepper, jarred or homemade (see page 233), cut into ½-inch-wide slices

12 littleneck clams, scrubbed

12 mussels, scrubbed and debearded

1 tablespoon finely chopped fresh parsley

4 (1-ounce) slices crusty whole wheat French bread

PER SERVING	(1½ CUPS STEW, 3 CLAMS, 3 MUSSELS, 1 OUNCE BREAD)
CALORIES	408
FAT	9.5 g
SATURATED FAT	2.5 g
CHOLESTEROL	124 mg
CARBOHYDRATE	35 g
FIBER	5.5 g
PROTEIN	44 g
SUGARS	11 g
SODIUM	979 mg

Season the fish and shrimp with the salt and black pepper. Heat a large, deep nonstick skillet over medium heat. Add the oil, chorizo, and shrimp and cook, stirring occasionally, until the shrimp is browned on both sides, about 3 minutes. Transfer the shrimp to a plate, leaving the chorizo in the skillet.

Add the onion and cook, stirring, until the onion is soft, about 5 minutes. Add the garlic and anchovies and cook, stirring, until the mixture is very fragrant, about 1 minute. Add the tomato and paprika and cook, stirring occasionally, 2 to 3 minutes. Add the chicken broth, tomato paste, bay leaves, and saffron; increase the heat to high; and bring to a boil. Add the peas and roasted pepper, cover, reduce the heat to low, and simmer until the flavors combine, about 10 minutes. Add the fish, cover, and let cook for 4 minutes. Add the clams and mussels, cover, and let cook until the clams and mussels have opened, about 5 to 7 minutes. Return the shrimp to the skillet, cover, and cook until the fish is opaque throughout and flakes easily, 1 minute. Remove the pan from the heat. Discard any unopened shells and the bay leaves. Garnish with the parsley.

To serve, ladle the fish and shellfish, along with the broth and vegetables, into 4 large bowls and serve with a crusty slice of bread.

skinny**scoop**

When purchasing clams and mussels, you want to make sure they are alive. The shells should be tightly closed and have no cracks or chips. They should smell like the ocean, not at all "fishy." When cooked, they should open; discard any that stay closed.

FOOD FACTS out-"musseling" depression
Mussels are a stellar source of vitamin B_{12}, which is essential for normal brain function. Just 3 ounces of the shellfish provide 1,000 percent of the RDA for B_{12}. And, according to research, falling short of the vitamin, as an estimated 20 percent of Americans do, could increase your chances for depression.

Roasting Bell Peppers

To roast bell peppers, place them directly over the burners of a gas burner on a medium-low flame, turning the peppers frequently, until the skin has turned completely black and has started to blister. If you don't have a gas stove, you can roast them in the oven: Preheat the oven to 400°F. Line a baking sheet with foil. Lay peppers on their sides on the baking sheet and roast 20 minutes. Using tongs, turn the peppers over, then place back in the oven for another 20 to 24 minutes, or until the skin is charred and soft, and the peppers look slightly collapsed. Transfer the peppers to a bowl, cover tightly with plastic wrap, and let steam for 10 minutes. Uncover the bowl and peel the skins off. Core or seed the peppers, then chop the flesh.

Skinny Shrimp, Chicken, and Sausage Gumbo

SERVES 6

(FF)

This makeover of a Cajun classic has so much flavor and comfort in every bite that you won't even miss all the fat of the original. My lightening techniques include simmering the "Holy Trinity" of Cajun cuisine—onions, celery, and bell peppers—to get them nicely caramelized, and then making a lighter roux with olive oil in place of butter and far less flour. Also, a key ingredient is Applegate's Organic Andouille Sausage. Made from turkey and chicken, it's leaner than traditional pork andouille, and it really adds great flavor and just the right amount of heat.

1 tablespoon canola oil

1 cup chopped onion

½ cup chopped green bell pepper

¼ cup chopped celery

¼ cup chopped fresh parsley

6 bone-in, skinless chicken drumsticks (3 ounces each)

1¼ teaspoons kosher salt

Freshly ground black pepper

2 tablespoons all-purpose flour

2 links Applegate's chicken and turkey andouille sausage, thinly sliced (6 ounces)

1 cup chopped tomato

1 cup frozen sliced okra

1 bay leaf

¾ pound peeled and deveined large shrimp

¼ cup chopped scallions

3 cups cooked brown rice

Heat a large, deep nonstick skillet over medium heat. Add the oil, onion, bell pepper, and celery. Cook until the vegetables are softened, 3 to 4 minutes. Add the parsley and cook 1 more minute. Push the vegetables to the edges of the skillet, add the chicken, and season with 1 teaspoon of the salt and black pepper to taste. Cook until browned, 2 to 3 minutes per side. Sprinkle the flour over the chicken and vegetables. Add 3 cups water, the sausage, tomato, okra, bay leaf, the remaining ¼ teaspoon salt, and black pepper to taste. Cover, reduce the heat to low, and simmer until the chicken is tender and cooked through, 30 to 35 minutes.

PER SERVING	(1¼ CUPS GUMBO + 1 DRUMSTICK + ½ CUP RICE)
CALORIES	400
FAT	12.5 g
SATURATED FAT	2.5 g
CHOLESTEROL	215 mg
CARBOHYDRATE	26 g
FIBER	3.5 g
PROTEIN	42 g
SUGARS	4 g
SODIUM	1,101 mg

Increase the heat to medium-high, uncover the pot, and add the shrimp. Cook until the shrimp are opaque throughout, about 3 minutes. Remove the bay leaf and sprinkle with the scallions.

To serve, put 1 drumstick and 1¼ cups of gumbo into 6 shallow bowls and top each with ½ cup brown rice.

skinny**scoop**

Bones add flavor and help make a rich broth, so when I make this, I always use skinless chicken on the bone. This recipe relies heavily on the smoky, spicy flavor of the andouille sausage. If you can't find it, substitute with a smoked turkey sausage or turkey kielbasa along with a few shakes of Tabasco to give you some heat.

Fishing for Heart Health

Talk about a real catch: Fish are high in protein, low in saturated fat, and a good source of heart-healthy omega-3 fatty acids. That's why the American Heart Association recommends eating fish, particularly fatty fish, at least two times (two servings) a week. Next time you go fishing, whether it's in the ocean or at the market, seek out these top fifteen omega-3 winners:

Atlantic salmon (farmed or wild)	Fresh tuna	Rockfish
	Halibut	Scallops
Blue crab	Lobster	Shrimp
Canned white or light tuna	Oysters	Swordfish
Coho salmon (farmed or wild)	Rainbow trout (farmed or wild)	Wild catfish
Flounder or sole		

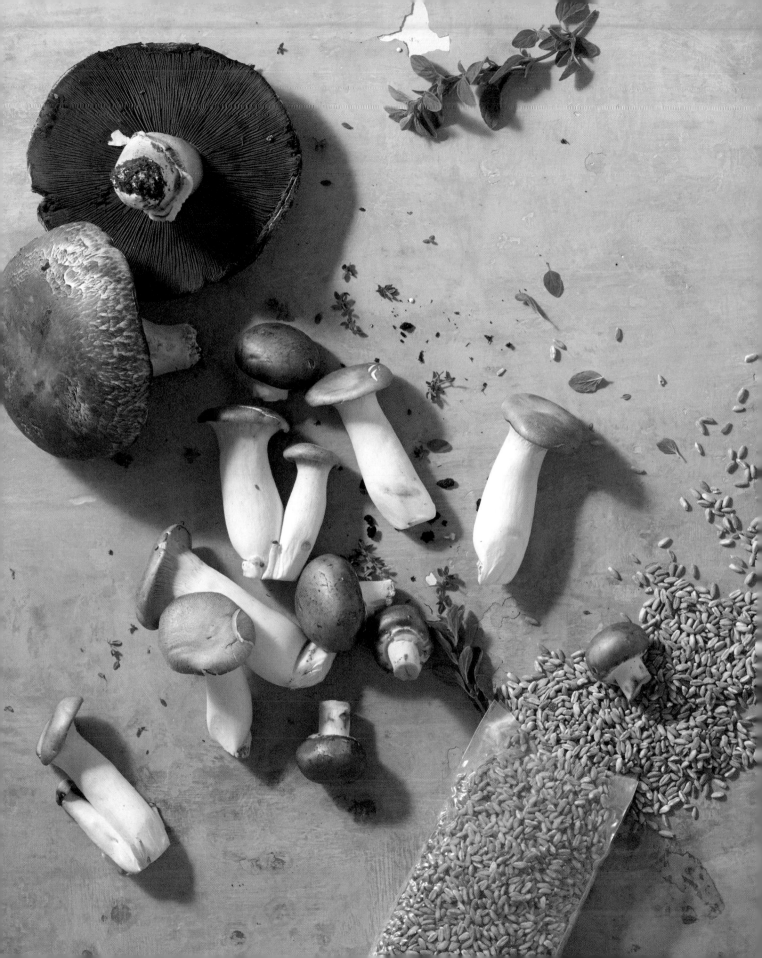

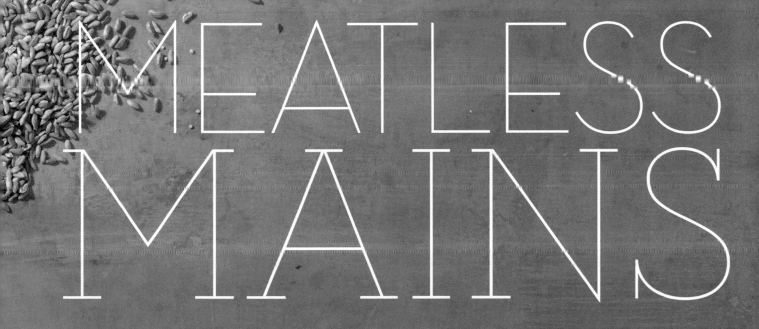

MEATLESS MAINS

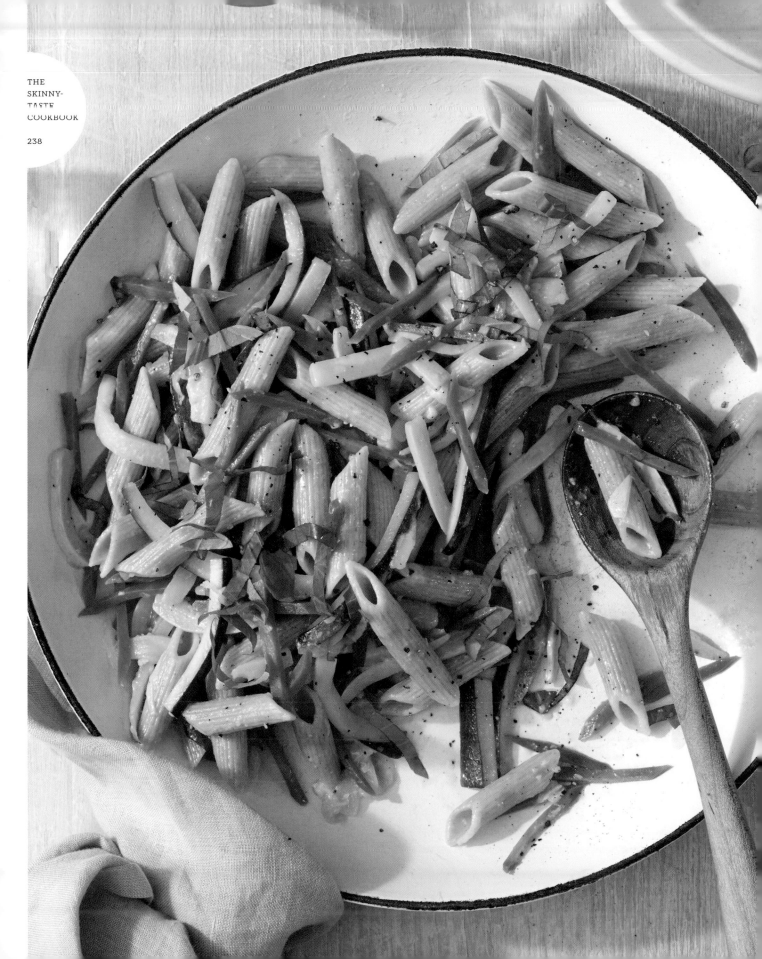

Tricolor Summer Penne

SERVES 4

Lots of wonderfully fresh vegetables are showcased in this quick pasta dish. Zucchini, yellow squash, and carrots, all loaded with disease-fighting antioxidants, are cut into matchsticks and tossed with pasta, garlic, and oil. I can't think of a better way to use up the summer's bounty. Once you have the veggies prepped, this dish takes less than 15 minutes to cook.

Kosher salt

8 ounces penne pasta (use brown rice* or quinoa pasta for gluten-free)

1 zucchini, seeded and cut into ¼-inch-thick matchsticks

1 yellow squash, seeded and cut into ¼-inch-thick matchsticks

1¼ cups shredded carrots

1 tablespoon olive oil

4 garlic cloves, thinly sliced

¼ cup grated Pecorino Romano cheese

Freshly cracked black pepper

2 tablespoons thinly sliced fresh basil

*Read the label to be sure this product is gluten-free.

Cook the pasta to al dente in a pot of salted boiling water according to package directions, adding the zucchini, squash, and carrots to the water in the last 2 minutes of cooking. Reserving ½ cup of the cooking water, drain the pasta.

Heat a large nonstick skillet over medium heat. Add the oil and the garlic and cook, stirring, until golden, 2 to 3 minutes. Quickly add the drained pasta and vegetables, ¼ cup of the reserved pasta water, the Pecorino Romano, ½ teaspoon salt, and black pepper to taste. Cook, tossing everything together well, for about 1 minute, adding the remaining ¼ cup pasta water if the mixture seems dry. Remove the pan from the heat, toss with the fresh basil, and serve hot.

skinny scoop

The quickest way to cut zucchini into matchsticks is to start by using a mandoline to slice the vegetables lengthwise ¼-inch-thick. Then use a knife to cut them crosswise into matchsticks about ¼ × ¼ inches thick. If you don't own a mandoline, you could also do this with a sharp knife.

PER SERVING	(1½ CUPS)
CALORIES	300
FAT	6.5 g
SATURATED FAT	1.5 g
CHOLESTEROL	6 mg
CARBOHYDRATE	50 g
FIBER	2 g
PROTEIN	13 g
SUGARS	4 g
SODIUM	266 mg

MEATLESS
MAINS

239

Crustless Swiss Chard Pie

SERVES 6

(V) (FF)

I'm a lover of all things green—spinach, kale, escarole, collards, you name it! But one green I downright adore is Swiss chard. It's ridiculously healthy and has a buttery flavor that stands up to sautéing, braising, and steaming. Unfortunately, not everyone in my home shares my sentiment, so when I want to prepare chard, I really need to get creative to showcase it in a way that even the pickiest of eaters will enjoy it. This savory crustless pie does just that.

Cooking spray or oil mister

1 small bunch Swiss chard, washed well

1 tablespoon unsalted butter

1 large white onion, cut into thin half moons (2 cups)

½ teaspoon kosher salt, plus more as needed

Freshly cracked black pepper

½ cup grated light Swiss cheese (2.5 ounces)

2 tablespoons grated Parmesan cheese

½ cup white whole wheat flour (I recommend King Arthur)

1 teaspoon baking powder

⅔ cup fat-free milk

1 teaspoon olive oil

2 large eggs, beaten

PERFECT PAIRINGS
This pie is perfect for brunch, lunch, or as a side or an entrée for dinner. As a main dish, you can pair it with a salad on the side such as **My House Salad, Made with Love (page 267)**.

Preheat the oven to 400°F. Lightly spray a 9-inch pie plate with oil.

Separate the stems from the leaves of the chard. Finely chop the stems. Roll up the leaves and slice them into thin ribbons.

In a 10-inch skillet, melt ½ tablespoon of the butter over low heat. Add the onion and a pinch each of salt and black pepper. Cook, stirring occasionally, until translucent, 8 to 10 minutes. Increase the heat to medium and cook until the onions caramelize, 8 to 10 more minutes. Transfer to a large bowl.

Increase the heat to medium-high, add the remaining ½ tablespoon butter and the chard stems. Cook, stirring, until tender, 3 to 4 minutes. Add the chard leaves and cook until wilted, 2 to 3 minutes. Season with ¼ teaspoon of the salt and black pepper to taste and add them to the bowl of onions. Add the cheeses and toss well.

PER SERVING	(1 WEDGE)
CALORIES	146
FAT	6 g
SATURATED FAT	3 g
CHOLESTEROL	74 mg
CARBOHYDRATE	15 g
FIBER	2.5 g
PROTEIN	9 g
SUGARS	4 g
SODIUM	354 mg

Sift the flour and baking powder into a medium bowl. Whisk in the milk, olive oil, eggs, and the remaining ¼ teaspoon salt. Pour into the bowl of Swiss chard and mix well. Pour the mixture into the prepared pie plate.

Bake until a knife inserted in the center of the pie comes out clean, 27 to 30 minutes. Let it stand at least 5 minutes before serving. Slice into 6 wedges.

FOOD FACTS super chard
Chard is famous for its nutrient density and mildly bitter and briny flavor, which hints at its ancestor, the sea beet. Small, young leaves are delicious raw, while sautéing subdues the stronger flavor found in mature leaves. Just 1 cup chard provides about 13 percent of the Daily Value for vitamin C, 44 percent for vitamin A, and a whopping 332 percent for vitamin K (talk to your doctor before adding it to your diet if you use a blood thinner).

Quinoa-Stuffed Peppers

SERVES 4

I LOVE stuffed peppers. I stuff them with just about anything—beef, turkey, and even my leftover Slow-Cooker Santa Fe Chicken (page 73). On nights when I want to go meatless, these Italian-inspired quinoa-stuffed peppers are simple to make, packed with protein, and delicious! For extra flavor, I like to cook my quinoa in broth, or water with a little salt, a garlic clove, and a sprig of parsley. This recipe can easily be doubled and frozen if you want to make an extra batch of meals for the month.

FILLING

½ cup quinoa

1 cup Pacific vegetable broth*

1 teaspoon extra-virgin olive oil

2 garlic cloves, chopped

¾ cup canned crushed tomatoes (I like Tuttorosso)

¼ teaspoon kosher salt

Freshly ground pepper

3 tablespoons grated Pecorino Romano cheese

½ cup chopped baby spinach

2 tablespoons chopped fresh basil

¼ cup shredded whole-milk mozzarella cheese (1 ounce)

PEPPERS

2 large red bell peppers

4 tablespoons canned crushed tomatoes

2 teaspoons grated Pecorino Romano cheese

¼ cup shredded whole-milk mozzarella cheese (1 ounce)

⅓ cup Pacific vegetable broth

Read the label to be sure this product is gluten-free.

For the filling: Rinse the quinoa under running water for about 2 minutes. Put the quinoa in a medium saucepan, add the vegetable broth, and bring to a rolling boil. Reduce the heat to low, cover, and cook until the liquid is absorbed, about 15 minutes. Remove the pan from the heat and let stand, covered, for 5 minutes. Fluff with a fork.

Preheat the oven to 350°F.

Heat a medium saucepan over medium heat. Add the oil and garlic and cook, stirring, until golden, about 1 minute. Add the tomatoes, salt, and black pepper to taste, and cook, stirring, for 5 minutes to develop the flavors. Remove the pan from the heat, add the cooked quinoa, Romano, spinach, basil, and mozzarella.

(recipe continues)

PER SERVING	(1 PEPPER HALF)
CALORIES	183
FAT	6 g
SATURATED FAT	2 g
CHOLESTEROL	11 mg
CARBOHYDRATE	25 g
FIBER	5 g
PROTEIN	8 g
SUGARS	6 g
SODIUM	411 mg

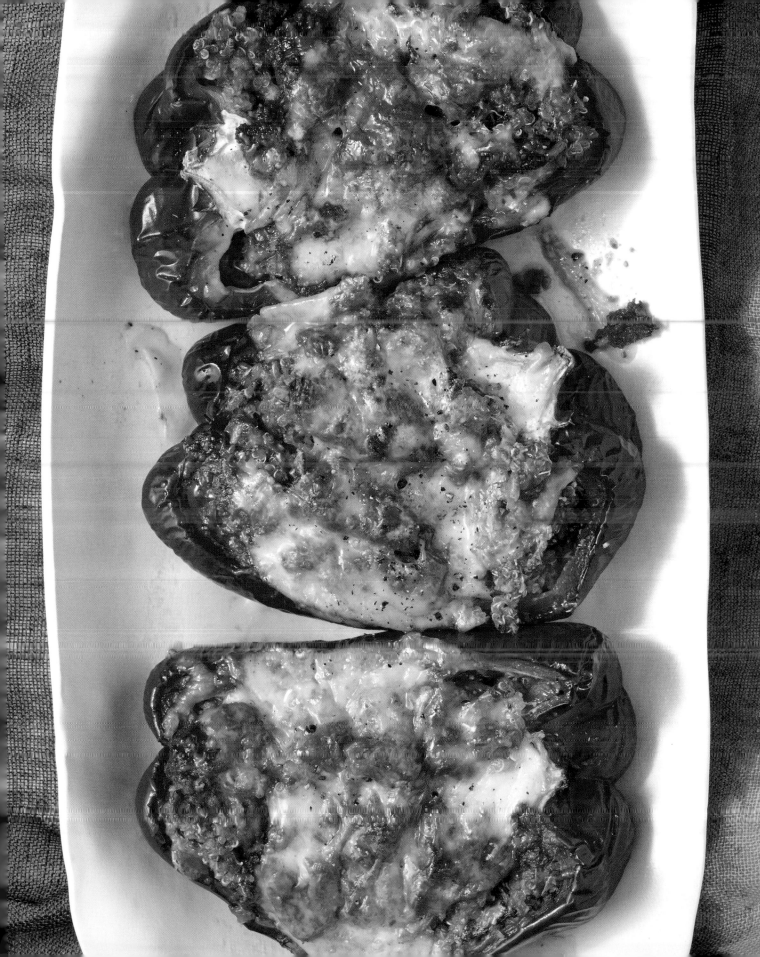

One serving is very filling, but if you want to serve this with a side dish, I recommend **My House Salad, Made with Love (page 267)**.

For the peppers: Halve the peppers lengthwise and remove the core, seeds, and stem. Place the peppers cut side up in a baking dish. Fill each pepper with ½ cup of the filling. Top each with 1 tablespoon crushed tomatoes, ½ teaspoon Romano, and 1 tablespoon mozzarella. Pour the broth into the bottom of the dish. Cover tightly with foil.

Bake until the peppers are soft, about 50 minutes. Remove them from the oven and let cool for 5 minutes before serving.

The Power of Protein

Strong, shiny nails? Sexy, sculpted shoulders? A leaner, meaner body? This powerhouse nutrient, which is found in every cell, tissue, and organ in your body, can help you build muscle, burn calories, and boost immunity. So how much is enough? The average healthy adult should get at least 0.8 grams of protein for every 2.2 pounds of body weight. For a 140-pound woman, that's 50 grams of protein each day.

To pump up your protein intake, eat a diet rich in meat, poultry, fish, dairy, eggs, legumes, and nuts. If you are a vegetarian and worrying about how to get enough protein in your diet, here's a list of protein-rich meat-free options:

Tofu (6 ounces)—15 grams	Split peas (½ cup cooked)—8 grams
Shelled edamame (½ cup)—8 grams	Chickpeas (½ cup cooked)—7 grams
Lentils (½ cup cooked)—9 grams	Chia seeds (1 ounce)—5 grams
Peanut butter (2 tablespoons)—9 grams	Peanuts (2 tablespoons)—5 grams
Black beans (½ cup cooked)—8 grams	Sesame seeds (1 ounce)—5 grams
Kidney beans (½ cup cooked)—8 grams	Quinoa (½ cup cooked)—4 grams

Creamy Carrot Farrotto

SERVES 4

Ⓥ

If you like creamy risotto as much as I do, then you'll love this creamy "farrotto," a healthier version that's made with pearled farro, a whole grain with a wonderful nutty flavor. This dish was inspired by an unforgettable carrot risotto that I enjoyed a few years ago at a quaint restaurant in Carmel, California. This version is a whole lot easier to make than the original, too, because you don't have to stand over it the whole time as you do when you use Arborio rice.

SALAD

1 medium carrot, peeled into ribbons

2 tablespoons fresh lemon juice

1 teaspoon extra-virgin olive oil

⅛ teaspoon kosher salt

Freshly cracked black pepper

1½ cups baby arugula

CARROT PUREE

1 tablespoon olive oil

½ cup minced shallots

3 garlic cloves, minced

1½ cups chopped carrots

2 cups Pacific low-sodium vegetable broth

½ teaspoon kosher salt

⅛ teaspoon freshly ground black pepper

FARROTTO

1¼ cups semi-pearled farro, rinsed

3 cups Pacific low-sodium vegetable broth, plus more if needed

½ teaspoon kosher salt

¼ cup grated Parmigiano-Reggiano cheese, plus 2 tablespoons freshly shaved, for garnish

For the salad: In a medium bowl, combine the carrot ribbons, lemon juice, olive oil, salt, and a pinch of black pepper to taste. Refrigerate until ready to serve.

For the carrot puree: In a large deep nonstick skillet, heat the oil over medium heat. Add the shallots and garlic and cook, stirring, until soft, 3 to 4 minutes. Add the carrots and vegetable broth and season with the salt and black pepper. Bring to a boil. Reduce the heat to medium-low, cover, and simmer until the carrots are soft, about 30 minutes. Remove the pan from the heat and let cool slightly.

Puree the carrots in a blender or with an immersion blender (be careful to keep the lid slightly ajar to release steam, and cover with a kitchen towel to catch any splatters). Set aside.

(recipe continues)

PER SERVING	(1 GENEROUS CUP + ⅓ CUP SALAD)
CALORIES	330
FAT	9 g
SATURATED FAT	3 g
CHOLESTEROL	8 mg
CARBOHYDRATE	53 g
FIBER	9.5 g
PROTEIN	10 g
SUGARS	11 g
SODIUM	560 mg

MEATLESS MAINS

245

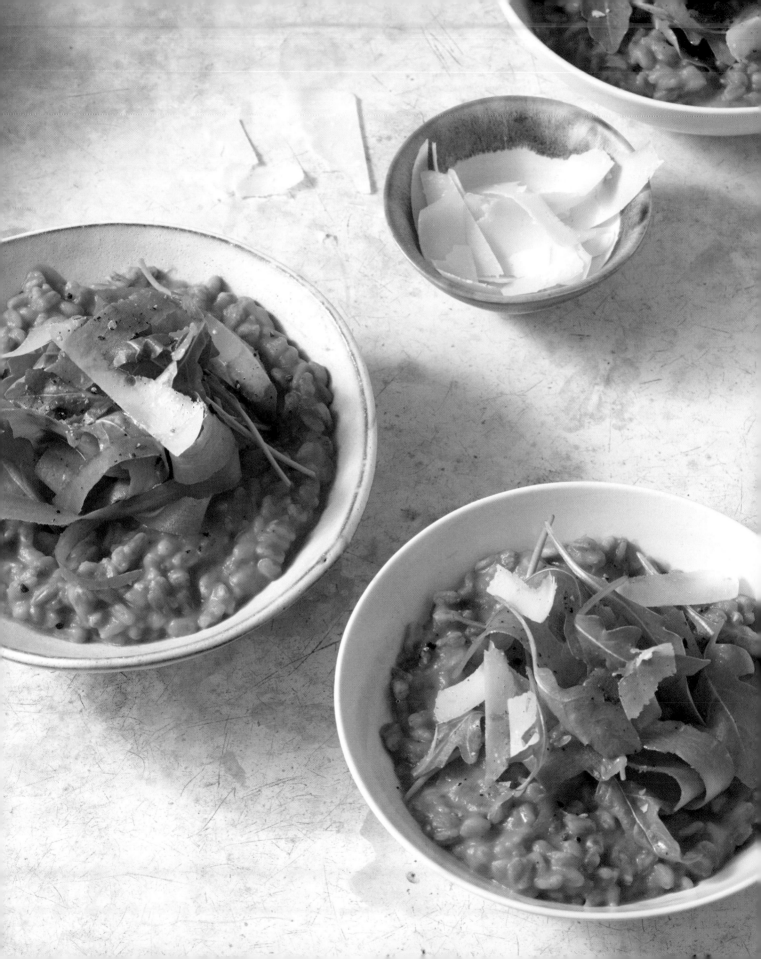

For the farrotto: In a large saucepan, combine the farro, vegetable broth, and salt. Bring to a low boil over medium-low heat and cook until the farro is al dente, 15 to 20 minutes or according to package directions. Drain and return the farro to the pan.

Add the carrot puree to the farro and cook over medium-low heat, stirring occasionally, until creamy, 4 to 6 minutes, adding more vegetable broth if needed. Stir in the grated Parmesan.

To serve, toss the arugula with the carrot ribbons. Divide the farrotto among 4 plates, sprinkle with the shaved Parmesan, and top with the carrots and arugula.

FOOD FACTS **fabulous farro**

Farro (also called emmer wheat) is a grain that's starting to gain popularity in the United States. It was a staple crop in ancient Rome, and was widely used in other countries up until the twentieth century, at which point it was replaced by other forms of wheat that are easier to harvest and hull. Farro is now making a comeback, thanks to its taste, firm and chewy texture, and nutrition profile. A study from scientists in Turkey found that farro had higher levels of antioxidants than other forms of wheat.

Butternut Squash Lasagna Rolls

SERVES 9

I have such fond memories of helping my mom make lasagna as a kid. I was in charge of layering the noodles, sauce, ricotta, and mozzarella. Today, my lasagna is a bit lighter than my mom's. Rather than making it as a large tray, I prefer to make rolls—which I load up with vegetables—for better portion control. And here I swap tomato sauce for a wonderfully savory butternut squash sauce with shallots, garlic, and Parmesan cheese.

BUTTERNUT SQUASH

1 pound peeled butternut squash, diced

1 teaspoon kosher salt

LASAGNA ROLLS

1 teaspoon olive oil

¼ cup minced shallots

2 cloves garlic, minced

½ teaspoon kosher salt

⅛ teaspoon freshly cracked black pepper

½ cup plus 2½ tablespoons freshly grated Parmesan cheese

10 ounces frozen chopped spinach, cooked according to package directions, cooled, and squeezed dry

1¾ cups (15 ounces) fat-free ricotta cheese

1 large egg

9 lasagna noodles, wheat or gluten-free,* cooked

9 tablespoons shredded part-skim mozzarella cheese (about 3 ounces)

*Read the label to be sure this product is gluten-free.

Preheat the oven to 350°F.

For the butternut squash: Place the squash in a large pot with enough water to cover the squash by 2 inches. Add the salt and bring to a boil. Cover and cook over medium-low heat until soft, about 12 to 14 minutes. Remove the butternut squash with a slotted spoon and place it in a blender with ¼ cup of the liquid it was cooked in. Reserve an additional 1 cup of liquid and set aside. Puree the squash.

For the lasagna rolls: In a medium nonstick skillet, add the oil and sauté the shallots and garlic over medium-low heat until soft and golden, about 4 to 5 minutes. Add the pureed butternut squash, the ¼ teaspoon salt, and a pinch of black

(recipe continues)

PER SERVING	(1 LASAGNA ROLL)
CALORIES	234
FAT	5 g
SATURATED FAT	2.5 g
CHOLESTEROL	32 mg
CARBOHYDRATE	29 g
FIBER	3 g
PROTEIN	17 g
SUGARS	3 g
SODIUM	449 mg

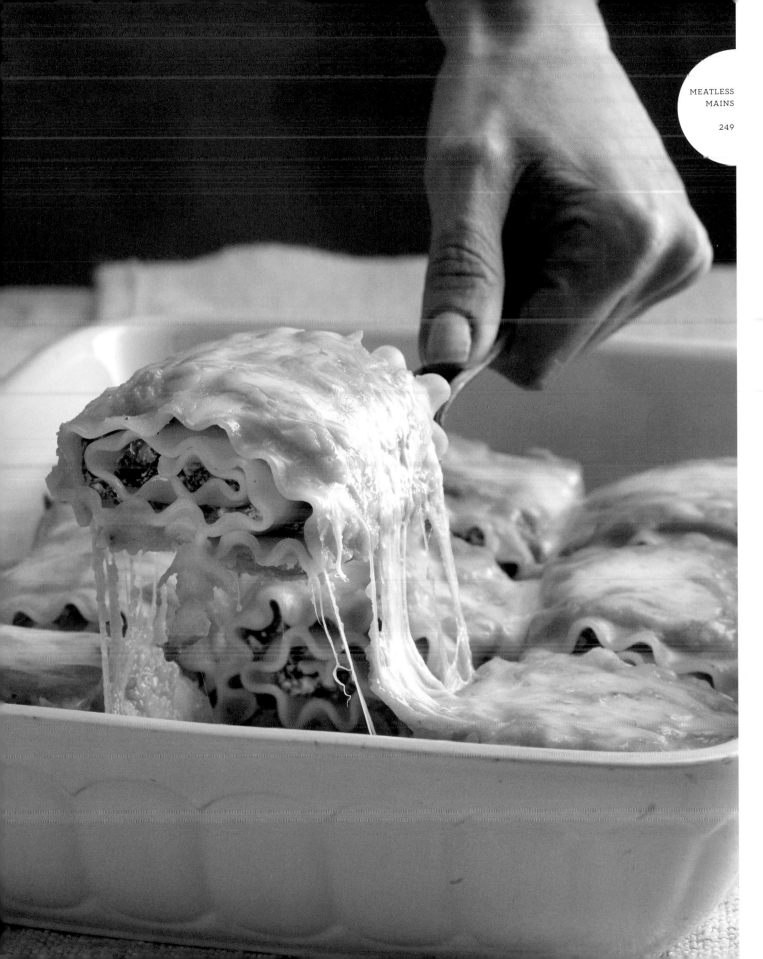

I always dish this up with **My House Salad, Made with Love (page 267)**.

skinny**scoop**

For best freezing results, freeze the lasagna rolls after you bake them in a freezer-safe zip-top bag or container. To reheat put the frozen lasagna rolls in a baking dish. Cover with foil and bake at 375°F for 45 to 50 minutes.

pepper, adding about ½ cup to ¾ cup of the reserved liquid to thin out the sauce until smooth. Stir in 2½ tablespoons of the Parmesan cheese and set aside.

In a medium bowl, combine the spinach, ricotta, the remaining ½ cup Parmesan, egg, ¼ teaspoon salt, and the black pepper.

Ladle about ½ cup of the butternut sauce into the bottom of a 9 × 13-inch baking dish.

Put a piece of wax paper on a work surface and lay the cooked lasagna noodles out on it. Make sure the noodles are dry. Spread ⅓ cup of the ricotta mixture over each noodle. Carefully roll them up and put them seam side down in the baking dish. Ladle the remaining sauce over the lasagna rolls and top each with 1 tablespoon mozzarella. Tightly cover the dish with foil.

Bake until the inside is heated through and the cheese is melted, about 40 minutes.

Black Bean Burrito Bowls

SERVES 5

(V) (GF)

When you consider my family's heritage—I'm half Colombian and my husband is half Puerto Rican—you can imagine how much we love rice and beans in my house. The funny thing is, as a kid I never cared much for beans. My mom always joked that I should have been Italian. But in my twenties, I grew to love beans and to appreciate all the varieties and different ways to prepare them. Black beans are one of my favorites, and when I have the time, I make a big pot from scratch using dried beans that I soak overnight and cook in my pressure cooker. It takes time and planning. On a busy weeknight, I'm not above using canned beans—if they're prepared correctly, they're wonderful.

RICE

¼ teaspoon kosher salt

1¼ cups long-grain brown rice

1 teaspoon olive oil

Juice of ½ lime (or more to taste)

3 tablespoons chopped fresh cilantro

SALSA

½ cup fresh or frozen corn kernels

2 tablespoons chopped red onion

1½ tablespoons fresh lime juice

⅛ teaspoon kosher salt

1 small tomato, chopped

1 small fresh jalapeño pepper, seeded and finely chopped (for hotter salsa, leave the seeds)

1 small garlic clove, minced

2 tablespoons chopped fresh cilantro

BEANS

2 teaspoons olive oil

⅔ cup chopped onion

2 garlic cloves, minced

2 scallions, chopped

2 tablespoons chopped red bell pepper

3 tablespoons chopped fresh cilantro

1 teaspoon red wine vinegar

1 (15-ounce) can black beans*

1 bay leaf

½ teaspoon ground cumin

¼ teaspoon dried oregano

¼ teaspoon kosher salt

Freshly ground black pepper

TOPPINGS

10 tablespoons shredded reduced-fat Cheddar-Jack cheese blend

1 Hass avocado, thinly sliced

1⅔ cups finely shredded romaine lettuce

*Read the label to be sure this product is gluten-free

For the rice: In a pot of salted boiling water, cook the rice according to the package directions. Transfer the rice to a large bowl and add the olive oil, lime juice, and cilantro. Toss well and set aside.

(recipe continues)

PER SERVING	(¾ CUP RICE + ½ CUP BEANS + TOPPINGS)
CALORIES	395
FAT	11 g
SATURATED FAT	2.5 g
CHOLESTEROL	10 mg
CARBOHYDRATE	53 g
FIBER	8 g
PROTEIN	17 g
SUGARS	3.5 g
SODIUM	245 mg

MEATLESS MAINS

251

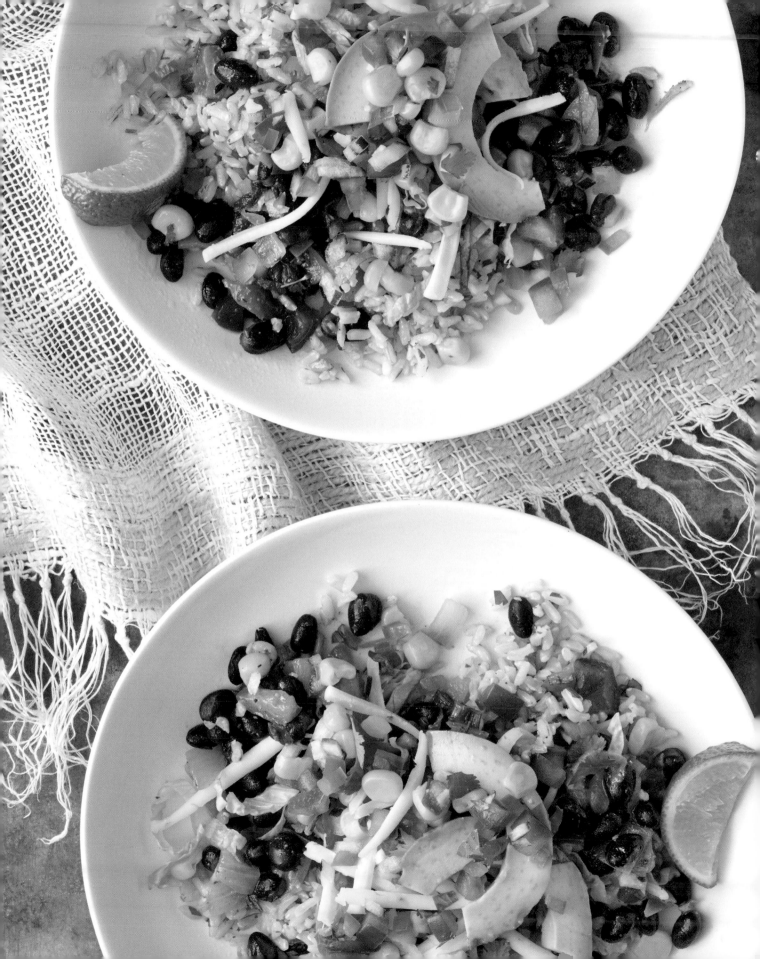

For the salsa: Cook the corn in a small pan of boiling water for 5 minutes. Drain and set aside to cool.

In a medium bowl, combine the red onion, lime juice, and the salt. Let sit for 5 minutes. Add the cooled corn, tomato, jalapeño, garlic, and cilantro.

For the beans: Heat a medium pot over medium heat. Add the olive oil, onion, garlic, scallions, bell pepper, and cilantro. Cook, stirring, until the vegetables are soft, 3 to 5 minutes. Add ½ cup water, the vinegar, beans, bay leaf, cumin, oregano, salt, and black pepper to taste. Bring to a boil. Reduce the heat to low, cover, and simmer, stirring occasionally, for 15 minutes to blend the flavors. Remove the bay leaf.

For the toppings: To serve, divide the rice equally among 5 serving bowls. Top each bowl with ½ cup black beans, 2 tablespoons shredded cheese, ¼ cup salsa, avocado slices, and romaine lettuce.

Cheesy Baked Penne with Eggplant

SERVES 8

(V) (GF) (FF)

One of my favorite dishes to make for my family is this baked pasta dish, with all its cheesy goodness and hidden bits of sweet eggplant. Picky eaters of all ages—and devout meat eaters, too—love this.

Olive oil spray or oil mister

1 cup (8 ounces) fat-free ricotta cheese

2 cups shredded part-skim mozzarella cheese (8 ounces)

½ cup grated Pecorino Romano cheese

¼ cup chopped fresh parsley

1 tablespoon olive oil

4 garlic cloves, roughly chopped

1 eggplant, cut into 1-inch cubes (16 ounces)

2 teaspoons kosher salt

Freshly ground black pepper

3½ cups canned crushed tomatoes

2 tablespoons chopped fresh basil

12 ounces penne rigate pasta, wheat or gluten-free*

skinny**scoop**

To freeze, let the pasta cool and then divide it into portions. Wrap the portions in plastic wrap and place them in a large freezer bag. The day before eating, transfer a piece to the refrigerator to thaw overnight.

*Read the label to be sure this product is gluten-free.

Preheat the oven to 375°F. Spray a 9 × 13-inch baking dish with olive oil.

In a medium bowl, combine the ricotta, 1 cup of the mozzarella, 6 tablespoons of the Romano, and the parsley.

In a large, deep skillet, heat the olive oil over medium heat. Add the garlic and cook, stirring, until golden, about 1 minute. Add the eggplant, ¾ teaspoon of the salt, and black pepper, and cook until golden, 4 to 5 minutes. Add the tomatoes, basil, ¼ teaspoon of the salt, and black pepper, reduce the heat to low, and cook until the eggplant is tender, about 5 minutes.

Add the remaining 1 teaspoon salt to a large pot of boiling water. Add the pasta and cook to 4 minutes less than al dente. Drain. Put half of the pasta into the prepared dish and top with one-third of the sauce. Spoon the ricotta mixture on top. Cover with the remaining pasta and sauce. Top with the remaining 1 cup mozzarella and 2 tablespoons Romano. Cover with foil.

Bake for 20 minutes. Remove the foil and bake until the mozzarella is melted and the edges are lightly browned, 6 to 7 minutes.

PER SERVING	(ABOUT 1½ CUPS)
CALORIES	325
FAT	9 g
SATURATED FAT	0 g
CHOLESTEROL	20 mg
CARBOHYDRATE	44 g
FIBER	4.5 g
PROTEIN	18 g
SUGARS	6 g
SODIUM	716 mg

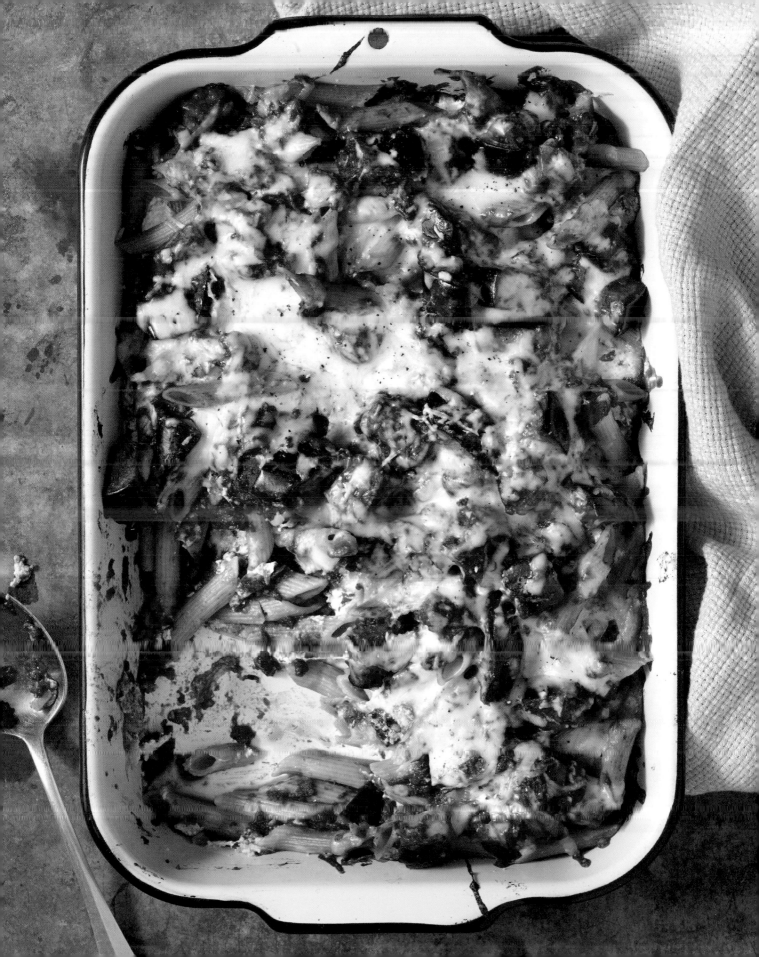

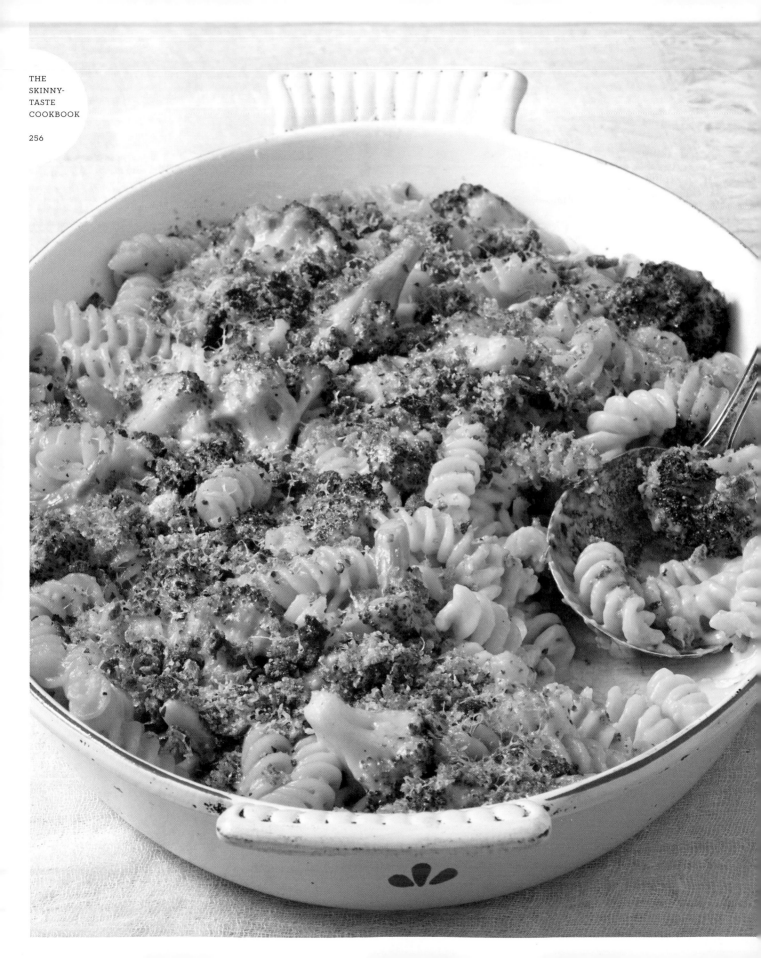

Skinny Broccoli Mac and Cheese

SERVES 8

(V) (FF)

Mac and cheese is the ultimate comfort food. Eliminating it from my diet was not an option, so early on I decided I would figure out a way to make it work. My secret weapon was to add some greens—broccoli, in particular, because it and cheese are a match made in heaven. I also developed a lighter cheese sauce to further ease the calorie guilt. I love that extra crunch you get from toasted bread crumbs, so I sprinkle a little on top just before I bake it.

Cooking spray or oil mister

Kosher salt

1 (12-ounce) bag broccoli florets

12 ounces rotini pasta

1½ tablespoons unsalted butter

⅓ cup finely chopped onion

¼ cup all-purpose unbleached flour

2 cups fat-free milk

1 cup Swanson 33% less sodium chicken broth (or vegetable broth)

Freshly cracked black pepper

2 cups shredded reduced-fat sharp cheddar cheese (8 ounces; I recommend Cabot 50%)

¼ cup seasoned whole wheat bread crumbs, homemade (see page 110) or store-bought

2 tablespoons grated Parmesan cheese

Preheat the oven to 375°F. Spray a 9 × 13-inch baking dish with oil.

Cook the broccoli and pasta to 3 minutes less than al dente in a large pot of salted boiling water according to package directions. Drain and set aside.

In a large nonstick skillet, melt the butter over medium-low heat. Add the onion and cook, stirring, until soft, about 2 minutes. Add the flour and cook, stirring, 1 minute. Whisk in the milk and broth, increase the heat to medium-high, and continue whisking until the mixture boils. Cook until the sauce is smooth and thick, 7 to 8 minutes. Season with ¼ teaspoon salt and black pepper to taste. Remove the pan from the heat and stir in the cheddar until melted. Add the pasta and broccoli and stir well. Pour into the prepared dish and top with the bread crumbs and Parmesan. Spray with oil.

Bake for 18 to 20 minutes. Increase the oven to broil and cook until the bread crumbs are golden, keeping an eye on them so they do not burn, about 2 minutes.

PER SERVING	(ABOUT 1 CUP)
CALORIES	312
FAT	8 g
SATURATED FAT	4.5 g
CHOLESTEROL	23 mg
CARBOHYDRATE	43 g
FIBER	2 g
PROTEIN	19 g
SUGARS	5 g
SODIUM	410 mg

MEATLESS MAINS

Spinach Falafel Lettuce Wraps

SERVES 4

(V) (GF) (Q)

My challenge: To create a healthier falafel that is quick and easy, skipping the deep-fry and soaking the chickpeas overnight. With a few smart swaps, I created my ideal falafels—using canned chickpeas, spinach, lots of fresh herbs and spices, and quinoa to bind them—that are light but packed with protein and a cinch to make. Also, instead of serving them in pita bread, I wrap the patties in crisp lettuce leaves.

TZATZIKI

¾ cup 0% Greek yogurt

¾ cup peeled, seeded, and grated cucumber

¼ teaspoon kosher salt

1 small garlic clove, crushed

1 tablespoon finely chopped fresh dill

1 tablespoon finely chopped fresh chives

1 teaspoon fresh lemon juice

Freshly ground black pepper

FALAFEL

1 cup loosely packed baby spinach

½ cup chopped scallions

½ cup chopped fresh parsley

⅓ cup chopped fresh cilantro

4 garlic cloves, minced

½ tablespoon ground cumin

1 teaspoon ground coriander

¾ teaspoon kosher salt

1 (15-ounce) can chickpeas,* rinsed and drained

⅓ cup cooked quinoa

1 large egg, beaten

1 teaspoon olive oil

Cooking spray or oil mister

4 large outer iceberg lettuce leaves

1 cup diced tomato

¼ cup shredded carrots

¼ cup shredded red cabbage

¼ cup hummus

8 teaspoons harissa, homemade (see page 206) or store-bought

Read the label to be sure this product is gluten-free.

For the tzatziki: Spoon the yogurt into a colander lined with a few sheets of paper towel and let drain for 10 minutes. Lightly sprinkle the cucumber with ⅛ teaspoon of the salt and set aside for 10 minutes to release some of its liquid. Using a paper towel, squeeze the excess moisture from the cucumber.

In a medium bowl, combine the yogurt, cucumber, garlic, dill, chives, lemon juice, the remaining ⅛ teaspoon salt, and a pinch of black pepper. Refrigerate until ready to serve.

PER SERVING	(1 WRAP)
CALORIES	293
FAT	8.5 g
SATURATED FAT	1 g
CHOLESTEROL	47 mg
CARBOHYDRATE	40 g
FIBER	4 g
PROTEIN	17 g
SUGARS	4 g
SODIUM	741 mg

For the falafel: In a food processor, combine the spinach, scallions, parsley, cilantro, garlic, cumin, coriander, and salt and process until smooth. Add the chickpeas and pulse 12 to 15 times, until coarsely mashed. Fold in the quinoa and egg. Form the mixture into 12 small flattened patties and refrigerate for 15 to 20 minutes.

Heat a large nonstick griddle or skillet over medium-high heat. Add the oil, swirling to coat the bottom of the pan. Put the patties in the skillet and cook until golden brown, 4 to 5 minutes. Lightly spray the tops with oil, flip, and cook until the second side is golden brown, 4 to 5 minutes.

To serve, put a lettuce leaf on each of 4 serving plates, spread each with ¼ cup tzatziki, and top each with 3 falafel patties, an equal amount of diced tomato, carrots, cabbage, and hummus, and 1 tablespoon harissa. Roll it up like a wrap and eat immediately.

PERFECT PAIRINGS
If you'd like to make a falafel platter, serve the patties with **Quinoa Tabbouleh (page 287)** and some hummus on the side.

skinny**scoop**

Quinoa has been called the "miracle grain" because it's nutritious, satisfying, and easy to prepare. Best of all, you can cook it and keep it in the fridge for up to 5 days, which makes it easy to throw together a weeknight meal. You can keep it in the freezer for up to 2 months, too!

Chickpea and Potato Curry

SERVES 6

When I worked in Manhattan, my good friend Tricia and I would have Indian for lunch once a week. It's probably what I miss most about working in the city. Often—but not intentionally—I found myself having a vegetarian meal, usually some type of curry. Whenever I make a pot of this rich, hearty dish of chickpeas, peas, and potatoes, the scent of the Indian spices brings me back to those memorable lunches.

1½ cups brown basmati rice

1 tablespoon coconut oil or canola oil

½ medium onion, finely chopped

5 garlic cloves, minced

½ teaspoon ground cumin

1½ teaspoons garam masala*

2 teaspoons curry powder*

1 (14.5-ounce) can petite diced tomatoes

1 (15-ounce) can chickpeas,* drained

1½ cups frozen green peas

2 medium Yukon Gold potatoes, peeled and cut into 1-inch cubes

¼ cup plus 2 tablespoons chopped fresh cilantro

1 fresh chile, chopped (optional)

1⅛ teaspoons kosher salt

PERFECT PAIRINGS
I serve this stew over brown basmati rice topped with fresh cilantro. Or you could pick up some Indian flatbread such as naan or roti, which are perfect for soaking up the sauce. This would also be wonderful with **Turmeric-Roasted Cauliflower (page 270)**.

*Read the labels to be sure these products are gluten-free.

Cook the rice according to package directions. Set aside.

Heat a large nonstick deep skillet over medium heat. Add the oil, onion, and garlic and cook, stirring, until soft, 2 to 3 minutes. Add the cumin, garam masala, and curry powder and cook 1 more minute. Add 1¼ cups water, the tomatoes, chickpeas, green peas, potatoes, 2 tablespoons of the cilantro, and the chile (if using). Season with the salt, cover, reduce the heat to low, and simmer until the potatoes are firm-tender, about 30 minutes.

To serve, divide the rice among 6 serving bowls. Divide the curry over the rice and top with the remaining ¼ cup cilantro.

PER SERVING	(1 CUP STEW + ¾ CUP RICE)
CALORIES	369
FAT	6 g
SATURATED FAT	2 g
CHOLESTEROL	0 mg
PROTEIN	12 g
CARBOHYDRATE	71 g
FIBER	7 g
SUGARS	6 g
SODIUM	531 mg

Spicy Black Bean Burgers with Chipotle Mayo

SERVES 4

(V) (FF)

One bite of this spicy burger, and you'll understand why all the adult carnivores in my home are big fans of it. When we want to go meatless, these burgers, which are loaded with fiber and protein, totally hit the spot. They're also very economical because they're made with canned beans, which are so inexpensive. And, they're pretty simple to make and have one small trick: The patties need to be frozen before you cook them so they keep their shape. You can even double the recipe and freeze burgers so you have them ready to go whenever you need a quick, healthy, last-minute dinner.

SPICY CHIPOTLE MAYO

3½ tablespoons light mayonnaise (I prefer Hellmann's Light)

1 tablespoon chopped chipotle chile in adobo sauce

BLACK BEAN BURGERS

1 (16-ounce) can reduced-sodium black beans, rinsed and drained

½ red bell pepper, roughly chopped

½ cup roughly chopped scallions

3 tablespoons roughly chopped fresh cilantro

3 garlic cloves

½ cup quick-cooking oats

1 large egg

1 teaspoon cayenne pepper hot sauce, such as Frank's

1 tablespoon ground cumin

¼ teaspoon kosher salt

Cooking spray or oil mister

4 whole wheat 100-calorie potato rolls (I recommend Martin's)

1 medium (4 ounces) Hass avocado, thinly sliced

For the spicy chipotle mayo: In a small bowl, combine the mayonnaise and chipotle. Set aside.

For the black bean burgers: Dry the beans well after rinsing (any extra moisture will keep the burgers from holding together well). Put the beans in a medium bowl and mash them with a fork or potato masher until thick and pasty.

(recipe continues)

PER SERVING	(1 BURGER)
CALORIES	347
FAT	10.5 g
SATURATED FAT	1 g
CHOLESTEROL	49 mg
CARBOHYDRATE	48 g
FIBER	17 g
PROTEIN	18 g
SUGARS	6 g
SODIUM	546 mg

PERFECT PAIRINGS
Try these with **Seasoned Sweet Potato Wedges (page 277)** for a healthier spin on the classic burgers-and-fries.

In a food processor, combine the bell pepper, scallions, cilantro, and garlic and pulse until finely chopped. Add the oats, egg, hot sauce, cumin, and salt and pulse a few times, until mixed well. Fold the mixture into the mashed beans. Form the mixture into 4 patties (using slightly oiled or wet hands helps) and put them on a baking sheet lined with wax paper. (If the mixture is too wet, refrigerate it for 30 minutes or add another tablespoon of oats.) Freeze for at least 2 hours before cooking.

To cook, heat a nonstick skillet over medium heat. Lightly spray the skillet with oil and cook the frozen burgers until browned, about 7 minutes per side. (Alternatively, preheat a grill to medium, lightly spray a sheet of foil with oil, put the burgers on the foil, and grill until browned, 7 to 8 minutes per side.)

To serve, place the burgers on the buns, and top with the spicy chipotle mayo and avocado slices.

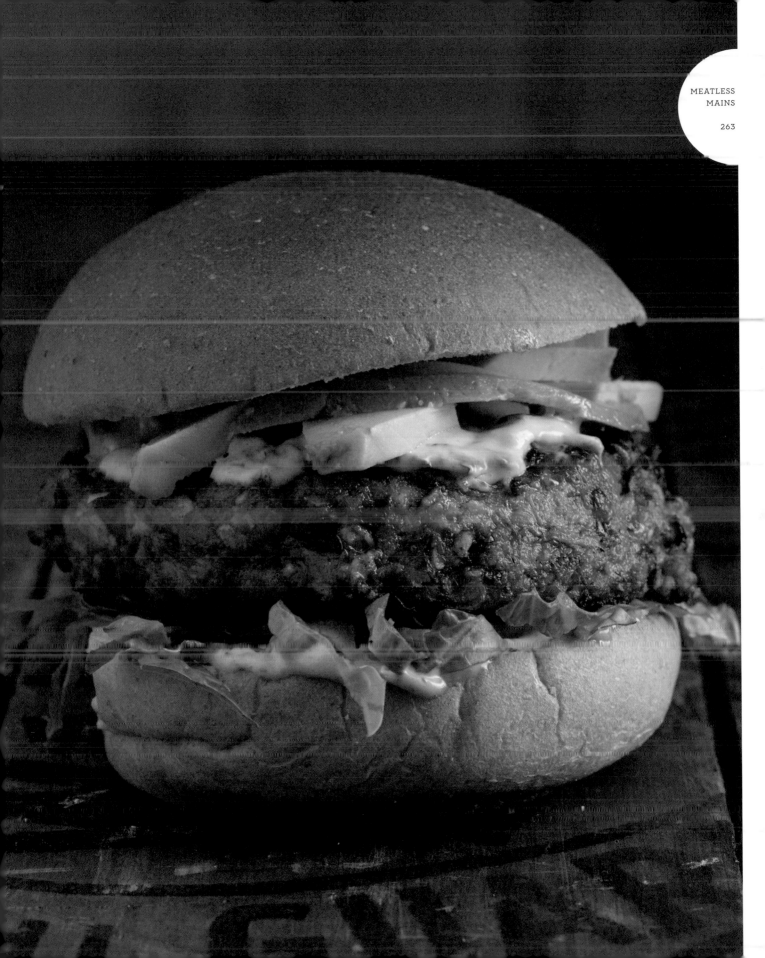

VEGGIE-LICIOUS SIDES

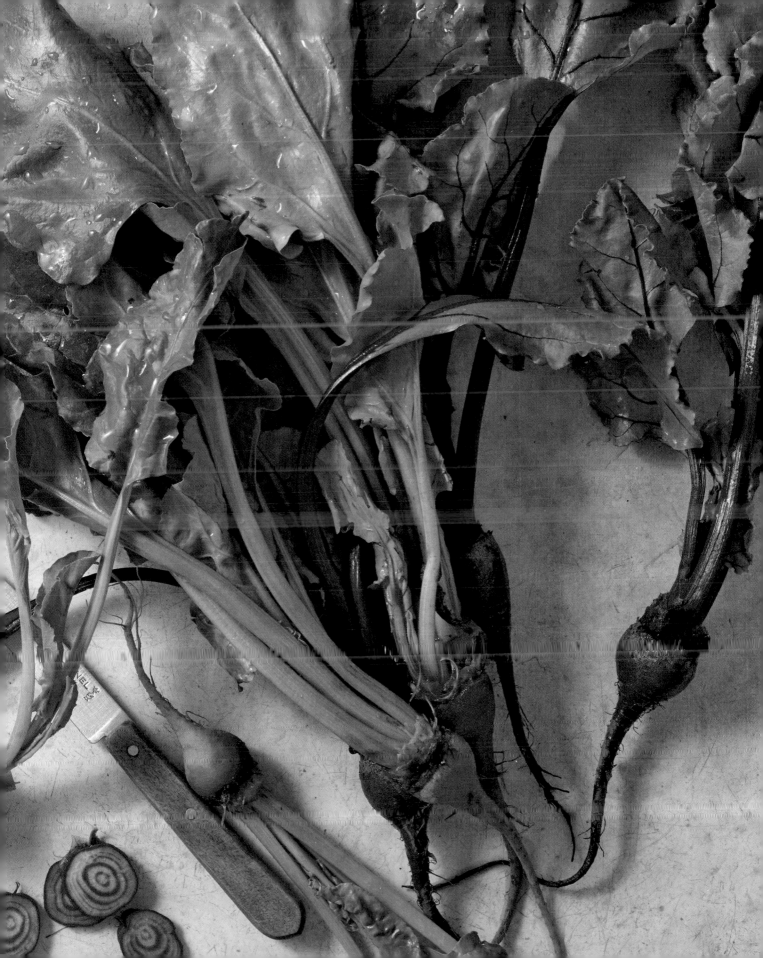

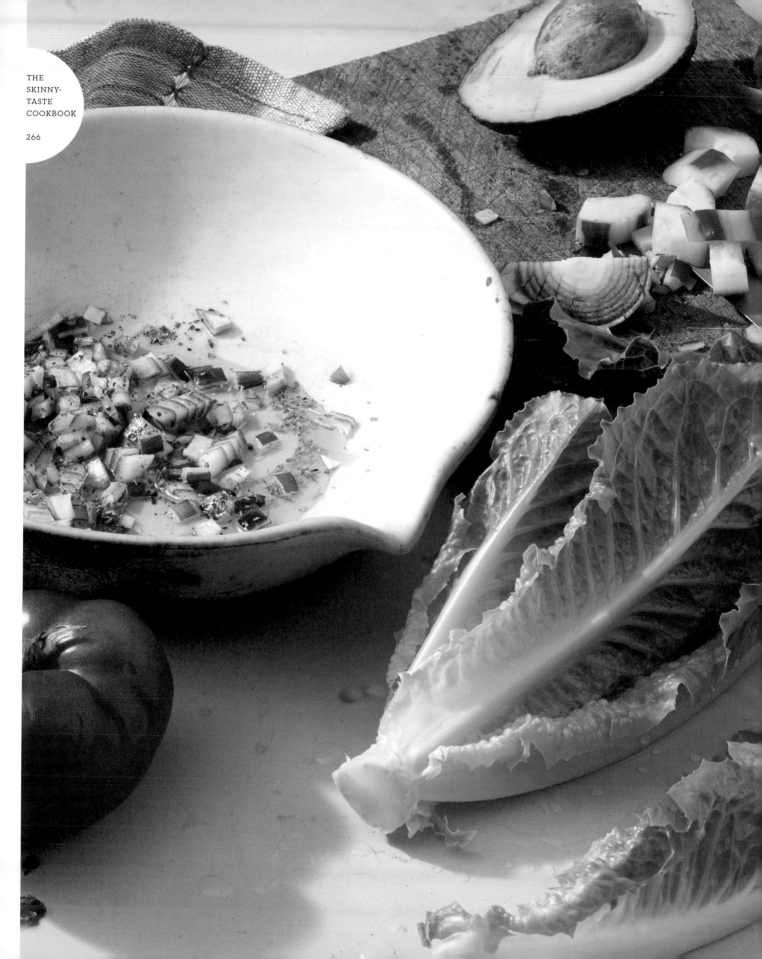

My House Salad, Made with Love

SERVES 4

(V) (GF) (Q)

This everyday salad is *my* special house salad. What makes it great isn't the ingredients but the love that goes into making it. I picked this up from my mother-in-law, who taught me how to make a truly tasty salad. She doesn't just combine all the ingredients at once with a quick toss. It's a process.

3 tablespoons roughly chopped red onion

1 tablespoon plus 1 teaspoon extra-virgin olive oil

1½ tablespoons apple cider vinegar (I love Bragg)

½ teaspoon kosher salt

Freshly ground black pepper

1 cup chopped tomato

⅛ teaspoon garlic powder

⅛ teaspoon dried oregano

1 cucumber, peeled and cut into 1-inch pieces (about 1½ cups)

1 medium (4 ounces) Hass avocado, chopped

3 cups chopped romaine lettuce

In a large bowl, combine the red onion with 1 tablespoon of the olive oil, 1 tablespoon of the vinegar, ¼ teaspoon of the salt, and black pepper to taste. Let sit until the onion flavor mellows, 5 minutes.

Add the tomato, garlic powder, oregano, the remaining ¼ teaspoon salt, and a pinch of pepper, and let sit for at least another 5 minutes. Add the cucumber and toss.

When ready to serve, toss in the avocado and lettuce, the remaining 1 teaspoon olive oil, and the remaining ½ tablespoon vinegar.

skinny**scoop**

Letting the chopped tomato sit a while with the onions and salt allows the juices to release and helps create a lighter dressing (a tasty way to cut back on oil).

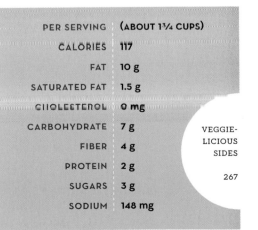

PER SERVING	(ABOUT 1¾ CUPS)
CALORIES	117
FAT	10 g
SATURATED FAT	1.5 g
CHOLESTEROL	0 mg
CARBOHYDRATE	7 g
FIBER	4 g
PROTEIN	2 g
SUGARS	3 g
SODIUM	148 mg

VEGGIE-LICIOUS SIDES

Squashta (Spaghetti Squash)

SERVES 5

(V) (GF) (Q)

I didn't grow up eating spaghetti squash. In fact, the first time I tried it was just a few years ago at a dinner at a friend's house. She served it as a side dish, roasted with a little olive oil, salt, and pepper. I thought it was great, and I have since played around with it in many different ways. Here are two basic ways to prepare it—a roasted method I often use when I'm not in a rush and a quick microwave technique I rely on when I have only 15 minutes. How you top it is completely up to you!

1 medium spaghetti squash (about 2¼ pounds)

Kosher salt and freshly ground black pepper

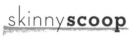

To serve, drizzle the squash with a little extra-virgin olive oil and sprinkle with grated Pecorino Romano. Top it with Quickest Marinara Sauce (page 94), or toss with some pesto. It's wonderfully versatile!

To roast in the oven: Preheat the oven to 400°F.

Halve the squash lengthwise and scoop out the seeds and fibers with a spoon. Season with a pinch of salt and black pepper and put the squash halves on a baking sheet, cut side down. Bake until the skin gives easily under pressure and the inside is tender, 50 minutes to 1 hour. Remove from the oven and let cool 10 minutes. Using a fork, scrape out the squash flesh—it will separate into spaghetti-like strands.

To quickly cook in the microwave: Using a sharp knife, poke holes all over the squash. Cook it in the microwave for 6 minutes on high. Turn the squash and cook until the shell is tender, 6 to 8 minutes. Remove it from the microwave and let cool for 8 to 10 minutes. Halve the squash lengthwise. (There should be no resistance, but if there is, microwave it a few more minutes.) Remove the seeds and use a fork to scrape out the spaghetti-like strands of squash. Season with a pinch of salt and black pepper.

SERVING SIZE	**1 CUP**
CALORIES	71
FAT	1.5 g
SATURATED FAT	0 g
CHOLESTEROL	0 mg
CARBOHYDRATE	16 g
FIBER	3.5 g
PROTEIN	1 g
SUGARS	6 g
SODIUM	53 mg

Cheesy Cauliflower "Mash"

SERVES 5

(V) (GF) (Q)

I love mashed potatoes just as much as the next girl, but I try to limit my carbs to just a few servings a day. That means if I have toast for breakfast and a sandwich for lunch, I try to skip the starches at dinner. To the rescue: mashed cauliflower, which is a lighter—but just as tasty—replacement for mashed potatoes. Adding cheese and fresh herbs makes them only better!

1 large head (7 cups) cauliflower, cut into florets

4 garlic cloves, crushed

⅓ cup 1% buttermilk

1 tablespoon unsalted whipped butter

¾ teaspoon kosher salt

Freshly cracked black pepper

1 tablespoon finely chopped fresh chives

⅓ cup shredded reduced-fat cheddar cheese

Bring a large pot of water to a boil. Add the cauliflower and garlic and cook until the cauliflower is soft, 15 to 20 minutes. Drain and return the vegetables to the pot. Add the buttermilk, butter, salt, and black pepper to taste. Using an immersion blender or a regular blender, puree the cauliflower. Stir in the chives and cheddar and serve hot.

PERFECT PAIRINGS

This is a great side dish to have with **Sunday Night Roast Beef and Gravy (page 211)**, **Skinny Salisbury Steak with Mushroom Gravy (page 201)**, roasted turkey breast, meatloaf, or any dish you'd normally serve with mashed potatoes.

PER SERVING	(GENEROUS ¾ CUP)
CALORIES	76
FAT	2 g
SATURATED FAT	1 g
CHOLESTEROL	6 mg
CARBOHYDRATE	10 g
FIBER	3.5 g
PROTEIN	6 g
SUGARS	4 g
SODIUM	281 mg

VEGGIE-LICIOUS SIDES

269

Turmeric-Roasted Cauliflower

SERVES 5

Once you've tasted roasted cauliflower, you'll never want to make it any other way—the vegetable becomes tender with slightly browned edges and a nutty taste that is pure yumminess. The garlic, cumin, and fresh cilantro give this side dish a fragrant finish with a warm, earthy tone. You'll also get a nice, vibrant color from the turmeric, which has been shown to have powerful curative properties.

6 heaping cups cauliflower florets (from a 1½-pound head cauliflower)

3 garlic cloves, smashed

¼ cup olive oil

1 teaspoon turmeric

1 teaspoon ground cumin

¼ teaspoon crushed red pepper flakes

½ teaspoon kosher salt

2 tablespoons chopped fresh cilantro (optional)

PERFECT PAIRINGS
Try this as a side dish to chicken or lamb, or my **Chickpea and Potato Curry (page 260)**.

Preheat the oven to 450°F.

Cut the cauliflower florets into 1-inch pieces and combine with the garlic in a large bowl. Drizzle with the olive oil and toss to coat.

In a small bowl, combine the turmeric, cumin, pepper flakes, and salt. Sprinkle over the cauliflower and toss to coat. Spread the cauliflower out on a large rimmed baking sheet.

Bake, stirring occasionally, until browned on the edges and tender, 23 to 27 minutes. Remove from the oven, sprinkle with the cilantro (if using), and serve hot.

PER SERVING	(SCANT ¾ CUP)
CALORIES	131
FAT	11 g
SATURATED FAT	1.5 g
CHOLESTEROL	0 mg
CARBOHYDRATE	7 g
FIBER	3 g
PROTEIN	3 g
SUGARS	3 g
SODIUM	150 mg

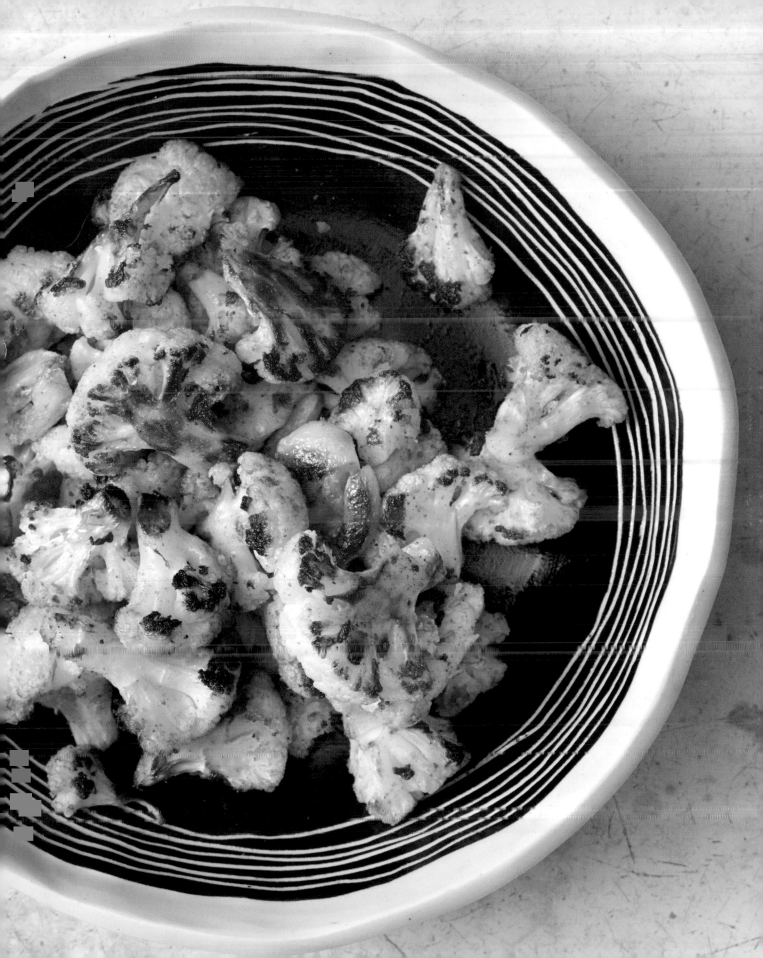

Roasted Sesame Green Beans

SERVES 4

In my opinion, green beans should never be mushy. They should be tender, but still crisp and slightly browned on the edges. The easiest way to achieve this is to roast or sauté them. To give them an Asian flair, I toss them with sesame oil and the popular Japanese condiment called *furikake*—a combination of sesame seeds, red shiso, and nori—that will take these string beans to a whole other level!

12 ounces green beans, trimmed

2 teaspoons sesame oil

¼ teaspoon garlic powder

1½ tablespoons furikake (I recommend Eden Shake)

⅛ teaspoon crushed red pepper flakes

Sea salt

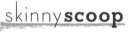

If you don't have furikake, you can replace it with sesame seeds and salt.

Adjust an oven rack in the lower third of the oven and preheat to 425°F. Line a large baking sheet with foil.

Arrange the green beans on the baking sheet and drizzle them with the sesame oil. Shake to coat evenly, then season with the garlic powder, furikake, pepper flakes, and a pinch of sea salt. Toss well.

Bake until browned on the bottom, about 10 minutes. Shake the pan or stir the beans and bake until golden and slightly browned on the edges, 5 to 6 more minutes. Remove from the oven and serve hot.

PER SERVING	(½ CUP)
CALORIES	67
FAT	4 g
SATURATED FAT	0.5 g
CHOLESTEROL	0 mg
CARBOHYDRATE	7 g
FIBER	3.5 g
PROTEIN	2 g
SUGARS	1 g
SODIUM	62 mg

Vegetable Fried Brown Rice

SERVES 5

When a craving for Chinese food strikes, I grab my wok and make my own takeout fake-out! I've perfected this healthier version of fried rice made with whole-grain rice and lots of veggies. The key to perfect fried rice is cold, day-old rice, so if I'm cooking rice the night before, I make a double batch of rice. I like to use short-grain brown rice, which stands up to reheating without turning to mush.

2½ tablespoons reduced-sodium soy sauce (or tamari* for gluten-free)

1 teaspoon fish sauce (omit for vegetarian)

1 large egg

3 large egg whites

⅛ teaspoon kosher salt

Freshly ground black pepper

Cooking spray or oil mister

1 tablespoon sesame oil

½ medium onion, chopped

½ cup chopped red bell pepper

6 scallions, white parts finely chopped and green parts cut into ¼-inch pieces

3 garlic cloves, minced

1 teaspoon finely chopped fresh ginger

1 cup frozen peas and carrots, thawed

3 cups cooked short-grain brown rice, cold (from 1 cup raw)

Read the label to be sure this product is gluten-free.

In a small bowl, combine the soy sauce and fish sauce (if using) and set aside. In a separate bowl, whisk together the whole egg, egg whites, salt, and black pepper to taste.

Heat a large nonstick wok over high heat. Spray with oil, add the eggs, and cook until scrambled, about 1 minute. Transfer to a plate.

Let the wok get really hot. Add the oil, then add the onion, bell pepper, and scallion whites. Cook, stirring, until lightly browned, about 2 minutes. Add the garlic and ginger and cook until fragrant, about 30 seconds. Add the peas and carrots and cook for 3 minutes. Add the cooked brown rice and toss, breaking up any clumps, then spread it over the surface of the wok. Let the rice cook undisturbed for about 2 minutes. Toss well, spread over the wok surface again, and let it cook undisturbed for 2 more minutes. Add the cooked egg and soy sauce mixture. Cook 1 minute, add the scallion greens, and cook, stirring, for 30 seconds. Serve hot.

skinny scoop

Prep all your vegetables before you start cooking because once the wok gets hot, this rice dish comes together in minutes. I like to use a nonstick wok when I make fried rice because it allows me to use less oil.

PER SERVING	(ABOUT 1 CUP)
CALORIES	218
FAT	5 g
SATURATED FAT	1 g
CHOLESTEROL	37 mg
CARBOHYDRATE	36 g
FIBER	4 g
PROTEIN	8 g
SUGARS	3 g
SODIUM	530 mg

VEGGIE-LICIOUS SIDES

273

Irresistible Vegetable Medley

SERVES 5

What's so irresistible about these vegetables, you may ask? Well, I do a little number on them that makes my family clamor for more. When the vegetables come out of the piping-hot oven, I top them with freshly shredded Parmigiano-Reggiano, which melts over the vegetables and gives them a wonderfully rich taste. Yum! The best part about roasting vegetables is that although they take a while to cook, the preparation time is pretty much nonexistent.

¾ pound (about 4 heaping cups) broccoli florets

¾ pound (about 4 heaping cups) cauliflower florets

1 large carrot, cut on an angle into ¼-inch-wide slices (½ cup)

1 small red onion, cut into 8 wedges

6 to 8 large garlic cloves, smashed

3 tablespoons extra-virgin olive oil

½ teaspoon kosher salt

Freshly cracked black pepper

¼ cup shredded Parmigiano-Reggiano cheese

Adjust an oven rack in the lower third of the oven and preheat to 450°F.

Put the broccoli, cauliflower, carrots, onions, and garlic in a 9 × 13-inch ceramic or glass baking dish and drizzle with the olive oil. Season with the salt and black pepper to taste and toss well.

Roast, stirring every 10 minutes or so, until the vegetables are tender and browned on the edges, 26 to 30 minutes. Remove the baking dish from the oven and top the vegetables with the Parmesan. Serve hot.

PER SERVING	(ABOUT 1 CUP)
CALORIES	149
FAT	10.5 g
SATURATED FAT	2.5 g
CHOLESTEROL	6 mg
CARBOHYDRATE	11 g
FIBER	2.5 g
PROTEIN	4 g
SUGARS	3 g
SODIUM	162 mg

Tangy Carrot Ribbon Salad

SERVES 4

Truth be told, I'm not a huge fan of carrots. I'm always amazed that my toddler can munch on raw carrots all day long. So I find it a bit bewildering that adding a little fresh lemon juice to carrots completely transforms the taste and balances out the sweetness with just the right amount of tang.

3 to 4 carrots (7 ounces), peeled

4 teaspoons extra-virgin olive oil

¼ cup fresh lemon juice

¼ teaspoon kosher salt

Freshly cracked black pepper

Using a vegetable peeler, shave the carrots into thin ribbons. You should end up with about 3 cups.

Put the carrot ribbons in a large bowl and drizzle with the olive oil and lemon juice. Season with the salt and black pepper to taste. Toss well and let sit for 10 to 15 minutes before serving. The salad can also be refrigerated in an airtight container for up to 2 days.

FOOD FACTS carrot crush
Carrots are one of those veggies that give you the biggest nutritional bang for the buck—literally. A cup gives you all the vitamin A you need for the day.

skinny**scoop**

You don't need a fancy tool to shave the carrots into ribbons—all you need is a simple vegetable peeler. If you want to add a little heat to the salad, you can even add a pinch of red pepper flakes.

PER SERVING	(¾ CUP)
CALORIES	64
FAT	4.5 g
SATURATED FAT	0.5 g
CHOLESTEROL	0 mg
CARBOHYDRATE	6 g
FIBER	1.5 g
PROTEIN	1 g
SUGARS	3 g
SODIUM	105 mg

VEGGIE-LICIOUS SIDES

275

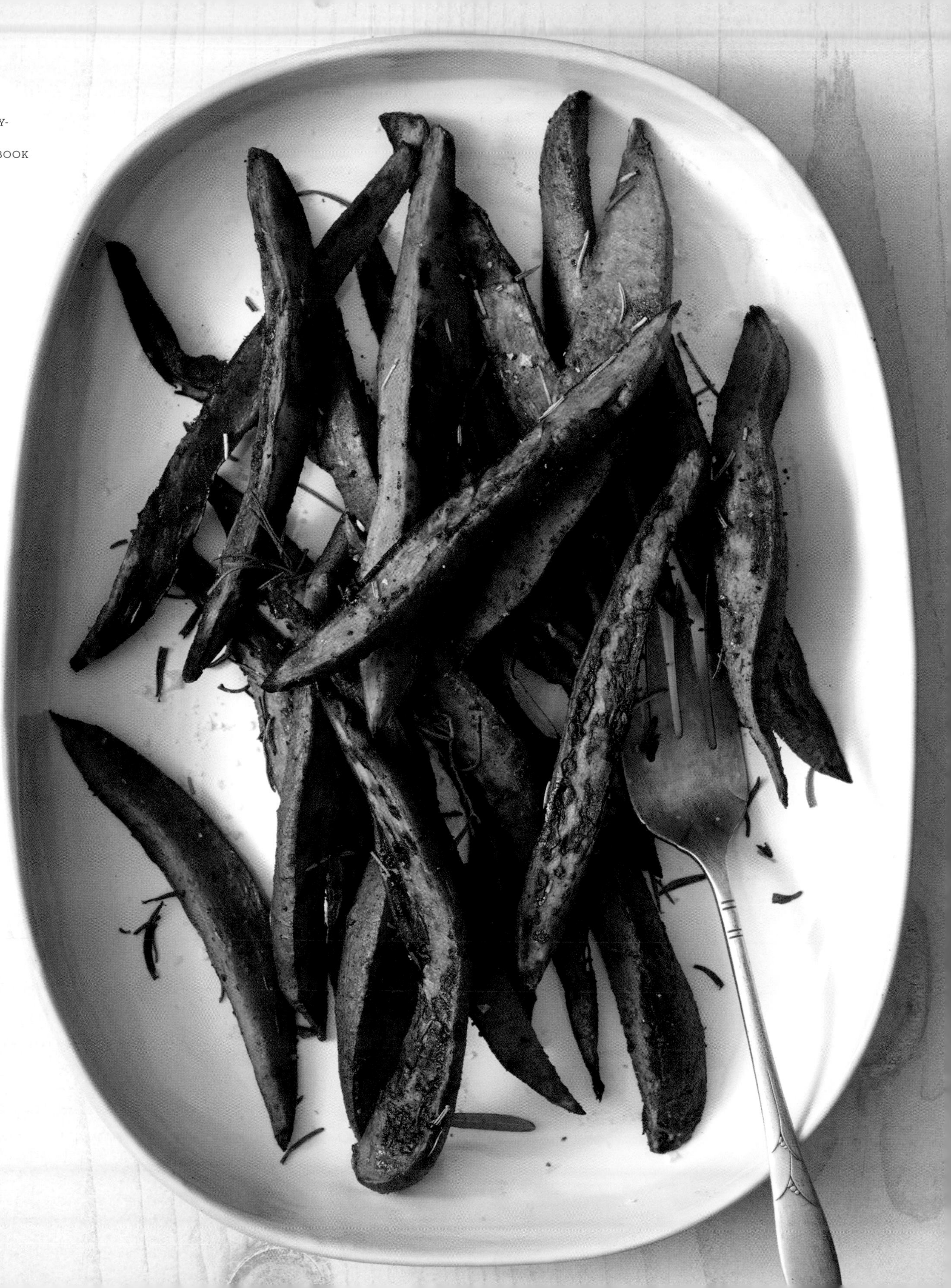

Seasoned Sweet Potato Wedges

MAKES 24 WEDGES · SERVES 4

Sweet and savory worlds collide with these deliciously seasoned sweet potato wedges. The seasoning is simple, but when combined with the sweet flavor of the spuds, it's pure harmony. Roasting the sweet potatoes at a high temperature ensures a soft interior and golden exterior. No need to fry in any added fat! Leave the skins on for added fiber.

Cooking spray or oil mister

4 medium sweet potatoes (1¾ pounds)

4 teaspoons olive oil

1 teaspoon garlic powder

¾ teaspoon sweet paprika

¾ teaspoon dried rosemary

Kosher salt

Preheat the oven to 425°F. Lightly spray a baking sheet with oil.

Halve the sweet potatoes lengthwise, put them cut side down on a cutting board, and carefully cut each half into 3 equal lengthwise wedges. You will have 24 wedges.

In a large bowl, toss the sweet potato wedges with the olive oil, garlic powder, paprika, rosemary, and ½ teaspoon salt. Put the wedges on the prepared baking sheet, flesh side down.

Roast until tender and golden, about 20 minutes, flipping over once halfway through. Finish with ⅛ teaspoon salt and serve hot.

PER SERVING	(6 WEDGES)
CALORIES	215
FAT	4.5 g
SATURATED FAT	0.5 g
CHOLESTEROL	0 mg
CARBOHYDRATE	41 g
FIBER	6 g
PROTEIN	3 g
SUGARS	8 g
SODIUM	285 mg

VEGGIE-LICIOUS SIDES

277

Lemon-Roasted Asparagus

SERVES 4

I love eating asparagus every which way, but roasting it with a little lemon juice and zest is one of my favorite quick sides. And it goes great with just about everything, from steak to pork to chicken (try it as a side with Chicken Cordon Bleu Meatballs on page 163). I prefer to use thinner spears when roasting asparagus because they're more tender, but if you use thicker spears, simply increase the cooking time. Look for asparagus with compact tips and firm stalks without wrinkles.

1 pound asparagus, tough ends trimmed

Olive oil spray or oil mister

¼ teaspoon kosher salt

Freshly cracked black pepper

1 teaspoon grated lemon zest

Wedge of lemon

Preheat the oven to 400°F.

Arrange the asparagus in a roasting pan in a single layer. Spray with olive oil and season with the salt and black pepper. Sprinkle the lemon zest over the asparagus. Roast until crisp-tender, 8 to 10 minutes. Squeeze a little fresh lemon juice on top and serve hot.

PER SERVING	(8 TO 9 MEDIUM SPEARS)
CALORIES	24
FAT	0 g
SATURATED FAT	0 g
CHOLESTEROL	0 mg
CARBOHYDRATE	5 g
FIBER	2.5 g
PROTEIN	3 g
SUGARS	2 g
SODIUM	2 mg

Roasted Winter Beets and Red Potatoes

SERVES 4

(V) (GF) (Q)

When I was younger, I remember that on occasion my mom would serve jarred pickled beets with dinner—blah! I wasn't a fan, and I completely wrote off beets until I discovered how great they are roasted. Slowly roasting beets turns them into candy, as all of their natural sugars become concentrated. For this dish, I slice the beets and potatoes thinly so that every bite is crispy and browned. This makes a wonderful winter side dish to beef or lamb (try it with the Grilled Lamb Chops with Mint Yogurt Sauce on page 202).

Olive oil spray or oil mister

2 medium peeled beets (10 ounces), greens and ends trimmed off

1 pound small red potatoes

2 tablespoons extra-virgin olive oil

¾ teaspoon kosher salt, plus more as needed

¼ teaspoon freshly cracked black pepper, plus more as needed

Preheat the oven to 425°F. Spray 2 large rimmed baking sheets with olive oil.

Halve the beets lengthwise, put them cut side down on a cutting board, and cut crosswise into ¼-inch-thick slices. Cut the slices in half.

Cut the potatoes into ¼-inch-thick slices, then cut the slices into quarters. Put the potatoes and beets in a bowl and toss with the olive oil. Arrange the vegetables in a single layer on the prepared baking sheets. Season with ¾ teaspoon of the salt and ¼ teaspoon of the black pepper, and toss well.

Bake until the vegetables are tender and the potatoes are golden, 24 to 28 minutes, flipping over with a spatula halfway through. Season with salt and black pepper to taste and serve hot.

FOOD FACTS why beets can't be beat

With nearly 4 grams of fiber, more than 30 percent of your daily folate needs, and a dose of vitamin C per cup, this root vegetable is a nutritional powerhouse. Its red color comes from the phytonutrient betalain, which may act as an antioxidant and have some anticancer powers.

skinny**scoop**

The trick to perfectly roasted vegetables every time is to be sure you cut all the vegetables uniformly so everything cooks evenly. Also, don't overcrowd the pan, or they won't crisp.

PER SERVING	(GENEROUS ½ CUP)
CALORIES	162
FAT	4 g
SATURATED FAT	0.5 g
CHOLESTEROL	0 mg
CARBOHYDRATE	29 g
FIBER	3 g
PROTEIN	4 g
SUGARS	3 g
SODIUM	138 mg

VEGGIE-LICIOUS SIDES

Sweet Maple-Roasted Acorn Squash

SERVES 4

(V) (GF)

I love all things fall: colorful gourds, cozy sweaters, changing leaves, and (of course!) spectacular autumn fruits and veggies. My soul just craves the sweet, buttery taste of this side dish when the weather starts to get cold. I also love how simple it is—in only 5 minutes, you can turn 4 ingredients into a scrumptious side dish. It doesn't get any easier than this.

4 teaspoons coconut oil

2 small acorn squashes, halved lengthwise, seeds scooped out

Kosher salt

2 tablespoons pure maple syrup

Preheat the oven to 400°F. Line a baking sheet with parchment paper.

Rub the coconut oil all over the flesh of the squash, then season with a pinch of salt. Put the squash halves cut side up on the prepared baking sheet, then drizzle with the maple syrup.

Bake until you can pierce the flesh with a fork, about 1 hour.

PER SERVING	(1 SQUASH HALF)
CALORIES	151
FAT	4.5 g
SATURATED FAT	4 g
CHOLESTEROL	0 mg
CARBOHYDRATE	29 g
FIBER	3 g
PROTEIN	2 g
SUGARS	6 g
SODIUM	25 mg

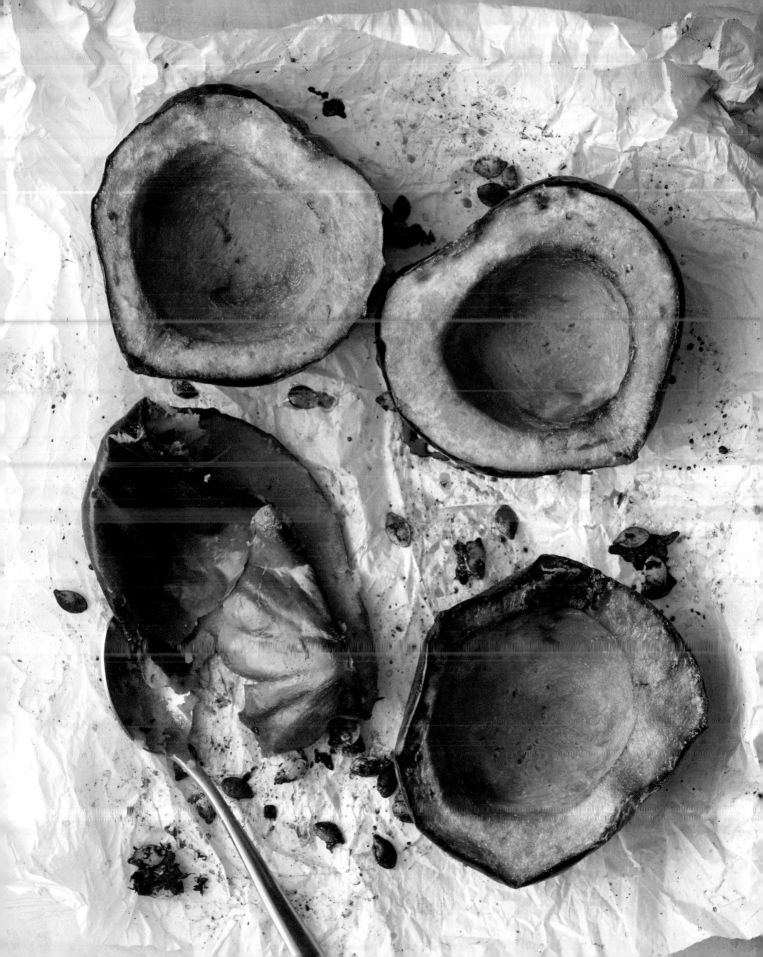

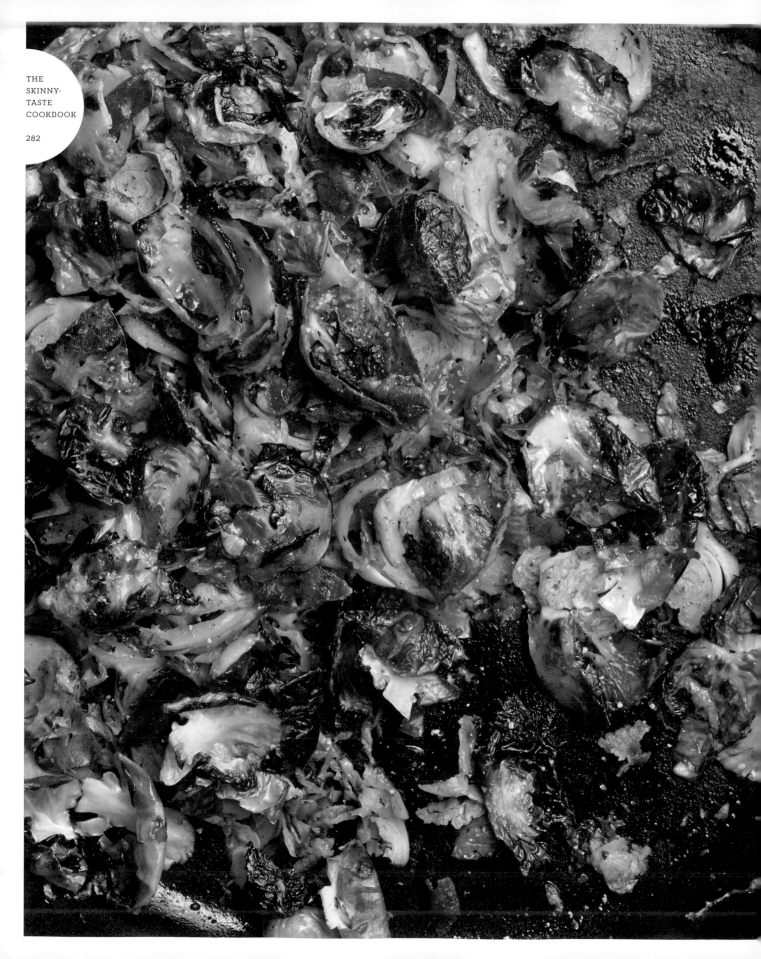

Shredded Brussels Sprouts with Prosciutto

SERVES 4

(GF) (Q)

Don't like Brussels sprouts? Well, this recipe may very well change your mind. In this dish, Brussels sprouts are shredded thin, sautéed until slightly browned, and cooked with thin slices of prosciutto and shallots—delish! Shredding the little cabbages makes all the difference, because the veggie can get thoroughly browned and seasoned.

12 ounces Brussels sprouts

2 teaspoons extra-virgin olive oil

¼ cup finely chopped shallots

2 thin slices prosciutto di Parma (1 ounce), chopped

¼ teaspoon kosher salt

Freshly ground black pepper

Using a large sharp knife, trim the stems off the Brussels sprouts, then thinly slice the sprouts.

Heat a deep 10-inch nonstick skillet over medium heat. Add the oil and shallots and cook, stirring, 30 to 40 seconds. Add the prosciutto and cook until the shallots are golden, 1 minute. Add the sprouts, season with the salt and black pepper to taste, and cook, stirring occasionally, until the sprouts are slightly browned and crisp-tender, about 5 minutes. Cover the skillet and cook until they begin to wilt, 1 minute. Remove the pan from the heat. Keep covered and let sit about 2 minutes to slightly wilt the leaves. Serve hot.

FOOD FACTS why brussels sprouts deserve a second chance
There's nothing stinky about sprouts! They're loaded with good-for-you nutrients, including vitamins, minerals, and powerful phytonutrients. A cup contains 3.3 grams of fiber and all your vitamin K needs for the day. It also nearly covers your daily vitamin C and A requirements, all for a mere 38 calories. As a member of the cruciferous vegetable family, Brussels sprouts also offer many of the same benefits of cauliflower and broccoli, including a reduced risk for cancer and other diseases.

PER SERVING	(ABOUT ½ CUP)
CALORIES	77
FAT	3 g
SATURATED FAT	0.5 g
CHOLESTEROL	5 mg
CARBOHYDRATE	9 g
FIBER	3.5 g
PROTEIN	5 g
SUGARS	3 g
SODIUM	284 mg

VEGGIE-LICIOUS SIDES

283

Sautéed Broccoli Rabe with Garlic and Oil

SERVES 4

(V) (GF) (Q)

Broccoli rabe (known as rapini in many parts of the world) is my all-time favorite vegetable. It's one of those vegetables that needs to grow on you, because of its slightly bitter taste. Blanching it before sautéing it with garlic and oil is the secret to mellowing out the bitterness, and it also sets its green color. Once cooked it can be served as a side or tossed with pasta and sun-dried tomatoes for a quick pasta dish. It's also one of my favorite pizza toppings and is wonderful in a panini with grilled chicken.

1 bunch broccoli rabe (about 16 ounces)

2 teaspoons kosher salt

1 tablespoon olive oil

5 garlic cloves, thinly sliced

¼ teaspoon crushed red pepper flakes

Trim 1½ inches off the stems of the broccoli rabe, discarding the trimmings, and cut it into 2-inch pieces.

Bring a large pot of water and 1 teaspoon of the salt to a boil. Add the broccoli rabe and cook until slightly tender and bright green, about 2 minutes. Drain well and set aside.

Heat a large, deep nonstick sauté pan over medium-high heat. Add the olive oil and garlic and cook, stirring, until golden, about 1 minute. Add the broccoli rabe, pepper flakes, and the remaining 1 teaspoon salt. Cook, stirring, until heated through, 2 to 3 minutes. Serve hot.

FOOD FACTS broccoli rabe makes a name for itself
This broccoli look-alike is actually a member of the turnip family, but it offers many of the same benefits as broccoli. It's rich in vitamin K and contains a compound called indole-3-carbinol, which has been shown to reduce the risk of cancer in animal studies.

PER SERVING	(½ CUP)
CALORIES	60
FAT	4 g
SATURATED FAT	0.5 g
CHOLESTEROL	0 mg
CARBOHYDRATE	4 g
FIBER	3 g
PROTEIN	4 g
SUGARS	0 g
SODIUM	318 mg

Confetti Slaw

SERVES 5

Naturally colorful food is not only beautiful, but it's also healthful. The different colors of foods indicate different phytonutrients and antioxidants, which help protect your body in a variety of ways. Put a multitude of hues on your plate (pictured on page 192) and you could very well color yourself healthy! And by the way, my kids love this.

4 cups coleslaw mix

½ cup thinly sliced red cabbage

½ cup julienne cut and peeled English cucumber

¼ cup thinly sliced yellow bell pepper

1½ tablespoons olive oil

1½ tablespoons apple cider vinegar (I recommend Bragg)

4 teaspoons fresh lime juice

½ teaspoon kosher salt

Freshly ground black pepper

In a large bowl, combine the coleslaw mix, cabbage, cucumber, bell pepper, olive oil, vinegar, and lime juice. Season with the salt and add a pinch of black pepper. Refrigerate for 10 to 15 minutes before serving.

PERFECT PAIRINGS
Serve this side dish with **Slow-Cooker Picadillo (page 193)**, **Buttermilk Oven "Fried" Chicken (page 151)**, barbecued meats, and sandwiches. It makes a perfect crunchy topping for tacos and tostadas, too.

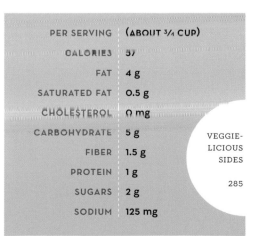

PER SERVING	(ABOUT ¾ CUP)
CALORIES	57
FAT	4 g
SATURATED FAT	0.5 g
CHOLESTEROL	0 mg
CARBOHYDRATE	5 g
FIBER	1.5 g
PROTEIN	1 g
SUGARS	2 g
SODIUM	125 mg

VEGGIE-LICIOUS SIDES

285

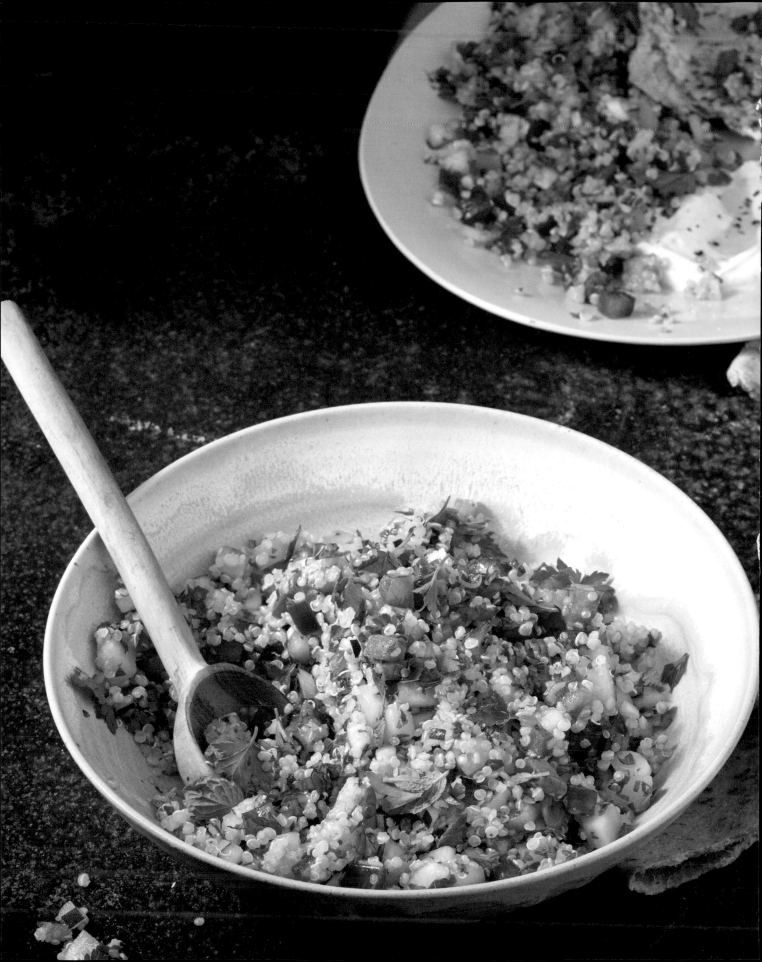

Quinoa Tabbouleh

SERVES 4

Tabbouleh is a wonderful Middle Eastern salad made with lots of chopped herbs, cucumbers, tomatoes, scallions, and bright flavors. It's typically made with bulgur, but I love using quinoa instead because it has a healthy dose of protein.

½ cup quinoa

Kosher salt

1 cup English cucumber, peeled and finely chopped

¾ cup finely chopped tomato

2 tablespoons finely chopped red onion

2 tablespoons sliced scallions

¼ cup finely chopped fresh parsley leaves

1½ tablespoons finely chopped fresh mint leaves

½ tablespoon extra-virgin olive oil

1½ tablespoons fresh lemon juice

1 tablespoon red wine vinegar

Rinse the quinoa under running water for about 2 minutes. Cook the quinoa in 1 cup of water with ⅛ teaspoon salt according to package directions. Set aside to cool.

When the quinoa is cool, put it into a large bowl and add the cucumber, tomato, red onion, scallions, parsley, mint, olive oil, lemon juice, and vinegar. Season with the remaining ¼ teaspoon salt and refrigerate until chilled, at least 20 minutes. Serve cold.

PERFECT PAIRING

If I'm grilling in the summer and I want to go with a Mediterranean theme, I make a big bowl of this salad and grill up some skewers, like my **Grilled Lamb Skewers with Harissa Dipping Sauce (page 206),** and serve everything with pita bread on the side.

PER SERVING	(¾ CUP)
CALORIES	110
FAT	3 g
SATURATED FAT	0.5 g
CHOLESTEROL	0 mg
CARBOHYDRATE	17 g
FIBER	2.5 g
PROTEIN	4 g
SUGARS	2 g
SODIUM	95 mg

VEGGIE-LICIOUS SIDES

Summer Pearl Couscous

SERVES 5

V **Q**

The first time I tried pearl couscous I instantly fell for it. Although it looks a lot like barley, it's actually small, toasted semolina pasta. Pearl couscous is a larger size of the grain that has a wonderful chewiness. This recipe is a fantastic hearty side for grilled chicken or fish, but I also love it as a meal in itself. Although I'm not usually a fan of the taste of whole wheat pasta, I don't mind it at all in this smaller shape. In fact, one way I like to trick picky vegetable eaters into not picking out the zucchini is to dice it so small that it matches the size of the cooked couscous (pictured on page 226).

Kosher salt

1 cup whole wheat pearl couscous

½ tablespoon extra-virgin olive oil

3 garlic cloves, minced

1⅔ cups diced zucchini, ¼-inch dice

1 cup cherry tomatoes, quartered

Freshly ground black pepper

2 tablespoons freshly grated Pecorino Romano cheese

Bring 1¼ cups water and ½ teaspoon salt to a boil in a small pot. Add couscous, cover, and simmer for 8 to 10 minutes, or according to the package directions.

Heat a large skillet over medium-high heat. Add the oil and garlic and cook, stirring, until golden, 1 to 2 minutes. Add the zucchini and tomatoes, season with ¼ teaspoon salt and a pinch of black pepper, and cook just until tender, about 2 to 3 minutes. Add the cooked couscous and Romano to the skillet and stir to combine; finish with ⅛ teaspoon salt and serve hot.

PER SERVING	(¾ CUP)
CALORIES	169
FAT	2.5 g
SATURATED FAT	1 g
CHOLESTEROL	0 mg
CARBOHYDRATE	30 g
FIBER	2.5 g
PROTEIN	6 g
SUGARS	2 g
SODIUM	204 mg

Grilled Mexican Corn Salad

SERVES 5

(V) (GF)

This vibrant side dish is a staple at backyard parties over the summer, when corn is at its sweetest. If I'm feeding friends, I make sure to double the recipe so there's enough for everyone. We love the smoky-sweet flavor you get from grilling the corn, which is livened up by the freshly squeezed lime juice and just the right amount of cilantro. And, of course, avocado is a must! Heck, I could pile this on a tostada, top it with queso fresco, and call it a meal!

3 medium ears corn, unhusked, or 1½ cups thawed frozen corn kernels

1 cup chopped tomatoes

¼ cup chopped red onion

1 fresh jalapeño pepper, finely chopped (optional)

¼ cup finely chopped fresh cilantro

1 small garlic clove, crushed

2 tablespoons fresh lime juice

1 teaspoon olive oil

½ teaspoon ground cumin

Kosher salt

Freshly ground black pepper

1 medium (4 ounces) Hass avocado, chopped

Preheat a grill to medium.

Soak the fresh unhusked corn in a large bowl of cold water for 30 minutes.

Remove the corn from the water and shake off any excess. Put the corn on the grill, close the lid, and grill, turning every 5 minutes, until the kernels are tender when pierced with a paring knife, 20 to 25 minutes. Let sit until cool enough to handle.

Increase the heat of the grill to high. Carefully remove the husks and silks from the corncobs, put the corn back on the grill, and cook, turning, until slightly charred, 2 to 4 minutes. Set aside to cool. When cooled, use a knife to cut the corn off the cobs.

In a large bowl, combine the grilled corn (or thawed frozen corn), tomatoes, red onion, jalapeño (if using), cilantro, garlic, lime juice, olive oil, cumin, ¼ teaspoon salt, and black pepper. Refrigerate for at least 20 minutes. Just before serving, toss in the avocado and finish with ⅛ teaspoon salt.

skinny**scoop**

To make this in half the time, you can use thawed frozen roasted corn, like Trader Joe's, instead of fresh grilled corn.

PER SERVING	(¾ CUP)
CALORIES	130
FAT	6 g
SATURATED FAT	1 g
CHOLESTEROL	0 mg
CARBOHYDRATE	17 g
FIBER	4 g
PROTEIN	3 g
SUGARS	5 g
SODIUM	99 mg

VEGGIE-LICIOUS SIDES

289

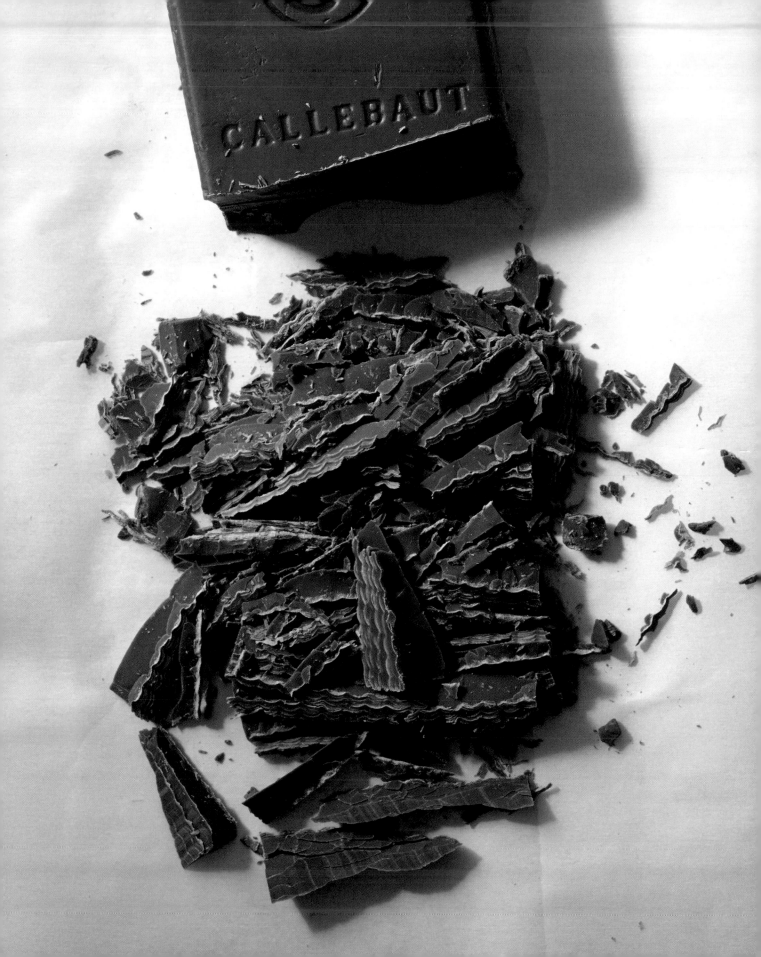

SKINNY SWEET TOOTH

Double Chocolate Chunk Walnut Cookies

MAKES 24 COOKIES

V **Q**

I've done some crazy, unconventional things in baking, but using avocados in place of butter may just be the craziest. Believe it or not, it works! For these chewy cookies made with chunks of chocolate and walnuts in every bite, I use absolutely no butter. They taste too good to be light—and you can't detect the taste of avocados at all. I tested these out on many unsuspecting adults, children, and teens, and everyone loved them. Karina, my college-age daughter, was the ultimate test—she's a true chocoholic. She thinks they're pretty awesome!

Cooking spray or oil mister (optional)

½ cup raw sugar

⅓ cup unpacked dark brown sugar

¼ cup mashed avocado

1 tablespoon unsweetened applesauce

1 large egg white

1 teaspoon pure vanilla extract

½ cup (65 grams) white whole wheat unbleached flour (I recommend King Arthur)

⅓ cup (50 grams) all-purpose flour

⅓ cup unsweetened cocoa powder (I use Trader Joe's)

¼ teaspoon baking soda

⅛ teaspoon kosher salt

⅓ cup semisweet chocolate chunks

½ cup finely chopped walnuts

skinny**scoop**

I love walnuts in my chocolate cookies, but if you have allergies, you can swap the walnuts for more chocolate chunks.

Preheat the oven to 350°F. Line 2 regular baking sheets with silicone baking mats (such as Silpats) or lightly spray nonstick baking sheets with oil.

In a large bowl, using an electric hand mixer, whisk together the sugars, avocado, applesauce, egg white, and vanilla until the sugar dissolves, about 2 to 3 minutes.

In a separate large bowl, whisk together the flours, cocoa powder, baking soda, and salt. Fold in the dry ingredients with a spatula in two additions. Using a spatula, fold in the chocolate chunks and walnuts. The dough will be very sticky. Cover the bowl with plastic wrap and refrigerate 15 minutes.

Drop the dough by tablespoonfuls about 1 inch apart onto the prepared baking sheets and smooth the tops.

Bake until almost set, 10 to 12 minutes. Let cool for 5 minutes on the pan, then transfer to wire racks to cool completely.

PER SERVING	(2 COOKIES)
CALORIES	152
FAT	5.5 g
SATURATED FAT	1.5 g
CHOLESTEROL	0 mg
CARBOHYDRATE	25 g
FIBER	2 g
PROTEIN	3 g
SUGARS	15 g
SODIUM	48 mg

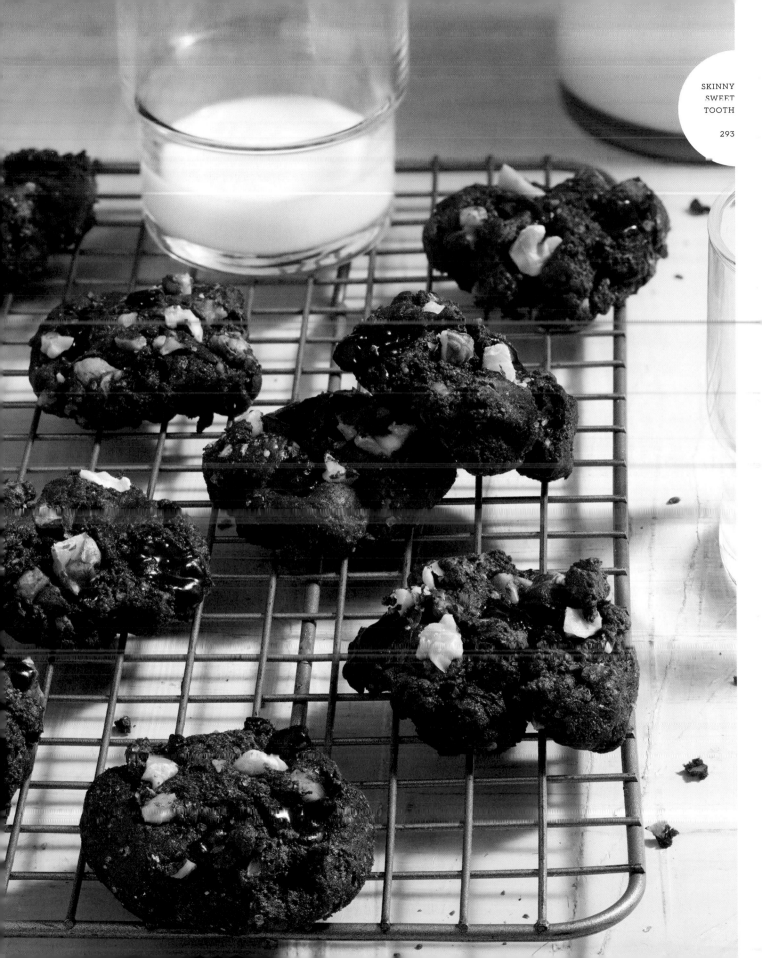

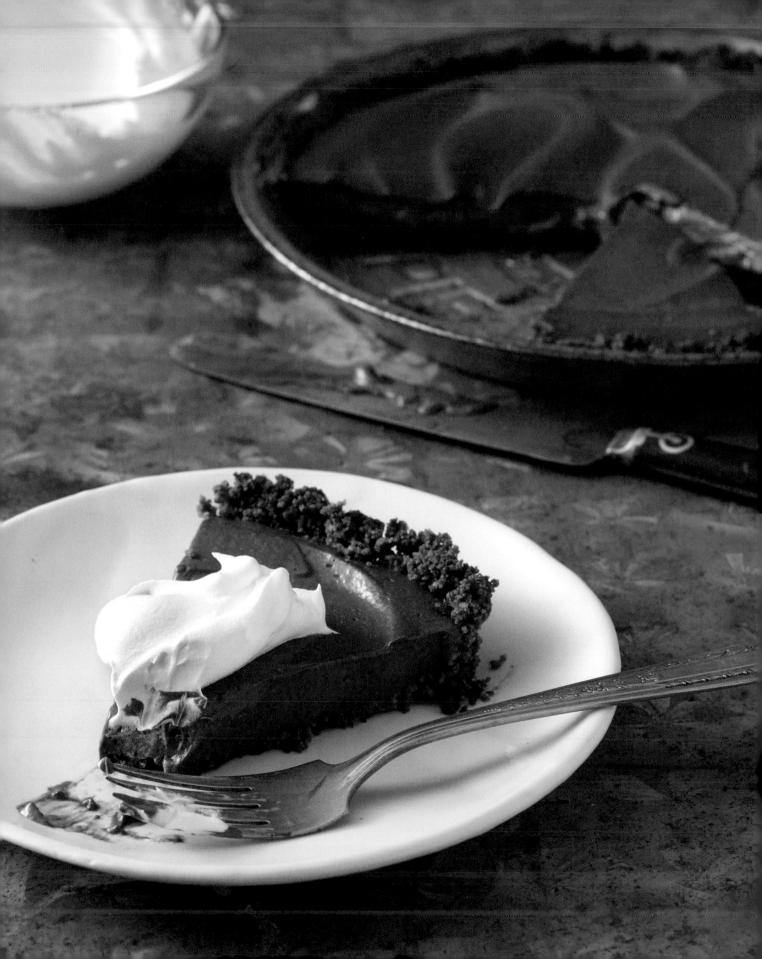

Silky Chocolate Cream Pie

SERVES 8

(V)

Chocolate lovers: This dessert is for you! You'll love the rich taste of this decadent, creamy chocolate pie. The secret to keeping it skinny is silken tofu, which has a light texture and a wonderful mouthfeel. Here, it has a puddinglike quality that will fool anyone.

CRUST

6 whole reduced-fat graham crackers, crushed

2 tablespoons raw sugar

3 tablespoons cold whipped butter

FILLING

1 (12.3-ounce) package firm silken tofu

¼ cup unsweetened almond milk

2 tablespoons raw sugar

5 ounces semisweet chocolate

For the crust: In a food processor, combine the crushed graham crackers, raw sugar, and butter. Pulse a few times, then add 1 tablespoon water. Pulse a few more times until it has the texture of coarse meal. Press the mixture into the bottom and up the sides of an 8-inch pie plate. Refrigerate for 30 minutes.

Preheat the oven to 375°F.

Bake the crust until the edges are golden, 8 to 10 minutes. Remove from the oven and let cool on a wire rack.

For the filling: Lightly mash the silken tofu with a fork and place it in a blender with the almond milk and raw sugar. Blend until smooth, about 1 minute.

Place the chocolate in a microwave-safe bowl and microwave on high for 30 seconds. Stir and microwave another 30 to 40 seconds. Repeat until the chocolate is completely melted. Pour the chocolate into the blender with the tofu and blend a few seconds until thoroughly combined.

Pour the filling into the cooled crust and refrigerate until set, about 2 hours. Serve chilled and cut into 8 slices.

skinny**scoop**

Silken tofu is usually packaged in aseptic boxes that do not require refrigeration. Because of this, it is sometimes sold in a different section of grocery stores than regular tofu, which is packed in water and requires refrigeration. When buying commercial tofu, look for organic, non-GMO brands like Nasoya.

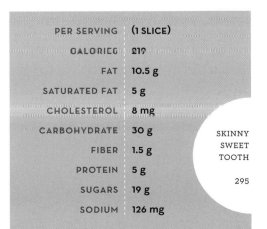

PER SERVING	(1 SLICE)
CALORIES	219
FAT	10.5 g
SATURATED FAT	5 g
CHOLESTEROL	8 mg
CARBOHYDRATE	30 g
FIBER	1.5 g
PROTEIN	5 g
SUGARS	19 g
SODIUM	126 mg

SKINNY SWEET TOOTH

Coconut Panna Cotta with Fresh Raspberries

SERVES 6

GF

This is one of my favorite desserts in the whole cookbook. Traditionally, panna cotta is made with heavy cream and milk, but with a little bit of tinkering, it can easily be adapted to work with just about any type of milk. I'm coconut-obsessed, so I like to make this dairy-free version with a combination of canned light coconut milk and coconut milk beverage, usually found in the refrigerated section of the supermarket.

¾ cup unsweetened coconut milk beverage

3½ teaspoons (12 grams) unflavored powdered gelatin

2 cups canned light coconut milk (I prefer Thai Kitchen)

¼ cup honey

Kosher salt

1½ cups raspberries

1 tablespoon grated lime zest (optional)

skinny**scoop**

Panna cotta is the perfect dessert to make when you have dinner guests. The reason: It needs to be made at least 4 hours in advance to set (it stays chilled in the refrigerator until ready to serve), which leaves you free to mingle with company instead of fussing in the kitchen. It can also be made a day or two ahead.

Pour the coconut milk beverage into a medium heavy-bottomed saucepan. Sprinkle the gelatin over the milk and let stand until the gelatin softens, about 10 minutes. Meanwhile, fill a large bowl with ice water.

Turn the heat under the saucepan to medium and whisk the gelatin until it has dissolved, but don't let the milk boil, about 3 minutes. Whisk in the light coconut milk, honey, and a pinch of salt. Cook, whisking, until the mixture is hot, but do not let it boil, 4 to 5 minutes. Transfer the milk to a clean, medium metal bowl. Put the bowl in the prepared ice bath and let cool, stirring slowly so no bubbles form, until the mixture begins to thicken, about 12 minutes.

Ladle about ½ cup into each of 6 small dessert bowls or parfait glasses. Cover each with plastic wrap and refrigerate until firm, 4 to 6 hours or overnight.

To serve, remove the plastic wrap and spoon the fresh berries over the panna cotta along with lime zest (if using).

PER SERVING	(1 PANNA COTTA + ¼ CUP BERRIES)
CALORIES	152
FAT	7.5 g
SATURATED FAT	4 g
CHOLESTEROL	0 mg
CARBOHYDRATE	19 g
FIBER	2 g
PROTEIN	2 g
SUGARS	13 g
SODIUM	29 mg

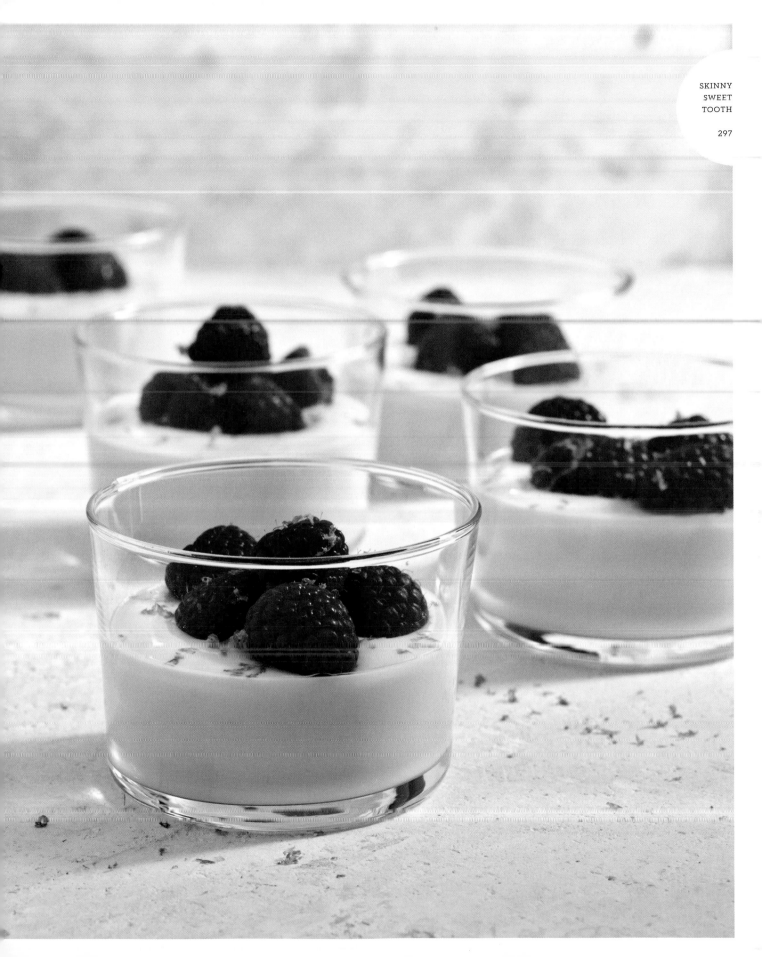

Warm Apple-Pear Crumble

SERVES 8

(V)

There's nothing better to me than a warm dessert on a chilly autumn evening. I'm all about hot desserts with cold toppings—a dab of fat-free frozen yogurt on top of something warm and sweet is enough to make me swoon. With this nutrient-packed dessert, you'll score an impressive 3 grams of filling fiber and 2 grams of satiating protein all for less than 200 calories. Good-bye, guilt!

Cooking spray or oil mister

FILLING

2½ cups peeled, sliced pears

2½ cups peeled, sliced Gala apples

¼ cup honey

1 tablespoon fresh lemon juice

1 tablespoon all-purpose flour

½ teaspoon ground cinnamon

TOPPING

¾ cup quick-cooking oats

¼ cup packed light brown sugar

¼ cup chopped walnuts

1 tablespoon all-purpose flour

¼ teaspoon kosher salt

3 tablespoons virgin coconut oil

skinny**scoop**

Coconut oil is a great substitute for shortening, butter, margarine, or vegetable oil. If you're not a fan of the taste of coconut, use expeller-pressed coconut oil, which has a neutral flavor, rather than cold-pressed, which tastes more like coconut

Preheat the oven to 325°F. Lightly spray a 9 × 9-inch baking dish with oil.

For the filling: In a large bowl, combine the pears, apples, honey, lemon juice, flour, and cinnamon. Pour the mixture into the prepared baking dish.

For the topping: In a separate bowl, combine the oats, brown sugar, walnuts, flour, salt, and coconut oil. Sprinkle the topping evenly over the filling.

Bake until browned and bubbling, 55 minutes to 1 hour. Serve warm.

PER SERVING	(½ CUP)
CALORIES	199
FAT	8 g
SATURATED FAT	4.5 g
CHOLESTEROL	0 mg
CARBOHYDRATE	32 g
FIBER	3 g
PROTEIN	2 g
SUGARS	21 g
SODIUM	75 mg

Baked Bananas Foster à la Mode

SERVES 4

(V) (GF) (Q)

We go *bananas* for this simple, slimmed-down dessert in my home. It's the perfect treat whenever you have ripe bananas sitting on your counter just begging to be used. And guess what? By baking them in the oven with just a little brown sugar, cinnamon, and vanilla, the bananas taste decadent with zero guilt. And bananas are available year-round, so you can make this any time you need a last-minute dessert. The fat-free vanilla frozen yogurt that I prefer is Stonyfield's Organic Gotta Have Vanilla, but you can use your favorite.

2 ripe medium bananas, sliced into ½-inch rounds

⅛ teaspoon ground cinnamon

1½ tablespoons light brown sugar

1 teaspoon pure vanilla extract

2 cups fat-free vanilla frozen yogurt

Preheat oven to 400°F.

Arrange the bananas in a 9 × 9-inch oven-safe dish and sprinkle them with cinnamon and brown sugar. Drizzle the vanilla extract over the bananas, wrap tightly with foil, and bake 10 to 12 minutes, or until the bananas are soft.

To serve, scoop ½ cup frozen yogurt into each of 4 dessert bowls. Divide the bananas among the bowls, and spoon the sauce that accumulates in the bottom of the baking dish over each. Serve immediately.

PER SERVING	(½ CUP FROZEN YOGURT + ¼ CUP BANANA WITH SAUCE)
CALORIES	173
FAT	0 g
SATURATED FAT	0 g
CHOLESTEROL	0 mg
CARBOHYDRATE	39 g
FIBER	1.5 g
PROTEIN	5 g
SUGARS	31 g
SODIUM	67 mg

SKINNY SWEET TOOTH

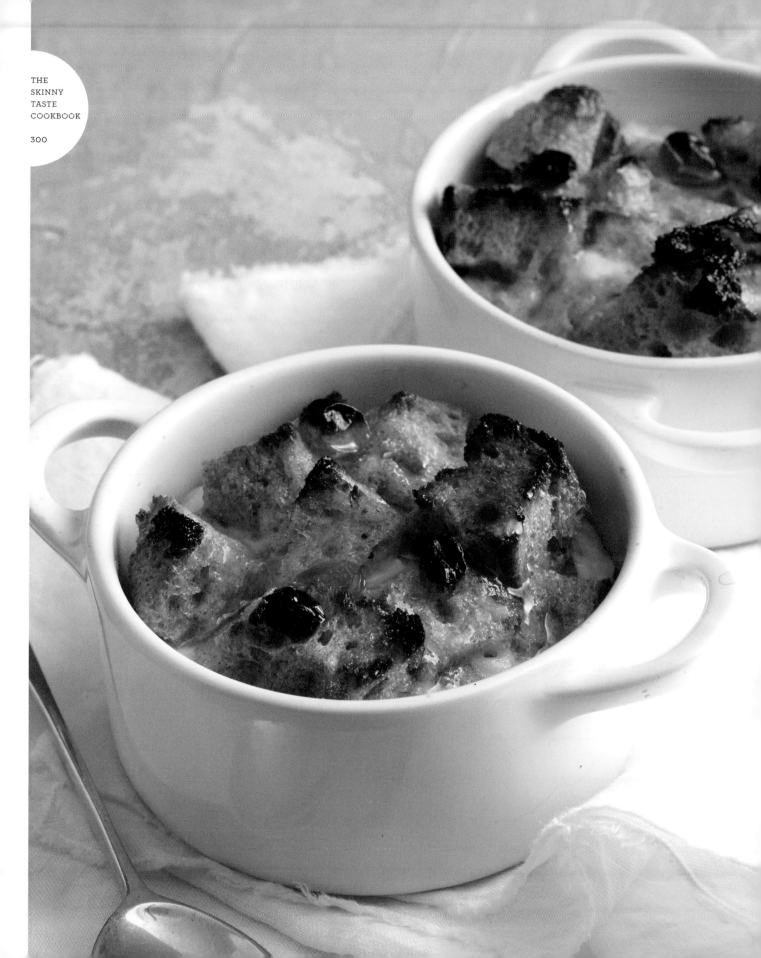

Almost Sinful Maple–Raisin Bread Pudding

SERVES 4

(V)

I've always found bread pudding pretty hard to resist, especially when it's still warm from the oven and topped with a touch of whipped cream. But how do you make a dessert that's based on bread and eggs a little less sinful? I swapped the white bread for whole wheat French bread, swapped the cream for fat-free milk, and cut back on the eggs. To sweeten it, I like to go natural, using pure maple syrup and raisins instead of refined sugar. But most important, I keep portions in check by baking them in individual ramekins, so I don't "accidentally" have more than my share.

2 cups (2½ ounces) whole wheat French bread, crusts removed, cut into ½-inch cubes

1 cup fat-free milk

¼ cup pure maple syrup

2½ teaspoons pure vanilla extract

2 large eggs

⅓ cup raisins

Cooking spray or oil mister

Preheat the oven to 350°F.

Arrange the bread cubes in a single layer on a baking sheet. Bake until golden, 5 to 6 minutes, stirring halfway through the cooking time. Let cool.

In a medium bowl, whisk together the milk, 3 tablespoons of the maple syrup, vanilla, and eggs. Stir in the raisins. Fold in the toasted bread cubes. Cover and refrigerate for at least 30 minutes or up to 4 hours.

Preheat the oven to 325°F. Spray 4 (5-ounce) ramekins with oil.

Divide the bread mixture equally among the prepared ramekins. Put the ramekins in an 8 × 8-inch baking pan and add 1 inch hot water to the pan.

Bake until set, 45 to 50 minutes. Drizzle with remaining tablespoon of maple syrup. Serve warm.

PERFECT PAIRINGS
For a little extra indulgence, I like to serve these with either a little fat-free frozen yogurt or light whipped topping.

PER SERVING	(1 RAMEKIN)
CALORIES	173
FAT	0.5 g
SATURATED FAT	0 g
CHOLESTEROL	1 mg
CARBOHYDRATE	35 g
FIBER	1 g
PROTEIN	6 g
SUGARS	23 g
SODIUM	143 mg

Piña Colada Chia Pudding

SERVES 4

V **GF**

Each spoonful of this healthy pudding offers a little taste of paradise. Chia pudding is one of my favorite guiltless desserts, because it's low in calories and is super easy because there's no cooking involved. Chia seeds (yes, the same seeds used to make chia pets) are the perfect "pudding" ingredient because they absorb any liquid you combine them with and expand to eight to nine times their weight. They end up with a nice texture that's similar to tapioca. Because the seeds have no flavor, they take on the taste of whatever liquid they absorb, like these delicious piña colada–inspired ingredients.

1 cup canned light coconut milk

1 cup unsweetened coconut milk beverage, such as So Delicious or Silk

1½ cups chopped fresh pineapple

¼ cup chia seeds

3 tablespoons sweetened shredded coconut

10 drops NuNaturals liquid stevia (or your favorite sweetener)

In a large bowl or container with a lid, combine the coconut milk, coconut milk beverage, pineapple, chia seeds, shredded coconut, and stevia. Cover, shake well, and let sit for 15 minutes. Shake again and refrigerate for 4 to 6 hours, or up to overnight. The pudding will keep in the refrigerator for up to 3 days.

Divide among 4 dessert bowls.

PER SERVING	(1 CUP)
CALORIES	161
FAT	9.5 g
SATURATED FAT	4 g
CHOLESTEROL	0 mg
CARBOHYDRATE	18 g
FIBER	6 g
PROTEIN	3 g
SUGARS	8 g
SODIUM	24 mg

Delightful Poached Pears with Yogurt

SERVES 4

(V) (GF)

My cousin Katia shared this recipe with me, and it's something she learned from her mom. It's a naturally light dessert option, but we played around with the original recipe to cut back on sugar—without losing any of the sweetness—by cooking the pears in a sweeter wine combined with pear nectar and pomegranate juice. The results were just lovely, and the yogurt adds a creamy finish that complements the sweet pears perfectly.

PEARS

2 peeled ripe Bosc pears

1½ cups Pink Moscato wine

1 cup pear nectar

¼ cup pomegranate juice

½ tablespoon vanilla extract

2 tablespoons raw sugar

½-inch piece fresh ginger, peeled and halved

2 cinnamon sticks

3 (2-inch) strips orange zest

¾ cup vanilla 0% Greek yogurt

For the pears: Halve the pears lengthwise, leaving the stems on, and remove the core and seeds. Put the pears, wine, pear nectar, pomegranate juice, vanilla, sugar, ginger, cinnamon sticks, and orange zest in a medium saucepan, with the cut sides of the pears facing up. Bring to a boil, reduce the heat to medium-low, cover, and simmer until the pears are soft but not falling apart, 30 to 40 minutes (or longer depending on the ripeness of the pears), carefully flipping the pears over halfway through.

Using a slotted spoon, transfer the pears to a 9 × 9 inch baking dish, reserving the liquid in the saucepan and discard the cinnamon sticks. Increase the heat under the saucepan to medium-high, bring to a boil, and cook until the liquid has reduced by half, about 5 minutes. Pour the liquid over the pears and let cool for 20 minutes. Cover and refrigerate until chilled, about 1 hour or overnight.

To serve, place a pear half, cut side up, on each of 4 small serving plates and drizzle each with ¼ cup of the sauce and 3 tablespoons of yogurt.

PER SERVING	(½ POACHED PEAR + ¼ CUP SAUCE + 3 TABLESOONS YOGURT)
CALORIES	230
FAT	0 g
SATURATED FAT	0 g
CHOLESTEROL	3 mg
CARBOHYDRATE	41 g
FIBER	3 g
PROTEIN	4 g
SUGARS	30 g
SODIUM	27 mg

SKINNY
SWEET
TOOTH

Summer Berry Cobbler

SERVES 6

(V)

Because cobbler is a favorite of mine, I've been playing around with this recipe for years. Traditional cobbler toppings are usually made with so much butter, but I've been able to cut down substantially by using sweet whipped butter. I use ramekins here for automatic portion control.

FILLING

½ cup raw sugar

1½ tablespoons cornstarch

Ground cinnamon

Kosher salt

1½ cups raspberries

1½ cups blackberries

1½ cups strawberries, cored and sliced

½ teaspoon grated lemon zest

1 tablespoon fresh lemon juice

TOPPING

¼ cup white whole wheat flour (I recommend King Arthur)

¼ cup unbleached all-purpose flour

2 tablespoons raw sugar

½ teaspoon baking powder

¼ teaspoon baking soda

Kosher salt

2 tablespoons cold unsalted whipped butter, cut into small pieces

⅓ cup low-fat buttermilk

1 tablespoon canola oil

2 teaspoons turbinado sugar

Preheat the oven to 375°F.

For the filling: In a large bowl, whisk together the raw sugar, cornstarch, and a pinch each of cinnamon and salt. Add the berries and gently mix to coat. Add the lemon zest and juice and divide the filling among 6 (8-ounce) ramekins. Put the ramekins on a rimmed baking sheet and bake until the berries are hot and bubbling on the edges, 22 to 24 minutes.

For the topping: In a bowl, whisk together the flours, raw sugar, baking powder, baking soda, and a pinch of salt. Cut in the butter using a pastry cutter or 2 knives until the butter pieces are the size of small pebbles. In a small bowl, combine the buttermilk and oil. Add to the dry ingredients and stir until just moistened.

Carefully remove the ramekins from the oven, and increase the oven temperature to 400°F. Spoon about 2 tablespoons of topping over the berries. Sprinkle with turbinado sugar. Bake until the berries are bubbling and the topping is golden and cooked through, 15 to 18 minutes. Remove from the oven and let cool for 15 to 20 minutes before serving.

PER SERVING	(1 RAMEKIN)
CALORIES	223
FAT	5.5 g
SATURATED FAT	2 g
CHOLESTEROL	7 mg
CARBOHYDRATE	43 g
FIBER	5 g
PROTEIN	3 g
SUGARS	27 g
SODIUM	163 mg

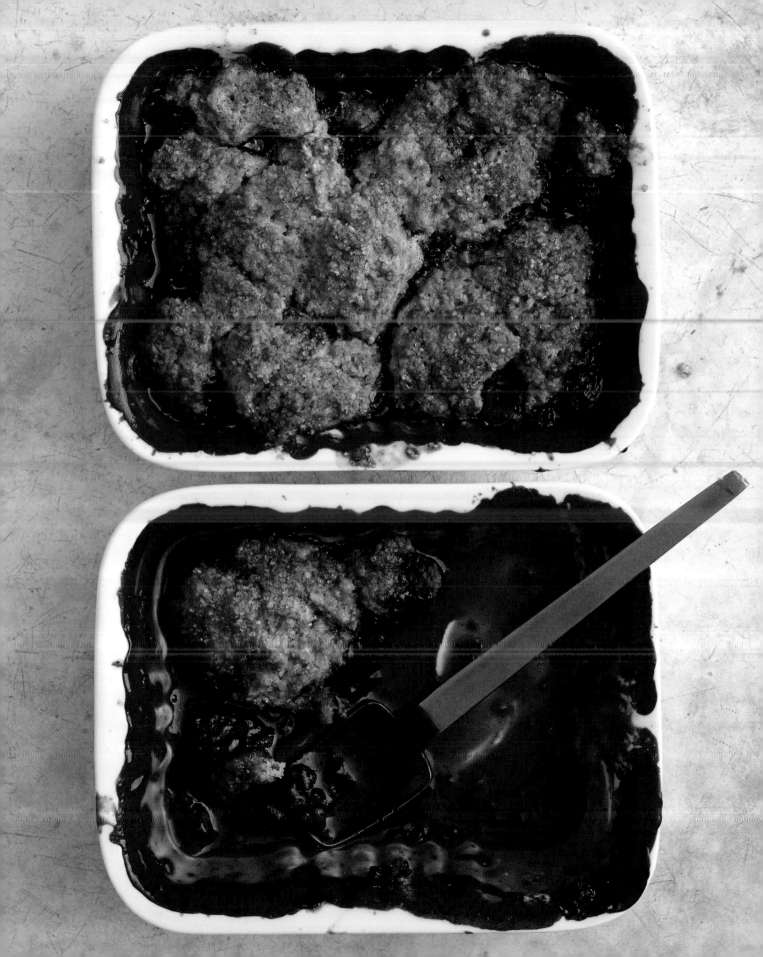

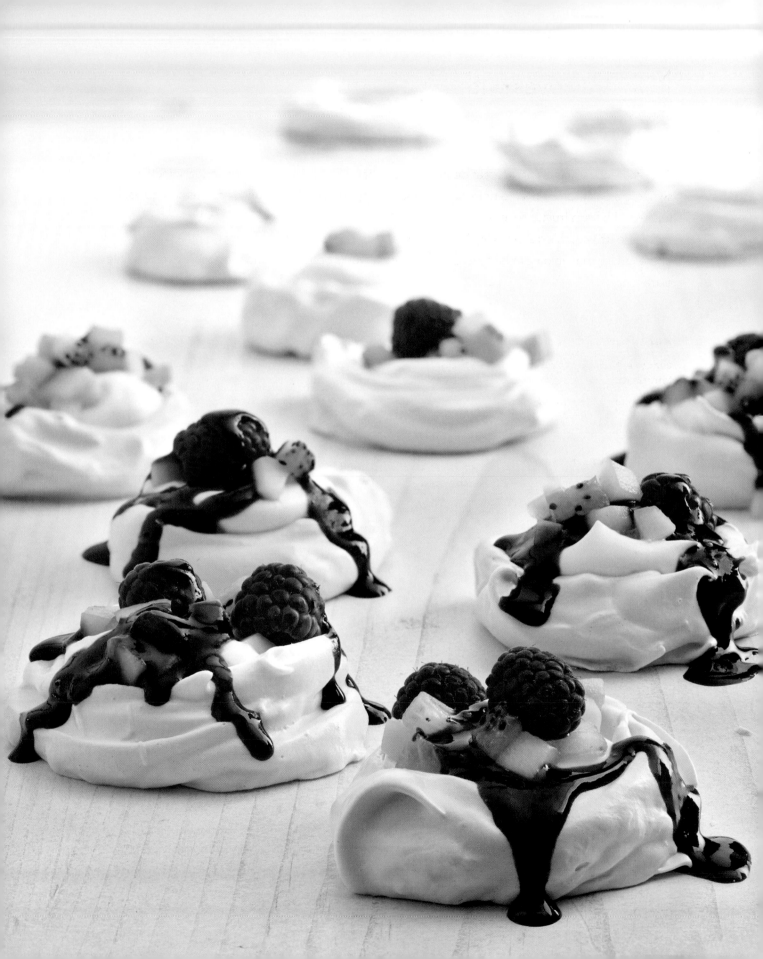

Mini Pavlovas with Fresh Fruit

SERVES 9

V GF

These sweet meringues are a great dessert if you're having company or want to bring something sweet to a party. Since they're nothing more than whipped egg whites, sugar, cornstarch, and vanilla topped with fresh fruit, they're naturally fat-free. But I do like to top them with a little fresh cream, so I came up with this delicious lighter alternative to full-fat whipped cream by whipping up only half of the cream, then folding in fat-free Greek yogurt. It works beautifully and the yogurt gives it a little extra tang.

MERINGUES

2 large egg whites, at room temperature

½ teaspoon pure vanilla extract

1 teaspoon cornstarch

⅛ teaspoon kosher salt

6 tablespoons sugar

FRUIT TOPPING

1¼ cups raspberries (1 pint)

2 tablespoons sugar

1 teaspoon fresh lemon juice

10 tablespoons finely chopped mango

2 small kiwifruits, finely chopped

LIGHTER WHIPPED CREAM

1 tablespoon sugar

¼ cup well-chilled heavy whipping cream

¼ teaspoon pure vanilla extract

¼ cup 0% Greek yogurt

Adjust the oven rack in the center of the oven and preheat to 200°F. Line a large rimmed baking sheet with parchment paper.

For the meringues: In the bowl of a stand mixer fitted with the whisk, beat the egg whites, vanilla, cornstarch, and salt at medium speed until foamy, 1 to 2 minutes. Increase the speed to medium-high and beat until the egg whites are soft and billowy, 2 to 3 minutes. Slowly add the sugar, 1 tablespoon at a time, beating until thick and glossy peaks form, 3 to 4 minutes.

Using a spatula, scoop ¼-cup mounds of meringue onto the prepared baking sheet, and use the spatula to make an indent in the center of each (like a bowl). You should have 9 meringues.

(recipe continues)

PER SERVING	(1 PAVLOVA)
CALORIES	92
FAT	1.5 g
SATURATED FAT	0.5 g
CHOLESTEROL	3 mg
CARBOHYDRATE	19 g
FIBER	2 g
PROTEIN	2 g
SUGARS	16 g
SODIUM	52 mg

SKINNY
SWEET
TOOTH

Bake until firm on the outside and smooth, about 1 hour 30 minutes. Turn the oven off and leave the meringues in the oven with the door closed until they are hard and dry, about 3 hours. Carefully remove the meringues from the paper. Immediately store them in an airtight container.

For the fruit topping: In a small saucepan, combine ¾ cup of the raspberries, the sugar, and lemon juice. Bring to a boil over medium heat and cook, stirring, for 2 minutes. Remove the pan from the heat and let sit about 10 minutes. Strain the mixture through a fine-mesh sieve into a bowl, using a spoon to press on the raspberries; discard the seeds. Refrigerate until ready to serve.

In a small bowl, combine the remaining raspberries with the mango and the kiwifruits.

For the lighter whipped cream: Put a metal bowl and the beaters of a hand mixer into the freezer for 10 to 15 minutes.

Remove the bowl and beaters from the freezer. Put the sugar, heavy cream, and vanilla into the bowl and beat with a hand mixer just until the cream reaches stiff peaks, 2 to 3 minutes. Fold in the yogurt.

Assemble the pavlovas by spooning 1 tablespoon light whipped cream into each meringue shell. Top each with 1 tablespoon of the fresh fruit, and 2 teaspoons raspberry sauce. Serve immediately.

Frozen Dark Chocolate–Almond Bananas

SERVES 4

I eat a banana just about every day, sometimes in my smoothie or oatmeal, other times as a quick snack on the go. But my favorite way to enjoy this potassium-filled pick, particularly in the summer when I need a chocolate fix, is frozen on a stick, dipped in dark chocolate, and sprinkled with chopped almonds. It's a guiltless frozen treat!

1 large ripe banana

4 Popsicle sticks

8 ounces dark chocolate*

1 teaspoon canola oil

3 tablespoons coarsely chopped dry-roasted almonds

*Read the label to be sure this product is gluten-free.

Line a baking sheet with wax paper.

Halve the banana lengthwise, then cut in half crosswise. Insert a Popsicle stick into each piece of banana and lay them on the prepared baking sheet. Freeze until completely frozen, at least 1 hour.

In a microwave-safe mug or bowl, combine the chocolate and oil. Melt the chocolate in the microwave on high, 30 seconds at a time, stirring until the chocolate is melted. Dip the bananas one at a time into the chocolate, scraping off the excess chocolate from the flat part of the banana, and put them on the baking sheet. Working quickly, before the chocolate sets, sprinkle the bananas with the chopped almonds. Put the bananas back into the freezer and freeze until the chocolate is hard, about 1 hour. Keep frozen until ready to serve.

Note: In order to coat the bananas with chocolate, you'll need to start with 8 ounces, but only 2 ounces will adhere to the bananas. The nutritional information accounts for 2 ounces of chocolate.

skinnyscoop

Don't let those browning bananas on your counter go to waste! They are perfect for this sweet treat!

PER SERVING	(1 POPSICLE)
CALORIES	133
FAT	7.5 g
SATURATED FAT	2.5 g
CHOLESTEROL	0 mg
CARBOHYDRATE	18 g
FIBER	2 g
PROTEIN	2 g
SUGARS	12 g
SODIUM	2 mg

SKINNY
SWEET
TOOTH

309

Watermelon Lime Granita

SERVES 4

Eating a sweet, juicy watermelon on a hot, summer day is hard to beat—but this Italian-ice-like dessert comes pretty darn close! And it's made with just three ingredients. Trust me, you'll want to make this all summer long! A granita is made by scraping frozen ice crystals as they form in the freezer. You don't need to own any fancy appliances or equipment—all you need is a blender, a metal baking pan, a freezer, and a fork!

4 cups chopped seedless watermelon

Juice of 1 lime

2 tablespoons sugar

In a blender, combine the chopped watermelon, lime juice, and sugar. Blend until smooth. Pour the puree into a 9 × 9-inch metal baking pan. Cover with plastic wrap and freeze for about 1½ hours. Using a fork, scrape the surface and mix it up. Return the pan to the freezer and freeze until almost set, about 2 hours. Using a fork, scrape the granita into chunky snowlike ice crystals. Freeze and repeat the scraping process until the entire mixture is frozen and shaved, 1 more hour.

Store, covered in plastic wrap, until ready to serve. To serve, spoon into 4 small glass bowls.

skinny**scoop**

For the sweetest results, always buy a whole, fresh watermelon instead of one that has already been cut. Look for a firm, symmetrical watermelon that's free of any bruises, cuts, or dents. The watermelon should be heavy for its size, and the underside of the watermelon should have a creamy yellow spot from where it sat on the ground and ripened in the sun. If it doesn't have that, it was picked too early and won't be as sweet.

PER SERVING	(GENEROUS 1 CUP)
CALORIES	72
FAT	0 g
SATURATED FAT	0 g
CHOLESTEROL	0 mg
CARBOHYDRATE	18 g
FIBER	0.5 g
PROTEIN	1 g
SUGARS	16 g
SODIUM	3 mg

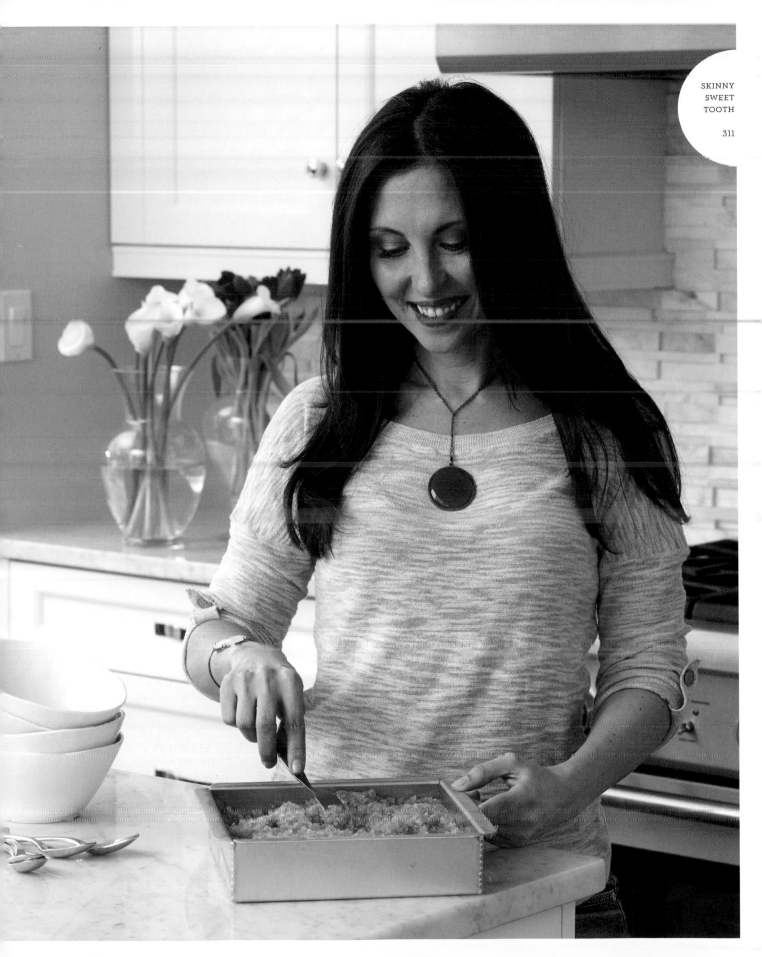

Sweet Plum Custard

SERVES 4

V GF

I love the taste and rustic simplicity of this French-inspired dessert. The sweet plums sink in to the batter, like purple crescent moons. The batter puffs up while it bakes in the oven and then collapses into a soft custard that's lightly dusted with powdered sugar just before eating. Use really ripe plums when you make these—they should be practically falling out of their skins. Other stone fruits, such as peaches or apricots, can be substituted, or try ripe pears in the fall.

Cooking spray or oil mister

1⅓ cups halved, pitted plums, cut into ¼-inch-thick wedges (about 4)

¼ cup raw sugar

2 tablespoons cornstarch

Kosher salt

2 large eggs, at room temperature

½ cup fat-free milk

1 teaspoon pure vanilla extract

Powdered sugar, for dusting

Preheat the oven to 375°F. Lightly spray 4 (6-ounce) shallow gratin dishes with oil.

Place the gratin dishes on a baking sheet and arrange the plums in each gratin dish in a single layer.

In a large bowl, whisk together the raw sugar, cornstarch, and a pinch of salt. Add the eggs, milk, and vanilla and whisk until smooth. Pour the egg and milk mixture over the plums.

Bake until lightly golden and a toothpick inserted into the center comes out clean, about 30 minutes. Transfer the gratin dishes to a wire rack and let cool until warm.

When ready to serve, dust with powdered sugar. Serve warm.

PER SERVING	(1 CUSTARD)
CALORIES	161
FAT	2.5 g
SATURATED FAT	1 g
CHOLESTEROL	94 mg
CARBOHYDRATE	30 g
FIBER	3.5 g
PROTEIN	4 g
SUGARS	20 g
SODIUM	54 mg

Matcha Milkshake

SERVES 2

I love the taste of matcha, a traditional Japanese green tea powder. It has a complex, rich flavor that's unique and easily dissolves in any liquid (no need to boil water). Matcha offers the same health benefits as green tea leaves, plus it has two amino acids (theophylline and L-theanine) that have both an energizing and calming effect—maybe this explains why Buddhist monks have been drinking matcha for centuries! My favorite fat-free frozen yogurt to use here is Stonyfield's Gotta Have Vanilla.

1 cup fat-free vanilla frozen yogurt

1 cup sweetened vanilla almond milk

4 teaspoons matcha powder

4 to 5 ice cubes

In a blender, combine the frozen yogurt, almond milk, matcha powder, and ice cubes and blend until smooth. Divide between 2 glasses.

skinny scoop

After opening, matcha should be refrigerated or kept in the freezer in an airtight container.

FOOD FACTS magnificent matcha

Green tea is famous for its health-promoting properties, many of which stem from one powerful antitumor antioxidant called epigallocatechin-3-gallate (EGCG). Matcha green tea, a powder made from ground tea leaves, has triple the EGCG found in traditionally steeped green teas. It also boasts the amino acids theophylline and L-theanine, which improve focus, reduce stress, and contribute to an energy boost.

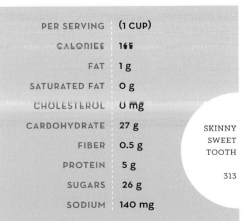

PER SERVING	(1 CUP)
CALORIES	165
FAT	1 g
SATURATED FAT	0 g
CHOLESTEROL	0 mg
CARBOHYDRATE	27 g
FIBER	0.5 g
PROTEIN	5 g
SUGARS	26 g
SODIUM	140 mg

SKINNY SWEET TOOTH

313

ACKNOWLEDGMENTS

Mom and Dad, we sat to eat together as a family every night; you're my inspiration and I am forever thankful for you both. My brother, Ivan, I can't imagine my life without you. To my loving and supportive husband, and my two favorite girls, Karina and Madison—thank you for being my official taste-testers; your honesty only made the recipes better. I love you!

A huge thank-you to Heather K. Jones, R.D., for all the time you poured into this book; your positive attitude lifted me up on those nights when I let self-doubt creep into my head; I couldn't have partnered with a better person and a true friend. To my aunt Ligia, thank you for your meticulous recipe testing and dedication. My editor, Ashley Phillips; you are sweet, brilliant, and talented. Thank you for guiding me through the process.

To the amazing photography team who inspired me every day on set: photographer Penny De Los Santos, who taught me that photos should always tell a story; Simon Andrews, thank you for your flawless food styling and for the invaluable lessons learned; Kaitlyn DuRoss, your positive energy and love of prop styling was contagious. Jay Kim, Stephanie Mungia, Barret Washburne, Idan Bitton—I couldn't have been in better hands. To the vendors who loaned their props: ABC Home, abchome.com; CLAM LAB ceramics, Brooklyn, NY, clamlab.com; Young In the Mountains, Boulder CO, younginthemountains.com; MONDAYS ceramics, Brooklyn, NY, mondaysprojects.com; and Looks Like White ceramics, Montreal Quebec, lookslikewhite.com. Thanks to Aloft Studios for making us feel at home.

To my girlfriends who came through for me when I needed them most, I love you all so very much: Denise H, Katia, Raquel, Doreen, Denise P, Kim, Gabbie, Nicole, and Julia—I am forever grateful for our friendship. My uncle and cousins, Rene, Nina, and Camila, who tasted most of these recipes in this book more than once. Jimmy and Maureen, neighbors extraordinaire who also doubled as taste-testers. Susan Hanover Designs, for letting me use your fabulous kitchen and wear your stunning jewelry. To Tara, for styling me, and Jacqueline Shepherd Makeup for making me pretty.

A special thank-you to Donna Fennessy, for polishing my writing. And Heather's nutrition team—Caroline Kaufman, M.S., R.D., Danielle Hazard, Juhie Bhatia, B.Sc., M.S.—as well as her nutrition interns: Hayley Morgan, Ryan Locke, Stephanie L. Leong, Kendall Wright, and Nicole Karetov.

And, of course, this book would not have been possible without my wonderful agent, Janis Donnaud, and the entire team at Clarkson Potter.

Last, a giant THANK-YOU to all my Skinnytaste, Facebook, Twitter, Pinterest, and Instagram fans who took part in naming the book, and helping me choose this winning cover design.

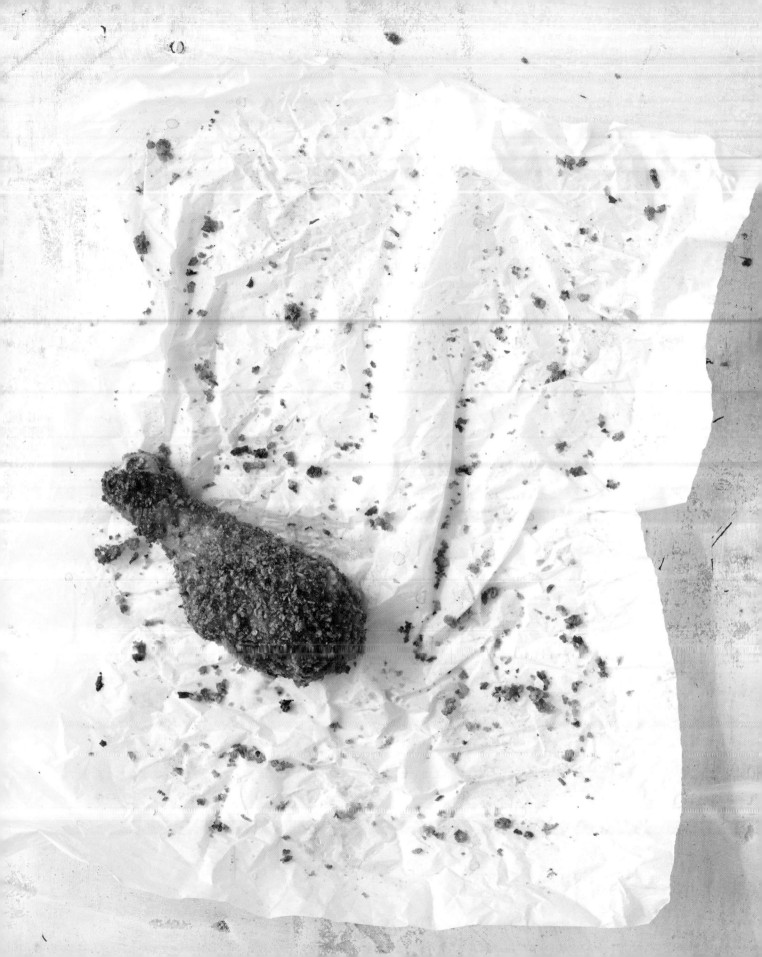

INDEX